Essentials
of Ophthalmology

Commissioning Editor: James Merritt
Project Development Manager: Andrea Deis
Project Manager: Kathryn Mason
Designers: Gene Harris, Bill Donnelly
Illustration Manager: Karen Giacomucci
Illustrators: James A. Perkins, Dartmouth Publishing Inc.
Marketing Managers: Jeremy Bowes (UK), John Gore (US)

Essentials of Ophthalmology

First Edition

Neil J. Friedman MD

Adjunct Clinical Associate Professor
Department of Ophthalmology
Stanford University School of Medicine
Stanford, California;
Private Practice
Mid-Peninsula Ophthalmology Medical Group
Palo Alto, California

Peter K. Kaiser MD

Director
Digital OCT Reading Center;
Staff
Vitreoretinal Section
Cole Eye Institute
Cleveland Clinic
Cleveland, Ohio

To Kathy — Hope this comes in handy. Best wishes! Neil

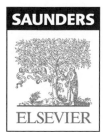

SAUNDERS

ELSEVIER

SAUNDERS
ELSEVIER

Saunders is an affiliate of Elsevier Inc.

© 2007, Elsevier Inc. All rights reserved.

First published 2007

No part of this publication may be reproduced, stored in a retrieval system, or transmitted in any form or by any means, electronic, mechanical, photocopying, recording or otherwise, without the prior permission of the Publishers. Permissions may be sought directly from Elsevier's Health Sciences Rights Department, 1600 John F. Kennedy Boulevard, Suite 1800, Philadelphia, PA 19103-2899, USA: phone: (+1) 215 239 3804; fax: (+1) 215 239 3805; or, e-mail: healthpermissions@elsevier.com. You may also complete your request on-line via the Elsevier homepage (http://www.elsevier.com), by selecting 'Support and contact' and then 'Copyright and Permission'.

ISBN-13: 978-1-4160-2907-6

British Library Cataloguing in Publication Data
A catalogue record for this book is available from the British Library

Library of Congress Cataloging in Publication Data
A catalog record for this book is available from the Library of Congress

Notice
Medical knowledge is constantly changing. Standard safety precautions must be followed, but as new research and clinical experience broaden our knowledge, changes in treatment and drug therapy may become necessary or appropriate. Readers are advised to check the most current product information provided by the manufacturer of each drug to be administered to verify the recommended dose, the method and duration of administration, and contraindications. It is the responsibility of the practitioner, relying on experience and knowledge of the patient, to determine dosages and the best treatment for each individual patient. Neither the Publisher nor the author assume any liability for any injury and/or damage to persons or property arising from this publication.
The Publisher

Printed in China
Last digit is the print number: 9   8   7   6   5   4   3   2   1

Contents

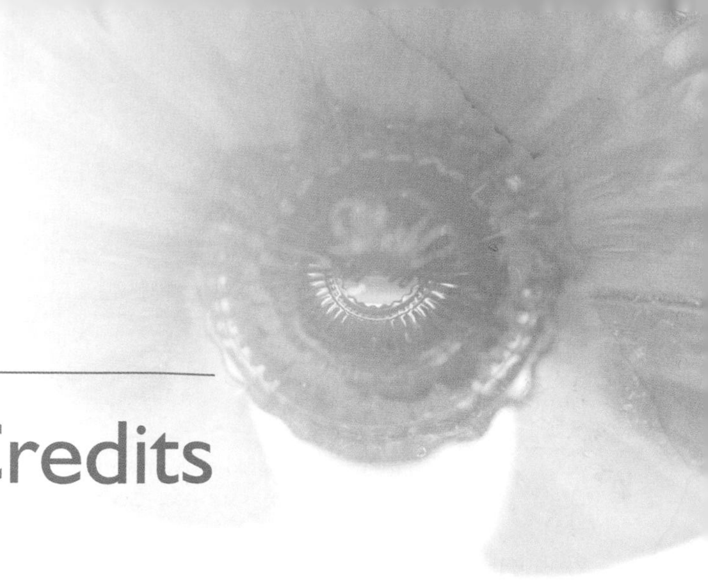

Figure Credits

From Albert D M, Jakobiec F A. (eds) 2000 Principles and Practice in Ophthalmology, 2nd edn. Saunders, Philadelphia.
Figures 2–8 and 14–11

From Asakura A. 1985 Histochemistry of hyaluronic acid of the bovine vitreous body as studied by electron microscopy. Acta Soc Ophthalmol Jpn 89: 179–191.
Figure 1–23

From Bajandas F J, Kline L B. 1988 Neuro-ophthalmology Review Manual. Slack, Thorofare, NJ.
Figures 5–8, 5–9, 5–11, 5–22, and 13–4

From Dutton J J. 1994 Atlas of Clinical and Surgical Orbital Anatomy. W B Saunders, Philadelphia.
Figures 1–2 and 1–9

From Friedman N J, Kaiser P K, Trattler W B. 2005 Review of Ophthalmology. Saunders, Philadelphia.
Figures 1–3, 1–4, 1–28, 1–29, 2–2 to 2–6, 3–1, 5–1, 5–4, and 6–42; Tables 1–1 to 1–3, 2–1, 3–1, 3–2, 6–1 to 6–3, and 11–1

Copyright Peter K. Kaiser, MD.
Figures 5–12, 5–14, 5–17, 5–19, and 5–20

From Kaiser P K, Friedman N J. 2004 The Massachusetts Eye and Ear Infirmary Illustrated Manual of Ophthalmology, 2nd edn. Saunders, St Louis.
Figures 4–1, 4–2, 4–4, 4–7, 4–12 to 4–16, 4–19, 4–20, 4–23, 4–25, 4–27, 5–16, 5–18, 5–21, 5–23 to 5–32, 6–1, 6–3 to 6–9, 6–11, 6–13 to 6–21, 6–23 to 6–26, 6–27 to 6–31, 6–33, 6–35 to 6–41, 6–44 to 6–46, 6–49 to 6–51, 7–2 to 7–19, 8–2, 8–4 to 8–28, 8–32 to 8–36, 8–38 to 8–41, 8–43, 8–44, 8–45, 8–47, 9–3 to 9–30, 9–32 to 9–43, 10–1 to 10–3, 10–5 to 10–12, 11–1 to 11–39, 12–2 to 12–14, 13–1, 13–3, 13–5 to 13–11, 13–13, 13–14, 14–1 to 14–4, 14–7 to 14–10, 14–12, 14–14 to 14–16, 15–1 to 15–22, 16–1 to 16–4, and 17–1 to 17–109

From Kanski J J. 2003 Clinical Ophthalmology: a Systematic Approach, 5th edn. Butterworth-Heinemann, London.
Figures 9–31, 13–2, and 14–5

From Kaufman P L, Alm A. (eds) 2003 Adler's Physiology of the Eye, 10th edn. Mosby, St Louis.
Figures 1–5, 1–11, 5–6, and 5–15

Courtesy of Robert Kersten, MD.
Figures 8–29, 8–42, and 8–46

From Krachmer J H, Palay D A. 1995 Cornea Color Atlas. Mosby, St Louis.
Figure 9–1

Courtesy of Timothy McCulley, MD.
Figures 6–34, 7–1, 8–3, and 8–30

From Palay D A, Krachmer J H. (eds) 2005 Primary Care Ophthalmology, 2nd edn. Mosby, Philadelphia.
Figures 1–17, 1–20, 1–21, 1–24, 2–7, 4–6, 4–8 to 4–11, 4–26, 4–28, 5–7, 6–10, 6–12, 6–47, 6–48, 8–37, 10–4, 13–12, and 13–15

Adapted from Parks M M. 1982 Extraocular muscles. In: Duane T D (ed) Clinical Ophthalmology. Harper and Row, Philadelphia.
Figure 1–16

From Parrish R K. (ed) 2000 Bascom Palmer Eye Institute Atlas of Ophthalmology, 2nd edn. Butterworth-Heinemann, Philadelphia.
Figures 6–2, 12–1, and 14–6

Courtesy of Julian Perry, MD.
Figures 6–32, 8–1, and 8–31

Adapted from Reed H, Drance S M. 1972 The Essentials of Perimetry: Static and Kinetic, 2nd edn. Oxford University Press, London.
Figure 5–3

From Schepens C L, Neetens A. 1987 The Vitreous and Vitreoretinal Interface. Springer-Verlag, New York.
Figure 1–22

Reprinted with permission from Slamovits T L. 1993 Basic and Clinical Science Course, Section 7: Orbit, eyelids, and lacrimal system. American Academy of Ophthalmology, San Francisco.
Figure 1–6

Reprinted with permission from Grand M G. 1999 Basic and Clinical Science Course, Section 2: Fundamentals and principles of ophthalmology. American Academy of Ophthalmology, San Francisco.
Figures 1–8 and 1–12

From von Noorden G K. 1977 Von Noorden–Maumenee's Atlas of Strabismus, 3rd edn. Mosby, St. Louis.
Figures 4–21 and 4–22

From Yanoff M, Duker J S. (eds) 1999 Ophthalmology. Mosby, London.
Figures 1–26, 5–13, 5–33, and 6–23

From Campolattaro B N, Wang F M. Anatomy and physiology of the extraocular muscles and surrounding tissues. In Yanoff M, Duker J S. (eds) 2004 Ophthalmology, 2nd edn. Mosby, St Louis.
Figures 1–7, 1–13, 1–14, 2–1, 5–2, 5–5, 5–10, and 6–43

From Yanoff M, Fine B. 2002 Ocular Pathology, 5th edn. Mosby, Philadelphia.
Figures 9–2 and 14–13

From Zide B W, Jelks B W. 1985 Surgical Anatomy of the Orbit, 10th edn. Raven Press, New York.
Figure 1–10

Preface

The goal of this book is to provide the basic information about the eye we believe all medical students and primary care physicians should know, as well as the common disorders encountered in clinical practice. This begs the question: what should physicians know about eye care? The answer is not clear, as evidenced by the various general ophthalmology texts that exist, most of which seem to be either overly simplistic or too detailed. Unfortunately, ophthalmology is not always learned during the clinical clerkships in medical school, so there is a considerable amount of variability in the general practitioner's knowledge on the subject. Thus, we sought to find a happy medium, combining critical ophthalmic knowledge with high-quality illustrations and schematic drawings, to create an introductory text rather than a comprehensive overview of the field. We have also included some less common ocular diseases that are vision-threatening or life-threatening, as an awareness of these entities is mandatory for all physicians.

In addition to deciding what diseases to cover, the other difficult issue in creating such a book is how to present the information in a manner that is easy to understand and access. There are numerous ways to organize such material, and we chose to do so according to the ocular structures and components of the eye exam rather than categories of disease. We have tried to make the format as straightforward and as readable as possible. The eye is a visual organ and its examination is almost entirely visual. Thus, illustrations are an essential part of any ophthalmology book, and for the new student of ophthalmology, they are also an invaluable learning aid. We have therefore included numerous pictures and schematic drawings throughout the text as well as helpful hints on diagnosis, management, and treatment. It is our hope that this book will provide a solid foundation of core ophthalmic knowledge. For further study, the reader is directed to the suggested readings.

Neil J. Friedman, MD

Peter K. Kaiser, MD

Acknowledgments

While writing this book, we relied on the help and support of numerous individuals, and we would like to say a special thank you here.

First of all, we are grateful to the students we teach at Stanford University and the Cole Eye Institute, Cleveland Clinic, as well as our internal medicine colleagues, for it is they who inspired us to create such a text. We also acknowledge the fine instruction and guidance from our ophthalmology mentors and peers, for without their tutelage this task could not have been undertaken.

There are also certain individuals to whom we are particularly indebted for making this book a reality. Foremost is our editor James Merritt for believing in this project from the start when it was just a simple idea and for supporting us through all stages of its development. Similarly, we are grateful to Andrea Deis, Kathryn Mason, and their colleagues at Elsevier for their dedication and expert assistance.

And of course, we reserve a special thank you for our families whose love and understanding are endless: Mae, Alan, Diane, Lisa, Maureen, Peter (PJ), Stephanie, Peter, Anafu, and Christine.

Neil J. Friedman, MD

Peter K. Kaiser, MD

CHAPTER ONE

Ocular Anatomy, Physiology, and Embryology

Introduction

The eyes function like cameras: images are focused by a "lens" (the cornea and lens) on to the "film" (photoreceptors which are special light receptors in the retina). The visual pathway (see Ch. 5) transmits these images to the brain where they can be interpreted or "seen." Knowing basic ocular anatomy, physiology, and embryology is important for understanding how this complex organ works and how it can be affected by disease.

Basic Ocular Anatomy and Physiology

The eye is a delicate sense organ that is surrounded by specialized structures and protected by the bony orbit, soft tissues, and eyelids. The globe itself is composed of three primary layers or "coats": the sclera, the uvea, and the retina. Anteriorly, the cornea covers the central area of the eye, and the conjunctiva covers the sclera. The iris, the ciliary body, and the choroid constitute the uvea. The crystalline lens separates the anterior and posterior chambers from the vitreous body. The optic nerve transmits images from the retina to the brain (Figure 1–1).

ORBIT

The orbit is a bony cavity that protects the eye. This pear-shaped socket is 40 mm wide, 35 mm high, and 45 mm deep, with a volume of 30 ml. The orbit has four sides composed of seven bones (Table 1–1; Figures 1–2 and 1–3).

The orbit contains a number of **apertures** that transmit vital nerves and vessels to the eye and surrounding tissues. The three major apertures are:

TABLE 1–1

Osteology		
Orbit	**Bones**	**Related structures/ miscellaneous**
Roof	Sphenoid (lesser wing) Frontal	Lacrimal gland fossa Trochlea Supraorbital notch (medial)
Lateral wall	Sphenoid (greater wing) Zygomatic	Lateral orbital tubercle of Whitnall Strongest orbital wall Lateral orbital rim at equator of globe
Floor	Maxilla Palatine Zygomatic	Contains infraorbital nerve and canal Forms roof of maxillary sinus
Medial wall	Sphenoid Maxilla Ethmoid Lacrimal	Lacrimal sac fossa Adjacent to ethmoid and sphenoid sinuses Posterior ethmoidal foramen Weakest orbital wall

1. **Superior orbital fissure**: located between the orbital roof and lateral wall, the superior orbital fissure separates the greater and lesser wings of the sphenoid, and transmits cranial nerves (CN) III, IV, V_1, and VI, the superior ophthalmic vein, and sympathetic fibers to the iris dilator muscle.

2. **Optic canal (orbital foramen)**: contained within the lesser wing of the sphenoid, the optic canal is 10 mm long and transmits the optic nerve (CN II), ophthalmic artery, and sympathetic nerves to the ocular and orbital blood vessels.

3. **Inferior orbital fissure**: bordered by the maxillary bone (medially), zygomatic bone (anteriorly), and the

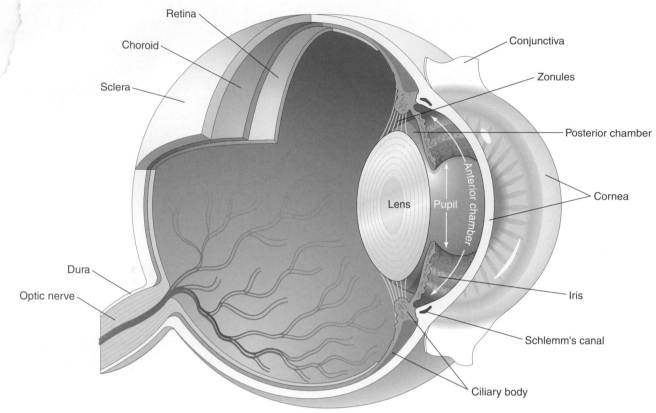

FIGURE 1–1
Basic anatomy of the eye.

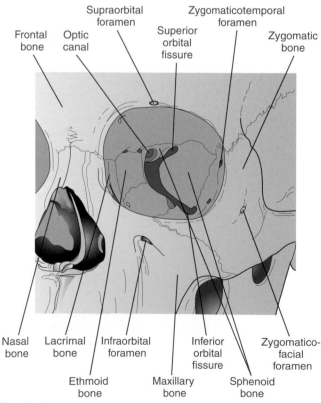

FIGURE 1–2
Bony anatomy of the orbit in frontal view.

greater wing of the sphenoid (laterally), the inferior orbital fissure transmits CN V$_2$, the zygomatic nerve, and inferior ophthalmic vein.

Orbital vasculature

The **ophthalmic artery**, which is the first branch of the internal carotid artery within the skull, gives rise to the **arterial system** (Figure 1–4), consisting of the:

- **Central retinal artery**, which enters the optic nerve behind the globe and supplies blood to the inner two-thirds of the retina.
- **Posterior ciliary arteries**: the long posterior ciliary arteries supply the anterior segment while the short posterior ciliary arteries supply the choroid and the optic nerve head.

The **venous system** consists of:

- The **superior and inferior ophthalmic veins**, which drain the superior and inferior vortex veins in the choroid, travel through the superior and inferior orbital fissures, respectively, and empty into the cavernous sinus.
- The **central retinal vein**, which emerges from the optic nerve behind the globe and joins the ophthalmic veins.

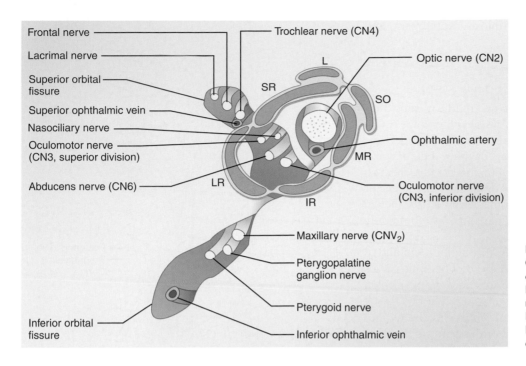

FIGURE 1–3

Orbital apex, superior and inferior orbital fissure. MR, medial rectus; IR, inferior rectus; LR, lateral rectus; SR, superior rectus; L, levator; SO, superior oblique. Note that the trochlear nerve lies outside the muscle cone.

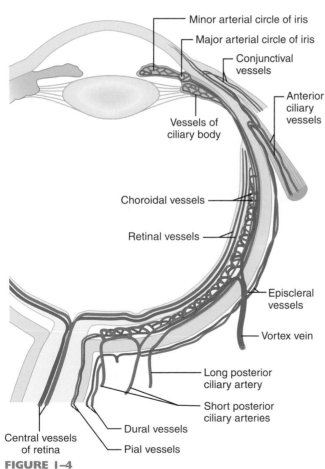

FIGURE 1–4

Vascular supply to the eye. All arterial branches originate with the ophthalmic artery. Venous drainage is through the cavernous sinus and the pterygoid plexus.

Orbital innervation

Sensory innervation of the orbit is provided by branches of the trigeminal nerve (CN V):

- **Ophthalmic division (V$_1$):** this has three branches:
  1. The **nasociliary nerve**, which enters the orbit within the annulus of Zinn and branches to form the short and long ciliary nerves. The short ciliary nerves pass through the ciliary ganglion without synapsing. The long ciliary nerves innervate the iris, cornea, and ciliary muscle.
  2. The **frontal nerve**, which enters the orbit above the annulus of Zinn and divides into the supraorbital and supratrochlear nerves, which innervate the medial canthus, upper eyelid, and forehead.
  3. The **lacrimal nerve**, which enters the orbit above the annulus of Zinn and innervates the upper eyelid and lacrimal gland.
- **Maxillary division (V$_2$):** this passes through the inferior orbital fissure and then branches into the infraorbital nerve, zygomatic nerve, and superior alveolar nerve.

Parasympathetic innervation synapses in the ciliary ganglion and enters the eye via the short ciliary nerves. The parasympathetics control accommodation (focusing), pupillary constriction, and lacrimal gland stimulation.

Sympathetic innervation follows the arteries and long ciliary nerves. These fibers control pupillary dilation, vasoconstriction, smooth-muscle function of the eyelids and orbit, and sweating (hidrosis). Dysfunction causes

Horner's syndrome (ptosis, miosis, anhidrosis, and vasodilation) (Figure 1–5).

Orbital sinuses

Four sinuses surround the orbits (Figure 1–6):

1. The **frontal** sinus drains into the middle meatus. This sinus is not radiographically visible before age 6.
2. The **ethmoid** is the first sinus to aerate and is composed of multiple thin-walled cavities. The anterior and middle air cells drain into the middle meatus, while the posterior air cells drain into the superior meatus. The lateral wall of this sinus is the medial wall of the orbit. Orbital cellulitis is most commonly caused by ethmoidal sinusitis.
3. The **sphenoid** sinus grows throughout childhood and becomes full-size after puberty. The optic canals are superior and lateral to the sphenoid sinuses, which drain into each nasal fossa.
4. The **maxillary** is the largest sinus and drains into the middle meatus. The roof of this sinus is the floor of the orbit and contains the infraorbital nerve.

Orbital soft tissues

The front of the orbit is protected by a dense fibrous sheath called the **orbital septum** that separates the orbit from the eyelids and maintains a barrier to the spread of infection. The septum originates from the periosteum of the orbital rims and inserts into the levator aponeurosis superiorly, lower eyelid retractors inferiorly, and lacrimal crest medially (Figure 1–7).

Most of the orbital contents are surrounded by adipose tissue divided by fine fibrous septa. The **preaponeurotic fat pads,** two in the upper lid and three in the lower lid, lie immediately posterior to the orbital septum.

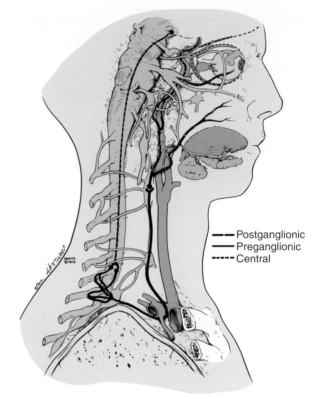

Postganglionic
Preganglionic
Central

FIGURE 1–5
Sympathetic innervation of the eye.

EYELIDS

The eyelids protect the surface of the eye and also contain glands that contribute components to the tear film. The upper eyelid (Figure 1–8) can be divided into two lamellae (layers): anterior (skin, orbicularis) and

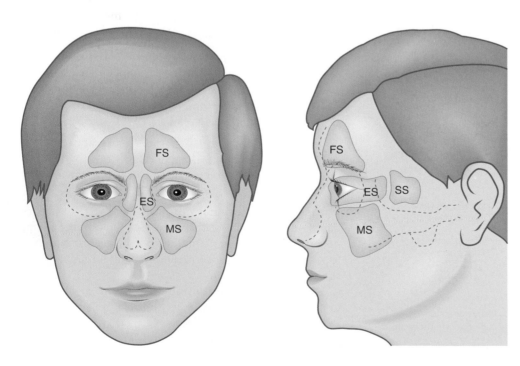

FIGURE 1–6
Relationship of the orbits to the paranasal sinuses. FS, frontal sinus; ES, ethmoid sinus; MS, maxillary sinus; SS, sphenoid sinus.

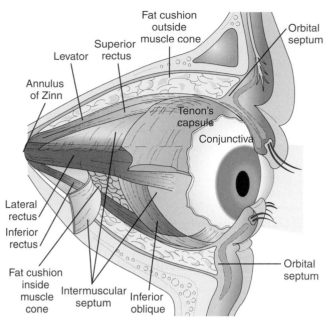

FIGURE 1–7
Orbital soft tissues.

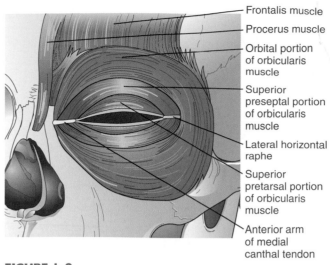

FIGURE 1–9
The orbicularis and frontalis muscles.

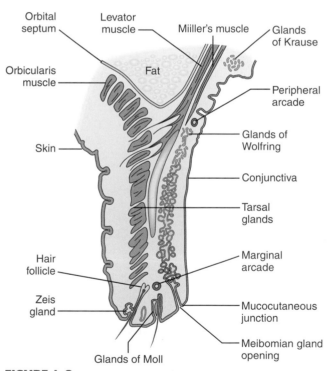

FIGURE 1–8
Cross-section of upper eyelid. Note the position of the cilia, tarsal gland orifices, and mucocutaneous junction.

posterior (tarsus, levator aponeurosis, Müller's muscle, palpebral conjunctiva).

Skin

The eyelid skin is the thinnest of the body and there is no subcutaneous fat. Sensory innervation is provided by CN V (V_1 to the upper lid and V_2 to the lower lid).

Orbicularis oculi

The orbicularis oculi is the main muscle that produces eyelid closure and is innervated by CN VII. It has three anatomic parts: the palpebral portion (pretarsal and preseptal) involved with involuntary blinking, and the orbital portion involved with voluntary, forced lid closure (Figure 1–9).

1. The **pretarsal** part overlies the tarsus and has superficial and deep heads. The superficial head contributes to the medial canthal tendon whereas the deep head contributes to the lateral canthal tendon, both of which fuse to the tarsal plates and help maintain apposition of the lids to the globe. The deep head also surrounds the canaliculi and thereby facilitates tear drainage by functioning as a lacrimal pump.
2. The **preseptal** part overlies the orbital septum.
3. The **orbital** part lies beneath the skin and is the thickest portion of the orbicularis. It interdigitates with the frontalis muscle superiorly at the eyebrow.

Eyelid retractors

The **upper eyelid retractors** (Figure 1–10) consist of the levator palpebrae, Whitnall's ligament, and Müller's muscle:

- The **levator palpebrae** originates from the lesser wing of the sphenoid above the annulus of Zinn and is innervated by CN III. The first 40 mm is muscular and the remaining 14–20 mm is the aponeurosis, which inserts into bone (laterally and medially), orbicularis (anteriorly), and the superior tarsus (posteriorly to form the upper eyelid crease), and divides the lacrimal gland into orbital and palpebral lobes.
- **Whitnall's ligament (superior transverse ligament)** is a condensation of the levator muscle sheath

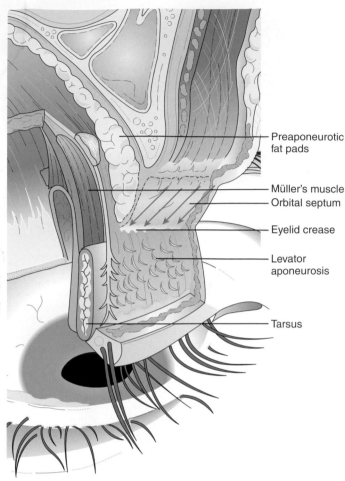

Preaponeurotic fat pads

Müller's muscle
Orbital septum

Eyelid crease

Levator aponeurosis

Tarsus

FIGURE 1–10
The orbital septum inserts into the levator aponeurosis (arrows). The preaponeurotic fat pads are located posterior to the septum. In downgaze, the lid crease becomes attenuated (weakened), and in a normal young eyelid, the fold is absent.

that acts as a check ligament to prevent excessive lid elevation.
- **Müller's muscle (superior tarsal muscle)** is located underneath the levator aponeurosis and is innervated by sympathetic fibers. It inserts into the upper border of the superior tarsus and helps raise the eyelid (2 mm). The peripheral arterial arcade of the upper eyelid is found between the aponeurosis and Müller's muscle.

The **lower eyelid retractors** include:
- **Capsulopalpebral fascia**, which is analogous to the levator aponeurosis. It arises from the inferior rectus muscle sheath, fuses with the orbital septum, and inserts into the inferior tarsus.
- **Lockwood's suspensory ligament**, which is analogous to Whitnall's ligament. It originates from fibrous attachments to the inferior rectus muscle and continues anteriorly as the capsulopalpebral fascia sending horns medially and laterally to form a suspensory hammock for the globe.

- **Inferior tarsal muscle**, which is analogous to Müller's muscle of the upper eyelid retractors. It originates from the capsulopalpebral fascia and has sympathetic innervation.

Tarsus

The **superior and inferior tarsi** (29 mm long, 1 mm thick, and 10 mm and 4 mm in height, respectively) are dense connective tissue plates that stabilize the eyelids and contain the Meibomian glands.

Eyelid margin

The eyelid margin has three distinguishing landmarks:
1. **Lash line**, which is located at the anterior lid margin and composed of 2–3 rows of eyelashes (100 in the upper and 50 in the lower lid).
2. **Gray line**, which is the border of the pretarsal orbicularis and represents the junction of the anterior and posterior lamellae.
3. **Meibomian gland orifices**, which are located at the posterior lid margin, there are 30 in the upper and 20 in the lower lid.

Eyelid vasculature

The eyelids have a rich **vascular supply**. Blood flows from the internal carotid artery to the ophthalmic artery to the superior marginal arcade in the upper lid, and from the external carotid artery to the facial artery to the angular artery to the inferior marginal arcade in the lower lid. Thus, the arcades allow for anastomosis between the internal and external carotids. The angular artery is an important surgical landmark that lies 6–8 mm medial to the medial canthus and 5 mm anterior to the lacrimal sac.

Venous drainage from the eyelids is divided into pre- and posttarsal systems. The pretarsal veins consist of the angular vein medially and the superficial temporal vein temporally, while the posttarsal veins include the orbital vein, anterior facial vein, and pterygoid plexus.

Lymphatic drainage is also split in the eyelids. The submandibular nodes drain the medial one-third of the upper lid and the medial two-thirds of the lower lid, while the preauricular nodes drain the lateral two-thirds of the upper lid and the lateral one-third of the lower lid. There are no lymphatic vessels or nodes within the orbit, but there are lymph vessels in the conjunctiva.

Eyelid glands

There are numerous glands in the eyelids (Table 1–2):
- **Eccrine**: secretion is by simple exocytosis.
- **Holocrine**: secretion is by release of the entire cellular contents (disruption of cell).
- **Apocrine**: secretion is by pinching or budding-off of a portion of the cytoplasm.

TABLE 1–2

Glands of the Eyelids

Gland	Location	Type	Function	Pathology
Lacrimal	Superotemporal orbit	Eccrine	Reflex tear (aqueous) secretion	Dacryoadenitis Tumors
Accessory lacrimal: Krause Wolfring	Fornix Just above tarsus	Eccrine	Basal tear (aqueous) secretion	Sjögren's syndrome Graft-versus-host disease Rare tumors (bone marrow transplantation)
Meibomian	Within tarsus	Holocrine	Lipid secretion Retards tear evaporation	Chalazion Sebaceous carcinoma
Zeis	Near lid margin Caruncle Associated with cilia	Holocrine	Lipid secretion Lubricates cilia	External hordeolum Sebaceous carcinoma
Moll	Near lid margin	Apocrine	Modified sweat glands Lubricates cilia	Ductal cyst Apocrine carcinoma
Sweat		Eccrine	Electrolyte balance	Ductal cyst Syringoma Sweat gland carcinoma
Goblet cells	Conjunctiva Plica Caruncle	Holocrine	Mucin secretion Enhances corneal wetting	Dry eye

The **lacrimal glands** consist of the main lacrimal gland and the accessory lacrimal glands. These eccrine glands produce the aqueous component of the tear film and are important in basal and reflex tear production (Figure 1–11).

- The **main lacrimal gland** is composed of two lobes, the orbital lobe and the palpebral lobe, which are separated by the levator aponeurosis. Ducts from both lobes pass through the smaller palpebral lobe and empty into the superior fornix. Innervation to the gland is secretomotor from CN VII and sensory from CN V. The blood supply is from the lacrimal artery.
- The **accessory lacrimal glands** are the glands of Krause and glands of Wolfring, located in the conjunctival fornices.

NASOLACRIMAL SYSTEM

The nasolacrimal system constitutes the tear drainage apparatus allowing tears to flow from the surface of the eye into the nose (Figure 1–12).

Punctum

The punctum is the small opening in the nasal aspect of each eyelid that allows drainage of the tear film from the eye. The puncta are slightly inverted against the globe

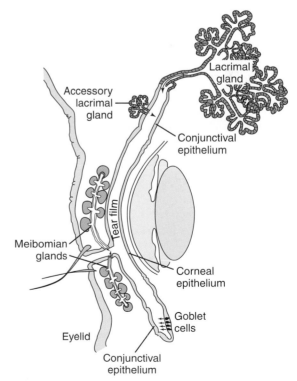

FIGURE 1–11

Glands and epithelia of the eye and ocular surface that contribute to the tear film.

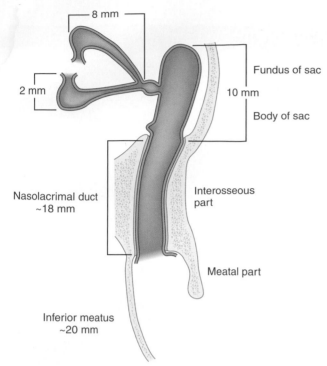

FIGURE 1–12
Excretory lacrimal system.

so that tears can gain access to the ampulla (see below). The puncta are attached to the canaliculi.

Canaliculi

The canaliculi are the drainage channels in the lids. They are 10 mm long (a 2 mm vertical segment (ampulla) and an 8 mm horizontal portion parallel to the lid margin). The upper and lower canaliculi combine to form a single common canaliculus in 90% of people. A small valve (the **valve of Rosenmüller**) at the distal end prevents the reflux of tears from the lacrimal sac back into the canaliculi.

Nasolacrimal sac

The nasolacrimal sac receives the tears from the canaliculi. It is 10 mm long and occupies the lacrimal fossa.

Nasolacrimal duct

The nasolacrimal duct spans 15 mm from the naso-lacrimal sac to the inferior meatus under the inferior turbinate by traveling inferiorly, posteriorly, and laterally within the nasolacrimal canal formed by the maxillary and lacrimal bones. The duct is partially covered by the **valve of Hasner**. A congenital nasolacrimal duct obstruction is usually due to an imperforate valve of Hasner.

FOREHEAD AND EYEBROW MUSCLES

The muscles that move the forehead and eyebrows are innervated by CNV. The **frontalis muscle** moves the scalp anteriorly and posteriorly and raises the eyebrows, the **corrugator muscle** pulls the medial eyebrow inferiorly and medially, producing vertical glabellar wrinkles, and the **procerus muscle** pulls the forehead and medial eyebrow inferiorly, producing horizontal lines in the nose.

EXTRAOCULAR MUSCLES

There are six extraocular muscles that control eye movements: four rectus muscles and two oblique muscles. The **annulus of Zinn** is a fibrous tissue ring arising from the periorbita that surrounds the optic canal. It is the origin of the four rectus muscles, which receive their blood supply from the ciliary arteries. The **intermuscular septum** is an extension of Tenon's capsule that connects the muscles. **Check ligaments** connect the muscles to the overlying Tenon's and insert on the orbital walls to support the globe (Table 1–3; Figures 1–13 and 1–14).

EYE

Conjunctiva

The conjunctiva is a clear, vascular, mucous membrane composed of non-keratinized epithelium with goblet cells and underlying loose stromal tissue (substantia propria).

Anatomically the conjunctiva is divided into two parts:

1. The **bulbar conjunctiva** covers the anterior sclera and is loosely adherent, except at its attachment to the corneal–scleral junction (the limbus), where it fuses with Tenon's capsule.

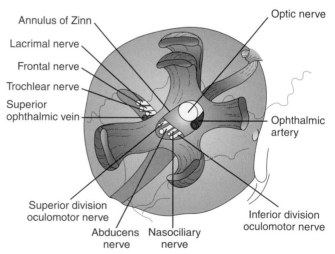

FIGURE 1–13
The annulus of Zinn and surrounding structures.

TABLE 1–3

Extraocular Muscles

Muscle	Anatomic insertion from limbus	Action from primary position	Origin	Innervation
Medial rectus (MR)	5.5 mm	Adduction	Annulus of Zinn	CN 3 (inferior division)
Lateral rectus (LR)	6.9 mm	Abduction	Annulus of Zinn	CN 6
Superior rectus (SR)	7.7 mm	1. Elevation 2. Intorsion 3. Adduction	Annulus of Zinn	CN 3 (superior division)
Inferior rectus (IR)	6.5 mm	1. Depression 2. Extorsion 3. Adduction	Annulus of Zinn	CN 3 (inferior division)
Superior oblique (SO)	Posterior to equator in superotemporal quadrant	1. Intorsion 2. Depression 3. Abduction	Orbital apex above annulus of Zinn	CN 4
Inferior oblique (IO)	Posterior to equator in inferotemporal quadrant	1. Extorsion 2. Elevation 3. Abduction	Behind lacrimal fossa	CN 3 (inferior division)

2. The **palpebral (or tarsal) conjunctiva** covers the inner surface of the eyelids, where it is firmly attached to the tarsal plates.

The **fornices** (superior fornix and inferior fornix) are the blind pouches where the conjunctiva reflects upon itself between the bulbar and palpebral surfaces. This prevents objects, like contact lenses, from traveling behind the eye.

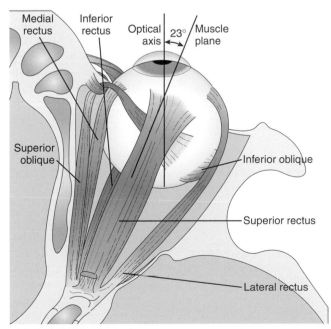

FIGURE 1–14
The extrinsic muscles of the right eyeball in the primary position, seen from above.

The **plica semilunaris** is a thickened fold of nasal bulbar conjunctiva adjacent to the caruncle. The **caruncle**, a small nodule of fleshy tissue at the medial canthus, is intermediate in structure between conjunctiva and skin, containing elements of both.

Tear film

The surface of the eye is bathed in tears. The tear film is composed of three layers:

1. The **lipid or outer layer** is produced by the meibomian, Zeis, and Moll glands and contains cholesterol and lipids. It is responsible for reducing evaporation of the tear film.
2. The **aqueous or middle layer** is produced by the lacrimal glands and contains 98% water, 2% protein (mainly lysozyme), and many other components, including lactoferrin, immunoglobulin A, and electrolytes. The aqueous layer provides oxygen to the cornea.
3. The **mucin or inner layer** is produced by conjunctival goblet cells (glands of Manz and crypts of Henle found primarily in the fornix) and is composed of glycoproteins. This layer reduces the surface tension of the tear film to allow the aqueous layer to spread evenly.

Cornea

The cornea is the clear window that covers the front of the eye. It is actually a complex structure that works like a lens in a camera, providing two-thirds of the focusing power of the eye. The cornea is slightly oval, with an average diameter of 12.5 mm horizontally and 11.5 mm

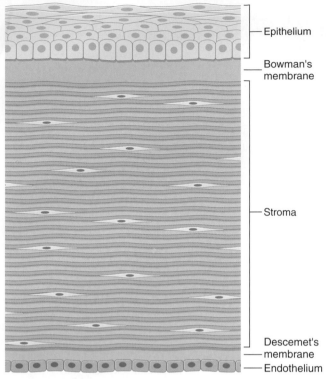

FIGURE 1-15
Anatomy of the cornea demonstrating the five histologic layers.

— Epithelium

— Bowman's membrane

— Stroma

— Descemet's membrane
— Endothelium

vertically. It is thinner (545 μm) and steeper centrally than it is peripherally (1.0 mm). Innervation to the cornea is via CN V_1. The cornea is composed of five layers (Figure 1–15):

1. **Epithelium** is a smooth refractive surface that also acts as a barrier against infection. Oxygen is absorbed from the tear film while the eye is open and from the eyelid vessels when the eye is closed. The epithelial cells that produce the epithelium originate from stem cells at the limbus, and turn over completely in 6–7 days. This is the reason for rapid healing of corneal abrasions. However, such epithelial defects are quite painful because of the abundant sensory nerve endings contained in this outer layer of the cornea.

2. **Bowman's membrane** is the thin, acellular structure to which the epithelium is attached. It is not a true basement membrane. If penetrated, it heals by scarring and does not regenerate.

3. **Stroma** makes up the majority (90%) of the corneal thickness. It is composed of highly organized collagen lamellae embedded in a mucopolysaccharide matrix that is mainly water, but also contains keratan sulfate and a variety of cells. The stroma is normally compact and clear, but it can swell like a sponge and become cloudy.

4. **Descemet's membrane** is the basement membrane of the endothelium and anchors it to the stroma.

Unlike Bowman's membrane, Descemet's membrane regenerates after damage if the overlying endothelium remains intact.

5. **Endothelium** is a monolayer of hexagonal cells joined by tight junctions and is responsible for transporting nutrients into the cornea and pumping fluid out of the cornea. This latter function is the most important as it keeps the cornea deturgesced and clear. Approximately half the endothelial cells are lost with aging. They do not regenerate; instead, adjacent endothelial cells stretch to bridge the gaps. The cells change in shape (pleomorphism) and size (polymegathism) as a response to various stresses (i.e., surgery, contact lens wear, medications, disease states). If the population of endothelial cells becomes too few or too weak, then it cannot adequately perform its pumping function and corneal edema results.

Limbus

The limbus is the 1–2 mm transition zone between the cornea and the sclera that roughly corresponds to the termination of Bowman's and Descemet's membranes. It is the location of the corneal epithelial stem cells and it is where the conjunctiva and Tenon's capsule are fused. This area also contains goblet cells, lymphoid cells, Langerhan cells, and mast cells.

Sclera

The sclera is the tough, avascular, outer fibrous layer of the eye that forms a protective coating. It is composed of dense collagen fibrils that are not highly organized (as opposed to the cornea), and thus this tissue appears white (rather than clear). The sclera is covered by fascia (**subconjunctival fascia** is known as **Tenon's capsule**) and conjuctiva anteriorly, and fat posteriorly. Anteriorly, Tenon's capsule fuses with the conjunctiva just behind the limbus, while posteriorly, it separates the orbital fat from the extraocular muscles and globe. The extraocular muscles insert into the sclera behind the limbus (Figure 1–16).

Uvea

The uvea refers to the pigmented layer of the eye and is made up of three distinct structures: the iris, the ciliary body, and the choroid (Figure 1–17).

The **iris** is the annular skirt of tissue in the anterior chamber that functions as an aperture to control the amount of light entering the eye. It is responsible for giving our eyes their "color." All irides have approximately the same number of melanocytes. The color of the iris is therefore determined by the amount of pigment in these melanocytes. The iris root attaches to the ciliary body peripherally. The pupil is the central opening in the iris. There are two muscles within the iris that control the size of the pupil: the circumferential sphincter at

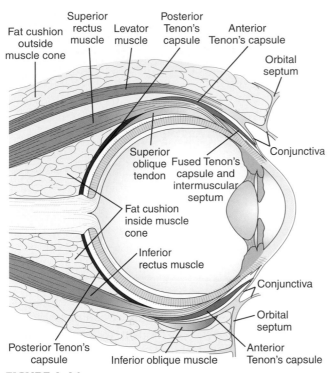

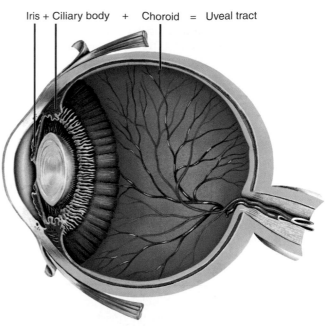

FIGURE 1–16
Sagittal section of orbital tissues through the vertical recti.

FIGURE 1–17
Uveal tract consists of the iris, ciliary body, and choroid (in red).

the pupillary border and the radial dilator in the mid-peripheral iris. The iris divides the anterior segment of the eye into two chambers: the anterior chamber (the space between the iris and cornea) and the posterior chamber (the space between the iris and lens).

The **ciliary body** is the 6 mm portion of uvea between the iris and choroid, and is attached to the sclera at the scleral spur. It is composed of two zones, the anterior

2 mm **pars plicata**, which contains the ciliary muscle, vessels, and processes, and the posterior 4 mm **pars plana**. The **ciliary muscle** controls accommodation (focusing) of the lens, while the **ciliary processes** suspend the lens (from small fibers called **zonules**) and produce the aqueous humor (the fluid that fills the anterior and posterior chambers and maintains intraocular pressure).

The **aqueous humor** drains from the eye through channels arising in the **anterior-chamber angle** (Figure 1–18). This ring of tissue between the cornea

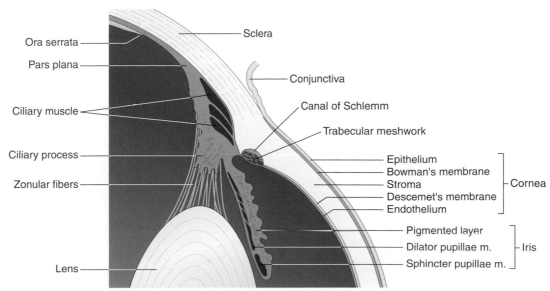

FIGURE 1–18
Anatomy of the anterior-chamber angle structures.

and ciliary body is called the **trabecular meshwork** and is only visible by examination with a special mirrored contact lens (gonioscopy). The aqueous filters through the pores of the meshwork into **Schlemm's canal** and then into collector channels and veins. If this outflow pathway becomes damaged or obstructed, intraocular pressure can rise, causing glaucoma.

The **choroid** is the tissue between the sclera and retina, and is attached to the sclera at the optic nerve and scleral spur. This highly vascular tissue supplies nutrition to the retinal pigment epithelium (RPE) and outer retinal layers. The layers of the choroid (from inner to outer) are: **Bruch's membrane**, the **choriocapillaris**, and stroma (Figure 1–19). Bruch's membrane separates the RPE from the choroid and is a permeable layer composed of the basement membrane of each, with collagen and elastic tissues in the middle.

A potential space, the suprachoroidal space, exists between the choroid and sclera. In certain disease processes, fluid or blood can fill this space, creating a choroidal detachment.

Lens

The **crystalline lens**, located between the posterior chamber and the vitreous cavity, separates the anterior and posterior segments of the eye. It is essentially a sac of gelatinous proteins surrounded by a basement membrane (the capsule) created by the lens epithelial cells. The lens grows by elongation and transformation of the epithelial cells into lens fibers (Figure 1–20).

Zonular fibers suspend the lens from the ciliary body and enable the ciliary muscle to focus the lens by changing its shape. This process is called **accommodation**. The lens works like a zoom lens of a camera, allowing us to see distant and near objects clearly. When the ciliary muscle is relaxed, the zonules are stretched tight and the lens is pulled into a flatter, thinner con-

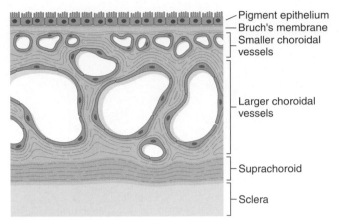

FIGURE 1–19
Anatomy of the choroid.

figuration to provide good distance vision. When we need to see up close, the ciliary muscle contracts, causing the zonules to loosen and the lens to assume a more spherical shape (Figure 1–21).

Vitreous

The **vitreous humor** is a viscous, gel-like substance that fills the posterior segment of the eye between the lens and retina. The vitreous is composed mainly of water, but also contains collagen fibers, mucopolysaccharide, and hyaluronic acid. The hyaluronic acid and associated water molecules serve as fillers between the collagen fibers. It is attached to the retina by collagen fibers at the vitreous base (which straddles the ora serrata and connects to the peripheral retina and the pars plana), macula, optic nerve, and retinal vessels, as well as at areas of degeneration and scarring. With aging, the vitreous liquefies, a process known as syneresis (Figures 1–22 and 1–23).

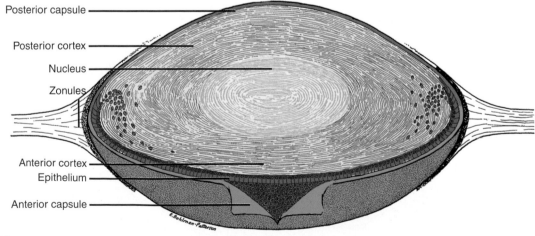

FIGURE 1–20
Normal lens anatomy.

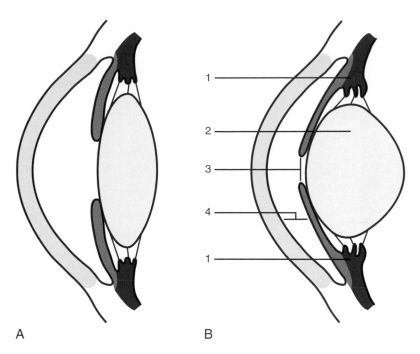

FIGURE 1–21

Cross-section of eye: (**A**) in non-accommodative state; and (**B**) during accommodation where the ciliary body (1) moves forward, relaxing the zonules, (2) thickening the lens, (3) constricting the pupil, and (4) shallowing the anterior chamber.

Retina

The retina is the delicate transparent light sensing inner layer of the eye that functions like film in a camera. Light travels through the retina to the photoreceptors in the outermost layer. These rod and cone photoreceptor cells convert the light into neural signals that pass back through the retina to the ganglion cells whose axons form the optic nerve (Figure 1–24).

The retina has nine distinct layers (Figure 1–25):

1. The **internal limiting membrane (ILM)** is the inner basement membrane.
2. The **nerve fiber layer (NFL)** contains unmyelinated ganglion cell axons that then form the optic nerve

FIGURE 1–22

Vitreous anatomy according to classic anatomic and histologic studies.

Egger's line forming Wieger's ligament (hyaloideo-capsular ligament)
Berger's space (retrolental space of Erggelet)
Ora serrata
Sclera
Choroid
Retina
Cloquet's canal
Area of Martegiani
Canal of Hannover
Pars plicata
Pars plana
Canal of Petit
Anterior vitreous cortex
Vitreous base
Secondary vitreous

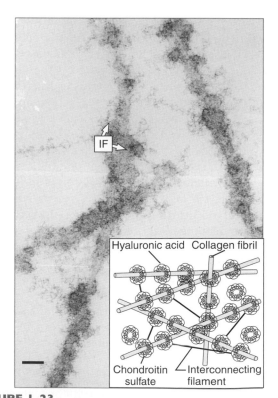

IF
Hyaluronic acid Collagen fibril
Chondroitin sulfate Interconnecting filament

FIGURE 1–23

Ultrastructure of hyaluronan–collagen interaction in the vitreous. IF, interconnecting filament.

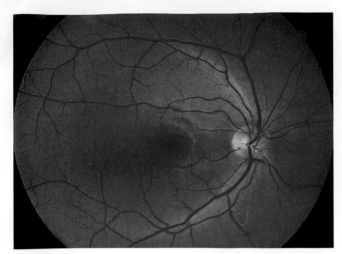

FIGURE 1–24
Normal fundus.

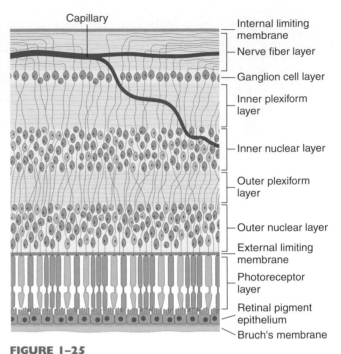

FIGURE 1–25
Anatomy of the retina, demonstrating the nine layers of the retina as well as the retinal pigment epithelium and Bruch's membrane.

and finally synapse with nuclei of cells in the lateral geniculate body.

3. The **ganglion cell layer** is composed of a single layer of ganglion cells, except in the macula, where it is multilayered.

4. The **inner plexiform layer** contains the synapses between the bipolar cells and ganglion cells or amacrine cells.

5. The **inner nuclear layer** contains the cell bodies of the bipolar, amacrine, horizontal, and Müller cells.

6. The **outer plexiform layer** contains the synapses between photoreceptors and the bipolar cells. This layer is also the location of the middle limiting membrane (MLM), which demarcates the different blood supplies to the internal and external retina: the central retinal artery supplies the retina internally (MLM to ILM), while the choriocapillaris supplies the retina externally (MLM to RPE). In the macula, the outer plexiform layer is called **Henle's fiber layer** and there is a radial orientation of fibers.

7. The **outer nuclear layer** is composed of the photoreceptor cell nuclei.

8. The **external limiting membrane (ELM)** is not a true basement membrane but rather consists of intercellular bridges that connect photoreceptor cells to Müller cells.

9. The **photoreceptor layer** contains the rods and cones. There are 120 million rods and 6 million cones; the macula has an equal number of each. The rods contain rhodopsin and are densest in a ring 20–40° around the fovea, while the cones contain three types of visual pigment (red, green, or blue) and are densest in the fovea.

The **peripheral retina** extends from the macula to the ora serrata and is defined as any area of the retina containing a single layer of ganglion cells.

The **macula** is the area in which the ganglion cell layer is more than one cell thick. The macula is located in the posterior pole, temporal to the optic nerve and bounded by the vascular arcades. It is 5–6 mm in diameter and is the region of the retina responsible for providing our sharpest vision. However, differentiation of the macula does not occur until age 4–6 months old (this is why infants are observed to have random eye movements and do not maintain steady fixation).

Within the macula is the **fovea**, a central depression of the inner retinal surface (1.5 mm in diameter) that corresponds to the foveal avascular zone where no retinal vessels traverse. This region contains taller RPE cells as well as xanthophyll pigment. The **foveola** is the central area of the fovea (350 μm in diameter) characterized by the absence of ganglion and other nucleated cells. The photoreceptors in the fovea are only cones (Figure 1–26).

Retinal pigment epithelium

The RPE is a vital monolayer of hexagonal cells between the retina and the choroid. The RPE performs a number of functions, including vitamin A metabolism and formation of the outer blood–retinal barrier.

The apices of these cells face the photoreceptors, creating a potential subretinal space. If liquefied vitreous enters the subretinal space, a retinal detachment occurs and the photoreceptors, no longer able to receive their blood supply from the choroid, can be damaged.

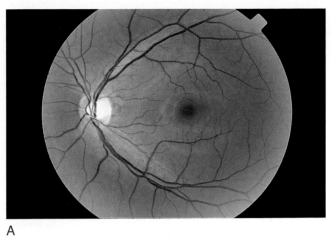

A

B

FIGURE 1–26
(**A**, **B**) Normal fundus with macula encompassed by major vascular arcades.

RPE cells are distinct in that they can undergo hypertrophy, hyperplasia, migration (into the retina to form bone spicules around blood vessels in retinitis pigmentosa, or through retinal holes to form preretinal membranes in proliferative vitreoretinopathy), and metaplasia (fibrous or osseous).

Optic nerve

The optic nerve is essentially a cable of many wires that transmits images from the eye to the brain where they can be interpreted. The nerve contains approximately 1.2 million axons formed from the retinal ganglion cells in the retina, and appears as a yellow-orange circle nasal to the fovea. This is the nerve head or **optic disc** and is actually an annulus of nerve tissue surrounding the **optic cup**, the central white area from which the retinal vessels emanate. The disc should appear flat with sharp margins, and the size of the cup with respect to the disc (the cup-to-disc ratio) should normally be less than 0.4 (Figure 1–27).

The appearance of the optic nerve changes in pathologic conditions. An elevated nerve head with blurred margins indicates optic disc edema, while an enlarged optic cup ("cupping") in relation to the disc may indicate glaucoma. The absence of retina at the optic nerve head results in an absolute scotoma (the physiologic blind spot) that is located 15° temporal to fixation and slightly below the horizontal meridian. The blind spot

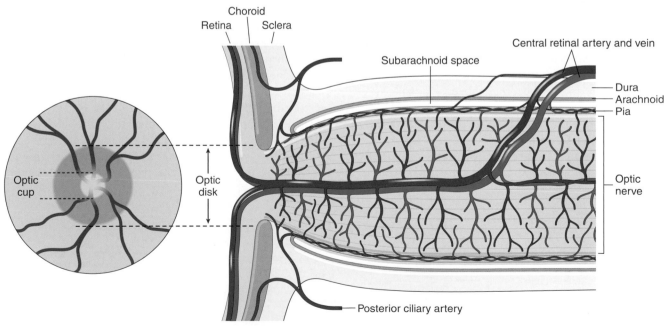

FIGURE 1–27
Anatomy of the optic nerve.

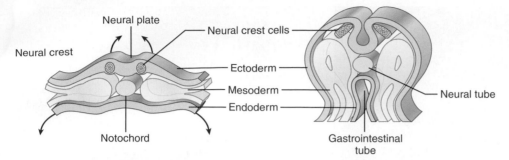

FIGURE 1–28
Neural tube formation.

can only be detected monocularly because the visual fields of the eyes overlap.

Embryology

The embryology of the eye begins with the embryonic plate and subsequent transformation to the neural plate from which the optic pit, vesicle, and cup develop. The embryonic plate contains ectoderm, mesoderm, and endoderm (Figure 1–28).

The **optic pit** forms at day 23 of gestation. On day 25, the **optic vesicle** pinches off from the primitive brainstem, as an outpouching that becomes the globe. Abnormalities of this process may result in congenital anomalies such as anophthalmia, cyclopia (synophthalmia), cystic eye, and non-attachment of the retina. The optic vesicle develops into a bilayered structure, the **optic cup** (Figure 1–29). The inner layer becomes the retina and the outer layer becomes the RPE. Between these layers is the subretinal space which was formerly the cavity of the neural tube and optic vesicle.

The **lens** starts to develop at day 27, when the surface ectoderm adjacent to the optic vesicle enlarges to form the **lens plate**. An indentation on the lens plate, the **lens pit**, invaginates to form a sphere, the **lens vesicle**. The surface ectoderm basement membrane, which forms the surface of this sphere, becomes the lens capsule.

The lens epithelial cells, located on the posterior part of the sphere, migrate and fill the core to become the embryonal nucleus at day 40.

The **embryonic fissure**, located on the undersurface of the optic cup, is the portal through which mesoderm enters the eye. When the fissure closes on day 33, the globe is formed. Incomplete closure of the embryonic fissure results in a coloboma or defect in one or multiple ocular tissues (usually the retina, choroid, iris, or optic nerve). However, an eyelid coloboma is not related to faulty closure of the embryonic fissure.

The **hyaloid artery** is the blood supply to the developing eye and enters the globe through the embryonic fissure. This artery nourishes the vitreous and lens and finally regresses by the 8th month, except for the portion that supplies the retina as the central retinal artery. Sometimes the hyaloid vasculature fails to regress completely and remnants can be seen in the eye as: **Bergmeister's papillae** (a glial tissue sheath at the optic nerve head), **peripapillary loop** (a vascular loop extending from the optic nerve head), **Mittendorf dot** (a small opacity on the central posterior lens capsule where the hyaloid artery attached to and formed the lens blood supply (posterior tunica vasculosa lentis)), and **persistent pupillary membrane** (remnants of the anterior tunica vasculosa lentis, appearing as thin iris strands that bridge the pupil and may attach to the lens capsule).

The **optic nerve head** develops from cells on the inner layer of the optic cup, and then ganglion cell axons grow through the disc. Myelination begins at the center of the nerve, reaching the chiasm at the 7th month, the lamina cribrosa at birth, and completion approximately 1 month after birth.

The **vitreous** is formed in stages by several tissues. The primary vitreous, produced by the hyaloid vascular system, is eventually replaced by secondary vitreous formed by the retina. If the regression of the primary

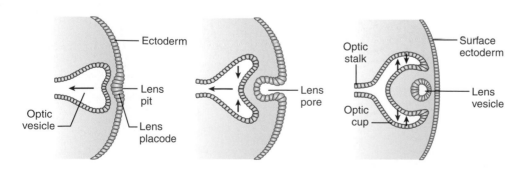

FIGURE 1–29
Optic cup formation.

vitreous fails to occur, the congenital abnormality persistent hyperplastic primary vitreous (PHPV) results. The tertiary vitreous is actually another name for the zonular fibers, which are formed from the ciliary processes and lens capsule.

The **retina** develops from neuroectoderm. The retinal vessels begin to form at 4 months, growing outward from the optic disc and reaching the nasal ora serrata during the 8th month and the temporal periphery 1–2 months later. The fovea is not mature until 4–6 months after birth.

The RPE is required for the development of the **choroid**. Neural crest cells form the choroidal stroma and vessel walls while mesoderm forms the vessel endothelium. The **sclera** is also formed from neural crest cells, except for a small temporal portion that is composed of mesoderm. The blue hue of the sclera at birth is due to its thinness, which enables the underlying uveal pigment to be seen.

The **cornea** forms from neural crest cells in two waves. The first wave grows between the epithelium and lens, forming the corneal endothelium. The second wave grows between the epithelium and endothelium, forming the stroma. Descemet's and Bowman's membranes develop at 4 and 5 months, respectively. Neural crest cells from the peripheral cornea differentiate into the **anterior-chamber angle** during the 5th week. In the 4th month, Schlemm's canal forms, and in the 8th month the angle is complete. The trabecular meshwork appears just before birth. Anterior-segment disorders such as congenital glaucoma and corneal endothelial dystrophies are due to neural crest abnormalities.

The rim of the optic cup grows around the lens to form the **iris**. The iris epithelium is derived from the inner and outer layers of the optic cup. In the 7th week, the iris stroma is formed from neural crest cells. The iris muscles develop from neuroectoderm in the 6th month, and during the following month, blood vessels enter the iris. Newborn babies typically have gray-blue eyes because the development of iris color may take months as stromal chromatophores continue to migrate into uveal tissue after birth. Similarly, the iris dilator muscle is still immature during infancy, causing a relative miosis or small pupils.

Formation of the **ciliary body** begins in the 3rd month with a fold in the optic cup, which becomes the epithelial layers of the ciliary processes. The ciliary processes develop in the 4th month, along with the zonules and blood vessels. During the 5th month, the pars plana forms, and neural crest cells adjacent to the cornea become the ciliary body stroma and ciliary muscle.

The **nasolacrimal system** starts to form at 6 weeks when surface ectoderm is buried in mesoderm between the maxillary and lateral nasal processes. This cord of tissue canalizes in the 3rd month. Defects in formation may result in an imperforate valve of Hasner, or rarely, absent puncta or canaliculi.

Formation of the **eyelids** begins at 8 weeks by fusion of adjacent processes (frontonasal for the upper lids; maxillary and nasal for the lower lids). The lid folds fuse at 12 weeks, and at 24 weeks separation occurs.

CHAPTER TWO

Basic Optics

Introduction

Since the eye functions like a camera, ocular structures are required to focus light and provide clear images of the world around us. In the eye, two structures focus light on the retina: the **cornea** provides most of the refractive power and the **lens** serves to fine-tune the focus at different ranges by the process of **accommodation** (focusing).

Knowledge of basic optics is necessary for an understanding of how the eye works. In particular, the properties of light and lenses are important principles that help explain refractive errors and their correction.

Properties of Light

Light behaves as both waves and particles (photons), but for the purpose of optics, it is easiest to only consider light as waves. The speed of a wave (v) is directly proportional to its wavelength (λ) and frequency (ν) ($v = \lambda\nu$), and in any given medium, the speed of light is constant ($v_{vacuum} = c = 3.0 \times 10^{10}$ cm/s). Thus, the wavelength and frequency of light are inversely proportional.

The energy of light is directly proportional to its frequency and inversely proportional to its wavelength ($E = h\nu = h(c/\lambda)$). Thus, light with shorter wavelengths has more energy than light with longer wavelengths.

INDEX OF REFRACTION

Light travels slower in any medium compared to its speed in air or a vacuum. The speed of light in a given medium depends on the density of the medium. This relationship is defined by the **index of refraction** (n), which is the ratio of the speed of light in a vacuum to the speed of light in the specific material ($n = c/v$). Air has an index of refraction of 1, water of 1.33 (which is the same as that of the aqueous and vitreous), cornea of 1.37, and crystalline lens of 1.42. When traveling through a substance, the frequency of light remains unchanged, but the wavelength becomes shorter (Figure 2–1).

REFLECTION AND REFRACTION

The behavior of a light wave as it encounters an optical interface (i.e., travels from one medium to another of different refractive index), can be described in a number of ways. The incoming or **incident ray** is partly reflected and partly refracted. The **reflected ray** bounces off the interface, and the greater the difference in refractive index between the two media, the greater the reflection. The direction of reflection depends on the angle of incidence. **Luminance** is the measure of reflected or emitted light (lumens/m^2), and the ability to detect small changes in luminance is called **contrast sensitivity**.

When the incident ray is not perpendicular to the surface (parallel to the normal), then the transmitted light is deviated or refracted. **Refraction** is the change in direction of light traveling across an optical interface. The direction of refraction is towards the normal when passing from a medium of lower index of refraction to a higher one, and away from the normal when passing from a denser to a less dense medium. This occurs because higher refractive index materials are harder for light to travel through, so light takes a shorter path (i.e., closer to the normal). **Snell's law** governs this behavior of light (Figure 2–2):

$$n \sin (i) = n' \sin (r)$$

where n = refractive index of material; i = angle of incidence (measured from normal); and r = angle of refraction (measured from normal).

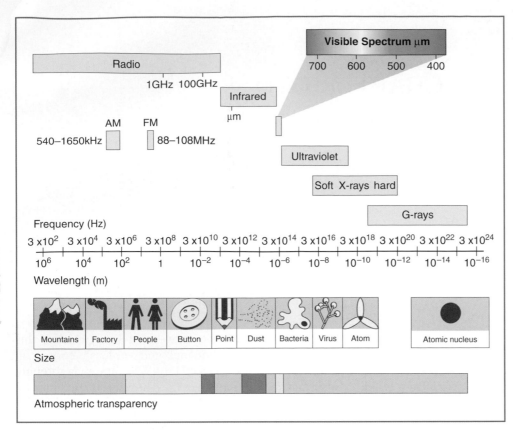

FIGURE 2–1
The electromagnetic spectrum. The pictures of mountains, people, buttons, viruses, and so forth are used to produce a real (i.e., visceral) feeling of the size of some of the wavelengths.

The angle at which incident light is bent exactly 90° away from the normal (when going from a medium of higher to lower n) and after which all light is reflected is called the **critical angle**. An interface between glass and air has a critical angle of 41°; the critical angle of the cornea is 46.5°. When the angle of incidence exceeds the critical angle and all the light is reflected back into the material with the higher index of refraction, then **total internal reflection** is said to occur. This happens at the cornea, preventing direct visualization of the angle structures without a special gonioscopy lens.

Transmission (the percentage of light penetrating a substance) varies with wavelength.

Light may also be scattered and diffracted. **Scattering** is the disruption of light by irregularities in its path. For example, an opacity in the cornea (scar) or lens (cataract) scatters light, causing glare and image degradation. This is a common complaint of patients with cataracts involving the visual axis. Shorter wavelengths scatter more than longer ones. Thus, particles in the atmosphere scatter blue light more than other wavelengths, causing the sky to appear blue.

Diffraction is the bending of light waves around the edge of openings. The amount of diffraction is related to wavelength (the shorter the wavelength, the less the change in direction) and the size of the aperture (the smaller the aperture, the greater the diffraction). This optical principle is best demonstrated by the pinhole test for measuring visual acuity. Looking through a pinhole reduces the patient's refractive error and improves vision by increasing depth of focus. However, the pinhole vision is limited by diffraction. The optimal aperture size of a pinhole is 1.2 mm, which may correct up to 3 D of refractive error. A smaller pinhole actually hinders visual acuity because the smaller the aperture, the greater the diffraction. Using a pinhole can also improve vision in eyes with corneal or lens irregularities, but it reduces

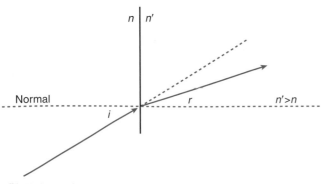

FIGURE 2–2
Refraction of light ray.

vision in eyes with retinal disorders. Squinting is a method of creating a natural pinhole to improve vision.

Properties of Lenses

VERGENCE

Lenses add vergence to light. Vergence is defined as the amount of spreading of a bundle of light rays (wavefront) emerging from a point source. The rays may come together (convergence), spread apart (divergence), or remain parallel. **Convergence** or plus vergence refers to converging rays, which are rare in nature and must be produced by an optical system. **Divergence** or minus vergence is the term for diverging rays. Parallel rays have zero vergence.

The focal length of a lens determines its converging or diverging effect. However, rather than working with lengths, it is easier to use power. Therefore, the unit of vergence is the **diopter (D)**: the reciprocal of the focal length of the lens (the reciprocal of the distance (in meters) to the point where the light rays are focused or intersect) (Figure 2–3).

A plus or convex lens is a converging lens because it adds vergence; a minus or concave lens is a diverging lens because it subtracts vergence. The effectiveness of a lens is a function of the lens power and its distance from the desired point of focus. Moving a lens away from the eye increases its effective plus power, so a plus lens becomes stronger and a minus lens becomes weaker. When a lens is held closer to the eye, more plus power is required to maintain the same distance correction.

ABERRATIONS

Lenses behave ideally near their optical axis, and aberrations occur peripheral to the optical axis. **Spherical aberration** is caused by the increasing prismatic effect of the lens periphery. Peripheral rays are refracted more than paraxial ones, producing a blur interval along the optical axis (Figure 2–4).

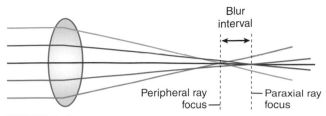

FIGURE 2–4
Spherical aberration.

The eye has compensatory mechanisms to reduce the spherical aberration of the crystalline lens: the size of the pupil (constriction eliminates peripheral rays), the shape of the cornea (progressively flatter in the periphery), and the index of refraction of the lens (higher centrally in the nucleus).

Coma is a comet-shaped image deformity from off-axis peripheral rays. **Curvature of field** occurs because a spherical lens produces a curved image of a flat object. **Astigmatism of oblique incidence** is the astigmatism induced by tilting a spherical lens since oblique rays encounter different curvatures at the front and the back lens surfaces. **Distortion** refers to the differential magnification from the optical axis to the lens periphery that causes straight lines to appear curved.

Chromatic aberration occurs because light of different wavelengths is refracted different amounts (shorter wavelengths are bent more).

PRISMS

Prisms displace and deviate light because their surfaces are not parallel. Light rays are deviated toward the base and the image is displaced toward the apex (Figure 2–5).

Lenses have a **prismatic effect**. Glasses induce prism by bending off-axis rays. Plus lenses act like two prisms placed base to base, while minus lenses act like two prisms aligned apex to apex (Figure 2–6).

This is why plus lenses cause convergence of peripheral rays toward the lens axis and are called converging lenses, and minus lenses produce divergence of peripheral rays away from the axis and are designated diverging lenses. The prismatic effect of glasses becomes stronger with increasing distance from the optical axis of the lens.

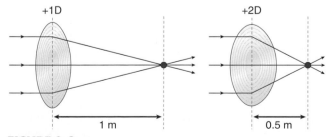

FIGURE 2–3
The principle of diopter and focal length demonstrated by 1 D and 2 D converging lenses.

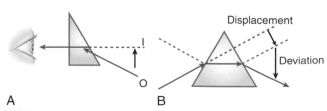

FIGURE 2–5
(**A**) Displacement of image toward apex. (**B**) Displacement and deviation of light by prism.

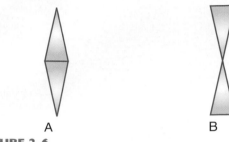

FIGURE 2–6
(**A**) Plus lenses act like two prisms base to base. (**B**) Minus lenses act like two prisms apex to apex.

Bifocal glasses cause unique prismatic effects depending on their shape. **Image jump** refers to the sudden upward shift of an image produced by the prismatic power of the bifocal segment. This is more bothersome than **image displacement**, which is the displacement of the image position by the total prismatic effect of the underlying lens and the bifocal segment.

Prismatic effect also varies with wavelength, so that shorter wavelengths are bent more than longer ones, resulting in **chromatic aberration**. This is the reason why white light shined through a prism produces a rainbow effect with blue rays closer to the base (bent most) and red rays closer to the apex.

The Eye as an Optical System

VISION MEASUREMENT

Vision can be measured with a variety of tests. Traditionally, vision is assessed with **Snellen acuity**. This is based on the angle that the smallest letter subtends on the retina. Each letter subtends 5 minutes of arc at a specific distance, represented by the denominator (i.e., the 20/40 letter subtends 5 minutes at 40 feet (12 meters), and the 20/20 letter subtends 5 minutes at 20 feet (6 meters)); the numerator is the testing distance, and each stroke width and space within the letter subtends 1 minute of arc. When measuring near acuity, the testing distance must be recorded. Legal blindness in the USA is defined as visual acuity of 20/200 or worse or a visual field of less than 20° in the better-seeing eye (Figure 2–7).

From the preceding discussion of optics, it is important to remember that acuity is influenced by pupil size. A larger pupil limits vision due to spherical and chromatic aberration, while a smaller pupil limits vision due to diffraction. The optimal pupil size is 3 mm.

Other components of vision can also be tested: **contrast sensitivity** is the ability to detect changes in luminance. Detecting the presence or absence of a stimulus is called the **minimum visible**, while **minimum discriminable** represents the resolving power of the eye. The smallest angle at which two separate

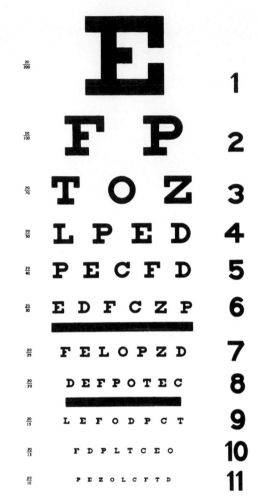

FIGURE 2–7
Snellen distance acuity chart.

objects can be discriminated, specifically the detection of a break in a line, is known as the **minimum separable**. **Vernier acuity** refers to spatial discrimination, that is, the ability to detect misalignment of two lines.

The eye is like a camera with a zoom lens: it can focus on objects at distance and near, from infinity to inches from the eye. The range of focus is defined as the interval between the **far point** and the **near point**. In the normal eye (**emmetropia** or no refractive error), an object at infinity is focused on the retina, which means that the secondary focal point of the eye is at the retina. To focus on a closer object, the lens changes shape to increase focusing power, a process known as accommodation. The near point, determined by the amount of accommodation, recedes with time. This decrease in accommodative amplitude with age, called **presbyopia**, is due to the loss of lens elasticity and becomes noticeable in our early 40s with symptoms of eyestrain during sustained near effort (**asthenopia**). As presbyopia progresses, reading glasses are needed to see clearly at near. Donder's table shows the relationship between accommodative power and age (Table 2–1).

TABLE 2–1

Donder's Table																
Age	8	12	16	20	24	28	32	36	40	44	48	52	56	60	64	68
Accommodation (D)	14	13	12	11	10	9	8	7	6	4.5	3	2.5	2	1.5	1	0.5

Up to age 40, accommodation decreases by 1 D every 4 years (starting at 14 D at age 8).
At age 40, accommodation is 6.0 D (± 2 D).
Between ages 40 and 48, accommodation decreases by 1.5 D every 4 years.
Above age 48, accommodation decreases by 0.5 D every 4 years

Various disorders can cause asthenopia as well as premature presbyopia. Asthenopia may result from conditions such as hypothyroidism, anemia, pregnancy, nutritional deficiencies, and chronic illness. Premature presbyopia is found in debilitating illness, diphtheria, botulism, mercury toxicity, head injury, cranial nerve III palsy, Adie's tonic pupil, and the use of tranquilizers. Subnormal accommodation is treated with glasses containing reading add and base-in prism to help convergence.

REFRACTIVE ERRORS

A refractive error exists when the secondary focal point of the eye is not located on the retina. If an object at infinity is focused in front of the retina, the eye is near-sighted (**myopic**), and if the object is focused behind the retina, the eye is far-sighted (**hyperopic**). Therefore, in myopia, the eye has too much converging power, while in hyperopia it does not have enough (Figure 2–8).

Hyperopia and myopia

Hyperopia and myopia can be classified as axial or refractive. In axial conditions, the power of the eye is normal but the length of the eye is too long (myopia) or too short (hyperopia). In refractive conditions, the length of the eye is normal, but the refractive power of the eye is too strong (myopia) or too weak (hyperopia).

Infants have an average of 2 D of hyperopia, but a myopic shift occurs between ages 8 and 13 years, so that most adults are emmetropic. Approximately 25% of the US population has myopia and 25% has hyperopia. After age 40, the incidence of hyperopia increases to 50%.

Acquired hyperopia results from disorders that decrease either the effective axial length of the eye, such as retrobulbar tumors, choroidal tumors, or central serous retinopathy, or the refractive power of the eye, like a change in lens position (posterior lens dislocation, aphakia, diabetes), drugs (chloroquine, phenothiazines, antihistamines, benzodiazepines), poor accommodation (tonic pupil, drugs, trauma), flattening of the cornea (contact lens), or intraocular silicone oil.

Processes that increase lens power, such as an osmotic effect (diabetes, galactosemia, uremia, sulfonamides), nuclear sclerotic cataracts, anterior lenticonus, changes in lens position or shape (medication (miotics), anterior lens dislocation, excessive accommodation), corneal power (keratoconus, congenital glaucoma, contact lens-induced corneal warpage), or axial length (congenital glaucoma, posterior staphyloma, retinopathy of prematurity, after scleral buckle surgery) may cause myopia.

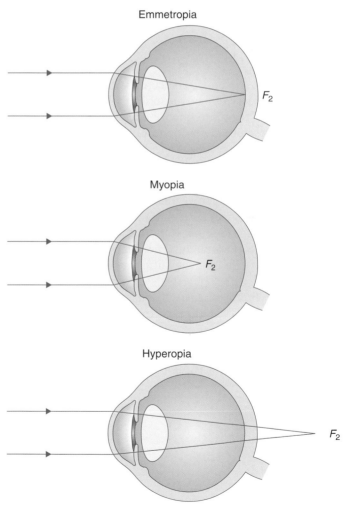

FIGURE 2–8

Emmetropia, myopia, and hyperopia. In emmetropia, the far point is at infinity and the secondary focal point (F_2) is at the retina. In myopia, the secondary focal point (F_2) is in the vitreous. In hyperopia, the secondary focal point (F_2) is located behind the eye.

Myopia also increases in the dark. This **night myopia** is related to several factors: pupil dilation (spherical aberration and irregular astigmatism increase), the Purkinje shift (spectral sensitivity shifts towards shorter wavelengths at lower light levels and chromatic aberration moves the eye's focal point anteriorly), and dark focus (there is no accommodative target in the dark, so the eye tends to overaccommodate for distance and underaccommodate for near).

Astigmatism

Astigmatism is the third type of refractive error and refers to unequal focusing of light in different meridians. Astigmatism is primarily caused by the cornea: if the corneal surface is not spherical (like a baseball) but is curved more steeply in one direction than the other (like a football), then two focal lines are produced on the retina rather than a single focal point.

Astigmatism may be induced by lid lesions (tumor, chalazion, ptosis), pterygium, limbal dermoids, corneal degenerations and ectasias, surgery (most commonly corneal and cataract), lenticular changes (cataract), and ciliary body tumors.

Correction of refractive errors

Refractive errors can be corrected with glasses, contact lenses, or surgery. When prescribing glasses or contact lenses, the strategy is to choose a lens with a focal point that coincides with the far point of the patient's eye. The basic types of lenses are:

- **Spherical**: a lens that has equal power in all meridians and moves the secondary focal point of the eye on to the retina so that images outside the eye's range of focus can be seen clearly.
- **Cylindrical**: a lens that is used to correct astigmatism and only has power in one meridian (perpendicular to its axis) to equalize the different curvatures of the cornea.
- **Spherocylindrical**: a lens that has greater power in one meridian than the other to correct both the spherical and cylindrical components of a refractive error.

A prescription for glasses may be written in one of two formats: plus cylinder or minus cylinder. If the lens is a spherical lens, then it is denoted by one number, which corresponds to the power of the sphere needed to correct the myopia (minus lens) or hyperopia (plus lens). On the other hand, a prescription for a spherocylindrical lens, which also corrects for astigmatism, contains a second and third number that describe the power of the cylinder and its orientation (axis). Depending on the sign of the cylinder, the prescription is designated plus cylinder ($+2.00 + 1.25 \times 60$) or minus cylinder ($+3.25 - 1.25 \times 150$). Any prescription can be written in either format. By convention, ophthalmologists use plus cylinder notation while optometrists and opticians work in negative cylinder. Converting from one format to the other is very easy and is called **cylinder transposition**. The three steps are:

1. new sphere = old sphere + old cylinder
2. new cylinder = magnitude of old cylinder but with opposite power
3. new axis = change old axis by 90°

(for example: $+2.00 + 1.25 \times 60 \rightarrow +3.25 - 1.25 \times 150$).

Magnifiers

The perceived size of any object depends on the size of its image on the retina, and this is determined by the angle the object subtends on the retina. To magnify objects, we naturally hold them closer to the eye. This maximizes the subtended angle and thus the retinal image size. We cannot bring an object closer than the near point of the eye without losing focus. However, a converging lens allows us to increase our accommodation and bring objects closer than the natural near point where they will subtend a bigger angle and therefore appear larger. Such a lens is called a **magnifier**.

The size of an image seen through glasses depends on the lens power and its distance from the eye (**vertex distance**). Minus-power lenses produce smaller images than plus lenses. Increasing the vertex distance increases the magnification of plus lenses and decreases the magnification of minus lenses. **Anisometropia** exists when there is a difference in power between the two eyes of more than 1 D. **Aniseikonia** is the difference in image size between eyes from unequal magnification of correcting lenses. Up to 6–7% (approximately 3 D of spectacle anisometropia) is usually well tolerated in adults, while children can adjust to much larger differences.

CHAPTER THREE

Ocular Pharmacology

Pharmacologic Principles

Most medications used in ophthalmology are topical. This route of administration provides good bioavailability to ocular tissues while minimizing systemic side-effects. Drugs in the tear film drain through the nasolacrimal duct, come into contact with mucosa, and enter the blood stream. Therefore topical eyedrops can have systemic side-effects because this system bypasses the hepatic first-pass metabolism.

The amount of drug absorption is related to corneal permeability and depends on concentration, rate of absorption, tissue binding, transport, metabolism, and excretion. The cornea also has barriers to penetration. Tight junctions contained in both the epithelium and endothelium limit the passage of hydrophilic drugs. Similarly, the water-rich stroma limits the passage of lipophilic drugs.

Despite these obstacles, absorption into the eye can be improved in a number of ways. Adding surfactants (preservatives like benzalkonium chloride) disrupts epithelial tight-junction integrity. Increasing the contact time, the frequency of drops, and the lipid solubility of the drug all raise the bioavailability. Occluding the lacrimal puncta decreases drainage from the ocular surface, as does closing the eyelids after drops are instilled. Prodrugs, ointments, sustained-release gels, and inserts have also been employed to increase absorption.

Even with these changes and frequent administration, topical medications often do not deliver sufficient drug levels in the eye. To increase bioavailability, drugs can be injected directly into (intravitreal) or around the eye (subconjunctival, subTenon's, retrobulbar, peribulbar), or given systemically. The subconjunctival or subTenon's route increases duration and concentration, bypasses conjunctival and corneal barriers, and avoids systemic toxicity. Retrobulbar or peribulbar injections are primarily used for surgical anesthesia. Intraocular administration is the most direct route but safety concerns, such as toxicity and the risk of infection, limit its use to retina specialists. It is, however, used intraoperatively and to treat macular edema, endophthalmitis, and choroidal neovascularization in macular degeneration. Oral and intravenous medicines are rarely employed for eye disease because systemic drugs have difficulty crossing the blood–ocular barrier (blood–aqueous for anterior segment and blood–retinal for vitreous). Thus, therapeutic tissue concentrations in the eye are rarely achieved and systemic toxicity becomes a concern. The exception is for the treatment of scleritis, severe uveitis, and various infections, for which systemic medicines are indicated.

Common Ophthalmic Medications

ANESTHETICS

Ophthalmic anesthetics are administered for eye exams and surgery. These drugs produce a reversible blockade of nerve fiber conduction by blocking sodium channels. Anesthetics are pH-dependent, working less effectively at low pH (i.e., in inflamed tissue).

There are two classes of anesthetic drugs, esters and amides, that do not necessarily have allergic cross-reactivity. The **esters** (cocaine, tetracaine, proparacaine, procaine, and benoxinate) are hydrolyzed by plasma cholinesterase and metabolized in the liver. The **amides** (lidocaine, mepivacaine, and bupivacaine), also metabolized in the liver, have a longer duration of action and less systemic toxicity.

Topical anesthetics

Topical anesthetics are used during exams to check the intraocular pressure (IOP), remove superficial foreign bodies, and relieve pain associated with corneal epithelial abnormalities (e.g., corneal abrasion). Most cataract and refractive surgery is also performed under topical anesthesia. These drugs all have corneal toxicity because they increase corneal permeability by disturbing inter-cellular junctions in the epithelium. Common topical anesthetics include the following:

- **Proparacaine (Ophthaine)** has a 10–30-minute duration and can cause allergic dermatitis (also common with atropine and neomycin). Interestingly, it does not necessarily have allergic cross-reactivity with tetracaine.
- **Tetracaine (Pontacaine)** is longer-acting and more toxic to the cornea than proparacaine.
- **Benoxinate** is similar to proparacaine and is often combined with fluorescein (Fluress) to use for tonometry.
- **Cocaine** provides excellent anesthesia but has the most epithelial toxicity. It is also used to test for Horner's syndrome because of its sympathomimetic effect.

Parenteral anesthetics

Parenteral anesthesia is necessary for many eye procedures because it also provides akinesia. It may be mixed with epinephrine (1:100 000) to increase duration since vasoconstriction reduces systemic absorption, or hyaluronidase (Wydase or Vitrase) to allow better tissue penetration. These drugs have durations of action between 30 minutes and 6 hours:

- **Procaine (Novocaine):** 30–45-minutes duration.
- **Lidocaine (Xylocaine):** 1-hour duration (2 hours with epinephrine).
- **Mepivacaine (Carbocaine):** 2-hours duration.
- **Bupivacaine (Marcaine):** 6-hours duration.

General anesthesia is sometimes required for ophthalmic surgery, especially for long operations and when the patient cannot cooperate.

AUTONOMIC SYSTEM MEDICATIONS

Both sympathetic and parasympathetic fibers innervate the eye. The **sympathetics** comprise an extensive system for mass response – the "fight or flight" response. Synapses are located near the spinal cord in the superior cervical ganglion, and the postganglionic nerves are long. The **adrenergic receptors** in the eye consist of α_1, α_2, and β_2 receptors, which regulate the following physiologic responses:

- α_1: smooth-muscle contraction of the arteries (decreases aqueous production by reducing ciliary body blood flow), iris dilator (dilates iris), and Müller's muscle (elevates upper eyelid).
- α_2: feedback inhibition (ciliary body decreases aqueous production).
- β_2: ciliary body (increases aqueous production), and trabecular meshwork (increases outflow).

The neurotransmitters are **acetylcholine (ACh)** at the preganglionic terminal, and **epinephrine** and **norepinephrine** at the postganglionic terminal.

The more limited **parasympathetic** system is homeostatic for discrete responses. The synapses are near the end-organ (ciliary ganglion), and the post-ganglionic nerves are short. Two classes of cholinergic receptors exist: (1) the **nicotinic** for somatic motor and preganglionic autonomic nerves, which innervate muscles outside the eye (extraocular muscles, levator, orbicularis); and (2) the **muscarinic** for postganglionic parasympathetic nerves, which innervate muscles inside the eye (iris sphincter and ciliary muscle). ACh is the neurotransmitter and is broken down by the enzyme acetylcholinesterase (AChE) (Table 3–1).

Adrenergic drugs

Adrenergic drugs include the sympathomimetics, which cause mydriasis, vasoconstriction, and decreased IOP (see section on glaucoma medications, below), and the sympatholytics, which cause decreased IOP.

The sympathomimetics are classified as:

- **Direct-acting α-agonists**: epinephrine, phenylephrine (Mydfrin), dipivefrine (Propine), apraclonidine (Iopidine), brimonidine (Alphagan-P), naphazoline (Naphcon), oxymetazoline (Afrin), tetrahydrozoline (Visine).
- **Direct-acting β-agonists**: epinephrine, isoproterenol, dopamine.

TABLE 3–1

Autonomic System Responses		
Organ/function	**Sympathetic (fight or flight)**	**Parasympathetic (homeostasis)**
Heart rate	Increase	Decrease
Blood pressure	Increase	Decrease
Gastrointestinal motility	Decrease	Increase
Bronchioles	Dilate	Constrict
Bladder	Constrict	Dilate
Vessels	Constrict	Dilate
Sweat	Decrease	Increase
Pupils	Dilate	Constrict
Eyelids	Elevate	Normal

- **Indirect-acting agonists**: cocaine, hydroxy-amphetamine, ephedrine.

The sympatholytics are classified as:

- **α-blockers** (reverse pupillary dilation): dapiprazole (Rev-eyes).
- **β-blockers** (lower IOP): timolol, levobunolol, betaxolol, metipranolol, carteolol.

Cholinergic drugs

Cholinergic drugs are divided into four categories: (1) direct-acting agonists; (2) indirect-acting agonists; (3) muscarinic agonists; and (4) nicotinic agonists.

Direct-acting agonists act on the end-organ and do not need intact innervation. These substances shallow the anterior chamber, disrupt the blood–aqueous barrier, and cause miosis, brow ache, and decreased IOP. Examples include ACh (Miochol; very short-acting and unstable, used intracamerally during surgery), carbacholine (Carbachol; also indirect-acting), and pilocarpine (resistant to AchE).

Indirect-acting agonists are anticholinesterases. These are the strongest agents. They cause miosis and decreased IOP, and can mimic an acute abdomen because of their gastrointestinal effects. The antidote is atropine. These drugs are **reversible** (physostigmine (Eserine; used to treat eyelid lice), edrophonium (Tensilon; for the diagnosis of myasthenia gravis), and carbacholine) or **irreversible** (ecothiophate (Phospholine Iodide; used to treat glaucoma and accommodative esotropia)). These agonists block the metabolism of succinylcholine (causing prolonged respiratory paralysis) and ester anesthetics. Other complications include cataracts and retinal detachment.

Muscarinic antagonists are the common anticholinergic drugs that are used to achieve mydriasis and cycloplegia for eye exams. They also deepen the anterior chamber and stabilize the blood–aqueous barrier. These eyedrops have increasing duration of action as follows: tropicamide (Mydriacyl; 4–6 hours), cyclopentolate (Cyclogyl; 24 hours; central nervous system side-effects may occur with the 2% solution, especially in children), homatropine (1–3 days), scopolamine (Hyoscine; 1 week; has more central nervous system toxicity than atropine), and atropine (1–2 weeks). Signs of anticholinergic toxicity are mental status changes (somnolence or agitation), hallucinations, tachycardia, urinary retention, flushing, dry mouth/skin, and fever. There is increased sensitivity in albinism, Down syndrome, and neonates. The antidote is physostigmine (1–4 mg IV).

Nicotinic antagonists can be **non-depolarizing** (gallamine, pancuronium), which do not cause muscle contraction, or **depolarizing** (succinylcholine, decamethonium), which do cause muscle contraction and elevated IOP, and are therefore contraindicated for use with general anesthesia in ruptured globe surgical cases because extraocular muscle contraction can cause extrusion of intraocular contents.

GLAUCOMA MEDICATIONS

Ocular hypotensive drugs lower IOP and are the mainstay of glaucoma therapy. There are many classes of agents with different mechanisms of action, but, in general, glaucoma medicines are intended either to decrease aqueous production or increase aqueous outflow. The former category includes the β-blockers, α-agonists, and carbonic anhydrase inhibitors (CAIs), while the latter one is composed of the miotics and the prostaglandin analogues.

Beta-blockers

The β-blockers reduce aqueous production by inhibiting the Na^+/K^+ pump. However, they lose effectiveness over time due to down-regulation of β-receptors, and they have systemic side-effects like bradycardia, heart block, bronchospasm, impotence, lethargy, depression, and headache. Cardioselective β-blockers have a greater affinity for β_1 than β_2 receptors and thus have fewer respiratory side-effects. They are indicated in patients with pulmonary problems who cannot tolerate a non-selective β-blocker, but patients with asthma *should not* be prescribed any β-blocker. Although these medications have traditionally been the gold standard of glaucoma therapy, the newer prostaglandin analogues are replacing them as first-line therapy. Therefore, any patient experiencing systemic effects from a β-blocker should be switched to a different glaucoma drop.

- **Non-selective β-blockers** (that bind to both β_1 and β_2 receptors): timolol (Timoptic), levobunolol (Betagan), metipranolol (Optipranolol), and carteolol (Ocupress).
- **Cardioselective β-blockers** (that have greater affinity for β_1 than β_2 receptors): betaxolol (Betoptic).

α₂-agonists

α_2-agonists reduce aqueous production. Side-effects include allergy, upper-eyelid retraction, miosis, lethargy, and headache. Brimonidine (Alphagan-P) is the only agent in this class that is routinely prescribed. Apraclonidine (Iopidine) is highly allergenic with sustained use and therefore is mainly used perioperatively for laser eye treatments in order to reduce the risk of a transient pressure spike, or to lower eye pressure acutely. Topical epinephrine and its prodrug Proprine are rarely used any more because of their poor efficacy.

- **α₂-agonists**: brimonidine (Alphagan-P), apraclonidine (Iopidine), epinephrine, Proprine.

Carbonic anhydrase inhibitors

CAIs reduce aqueous production and are available in systemic and topical formulations. Systemic CAIs are now only used temporarily to stabilize uncontrolled elevated IOP since they can cause metabolic acidosis, hypokalemia, paresthesias (in the hands, feet, and lips), gastrointestinal upset, diarrhea, lethargy, loss of libido, metallic taste, aplastic anemia, Stevens–Johnson syndrome, and transient myopia. The topical CAIs are much safer and better tolerated for longer-term IOP control, but can still produce metallic taste, paresthesias, malaise, and skin rash. CAIs are sulfonamide derivatives and should not be administered to patients with a sulfa allergy.

- **Systemic CAIs:** acetazolamide (Diamox; PO or IV), methazolamide (Neptazane PO; more lipid soluble, less toxicity).
- **Topical CAIs:** dorzolamide (Trusopt), brinzolamide (Azopt).

Miotics

Miotics are cholinergic drugs (direct- and indirect-acting agonists) that increase aqueous outflow by contraction of the ciliary muscle, which opens the trabecular meshwork. These medications are rarely used any more because of their side-effects. Pilocarpine, an ACh agonist, may produce headache, accommodative spasm, miosis (with resultant dimming/reduction of vision), myopia, and possible pupillary block (due to a forward shift of the lens and iris), follicular conjunctivitis, and dermatitis. Carbachol, an ACh agonist and AChE inhibitor, has a stronger effect and longer duration of action. Ecothiophate (Phospholine Iodide), a cholinesterase inhibitor with a 3-week duration, is also used to treat accommodative esotropia, but causes more orbicularis, ciliary, and iris muscle spasm, cataracts, and iris cysts in children (prevented by concomitant administration of topical phenylephrine).

- **Miotics:** pilocarpine, Carbachol, ecothiophate (Phospholine Iodide).

Prostaglandin analogues

Prostaglandin analogues are the most effective and safest pressure-lowering drops available. They are prostaglandin $F_{2\alpha}$ analogues that increase uveoscleral outflow. Side-effects are local and include conjunctival hyperemia, eyelash growth, iris and eyelid pigmentation, reactivation of herpes simplex virus (HSV) keratitis, macular edema at the time of cataract surgery, and, rarely, flu-like symptoms.

- **Prostaglandin analogues:** latanoprost (Xalatan), bimatoprost (Lumigan), and travoprost (Travatan).

Hyperosmotic agents

Hyperosmotic agents are a special group of glaucoma medications that decrease IOP by reducing the vitreous volume. These low-molecular-weight substances increase serum osmolality to draw fluid out of the eye. Hyperosmotic agents, like oral CAIs, are systemic drugs reserved for the temporary control of acute IOP rises, particularly for treating angle-closure attacks. Side-effects such as headache, thirst, nausea, vomiting, diarrhea, diuresis, and dizziness limit their usefulness. Mannitol (Osmitrol) is the most potent but may exacerbate congestive heart failure. Glycerin (Osmoglyn) may cause hyperglycemia in diabetics. Isosorbide (Ismotic) is not metabolized (so it can be used in diabetics) but often causes nausea and emesis.

- **Hyperosmotic agents:** mannitol (Osmitrol; IV; 20% solution), glycerin (Osmoglyn; PO; 50% solution), isosorbide (Ismotic; PO).

ANTI-INFLAMMATORY DRUGS

Non-steroidal anti-inflammatory drugs (NSAIDs) and steroids block the production of inflammatory mediators by interfering with the inflammatory cascade (Figure 3–1).

NON-STEROIDAL ANTI-INFLAMMATORY DRUGS

NSAIDs inhibit the cyclooxygenase pathway. Topical preparations are used to treat allergic conjunctivitis, corneal pain, postsurgical inflammation, and cystoid macular edema, as well as to prevent miosis during intraocular surgery. Oral NSAIDs are prescribed for the treatment of scleritis and some forms of uveitis.

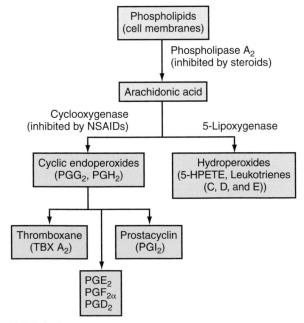

FIGURE 3–1

The inflammatory pathway. NSAIDs, non-steroidal anti-inflammatory drugs; PG, prostaglandin; 5-HPETE, 5-hydroperoxyeicosatetraenoic acid.

- **Topical NSAIDs**: diclofenac (Voltaren), ketorolac (Acular), suprofen (Profenal), flurbiprofen (Ocufen), bromfenac (Xibrom), nepafenac (Nevanac).

Steroids

Steroids inhibit the first step in the inflammatory pathway and are therefore the most potent anti-inflammatory drugs available. They also inhibit release of lysosomal enzymes, prevent macrophage migration, interfere with lymphocyte function, decrease fibroblast activity, inhibit neovascularization, and reduce capillary permeability. Topical steroids are available in three forms: phosphate, alcohol, and acetate. The type of preparation influences corneal penetrability and thus potency of the drop. Phosphates are hydrophilic with poor penetration of intact corneal epithelium, alcohols are biphasic and able to penetrate intact cornea, and acetates are more biphasic with the best corneal penetration.

Altering the molecular structure of steroids also affects the potency (increased by 1–2 double bond, 9 fluorination, 6 methylation, O at C11), as well as the tendency for the drop to increase IOP (deoxygenation at C21). Derivatives of progesterone (FML, medrysone) are weaker and are less apt to cause an IOP rise. The IOP-elevating potential of steroids is as follows: dexamethasone > prednisolone > fluoromethalone > hydrocortisone > tetrahydrotriamcinalone > medrysone (after 6 weeks of dexamethasone therapy, 42% have IOP >20 mmHg and 6% have IOP >31). The steroids with low IOP-elevating potential are fluoromethalone (FML), rimexolone (Vexol), and loteprednol (Lotemax, Alrex). In addition to elevated IOP, other ocular side-effects of steroids are cataract formation, delayed wound healing (corneal re-epithelialization), and secondary infections (bacterial, fungal, or reactivation of HSV keratitis).

Conjunctivitis, keratitis, scleritis, uveitis, hyphema, and cystoid macular edema are all indications for prescribing steroids. In certain circumstances, topical eyedrops are not sufficient. Other routes of administration include subconjunctival/subTenon's steroid injections (which produce higher ocular concentrations and longer duration) and systemic (oral and intravenous). An oral dose of 7.5 mg dexamethasone results in an intravitreal concentration of therapeutic levels. However, the patient must be warned of the potential systemic adverse effects: adrenal insufficiency, hyperglycemia, hypertension, hypokalemia, peptic ulcer, delayed wound healing, super-infection, emotional lability, psychosis, growth retardation, muscle atrophy, osteoporosis, aseptic necrosis of the hip, hirsutism, weight gain, cushingoid appearance, and pseudotumor cerebri.

- **Steroids**: dexamethasone, prednisolone, hydrocortisone, tetrahydrotriamcinalone, medrysone, fluoromethalone (FML), rimexolone (Vexol), loteprednol (Lotemax, Alrex).

ANTIALLERGY MEDICATIONS

Many allergy remedies are available for the relief of itchy eyes. These agents are categorized by their mechanism of action, which includes one or more of the following: antihistamine, vasoconstrictor, mast cell stabilizer, and eosinophil suppressor.

- **Antihistamine/vasoconstrictors** (over-the-counter eyedrops): Ocuhist, Opcon-A, Naphcon-A, Vasocon-A.
- **Mast cell stabilizers**: cromolyn (Crolom; Opticrom), nedocromil (Alocril), pemirolast (Alamast).
- **Mast cell stabilizer/eosinophil suppressor combination**: lodoxamide (Alomide).
- **H_1-blockers** (inhibit itching): levocabastine (Livostin), emedastine (Emadine).
- **H_1- and H_2-blocker/mast cell inhibitor combination**: olopatadine (Patanol), ketotifen (Zaditor), azelastine (Optivar), epinastine (Elestat).

IMMUNOSUPPRESSIVE AGENTS

Immunosuppressives are potent systemic agents used to treat severe forms of uveitis and scleritis. These drugs are divided into a number of classes. The **cytotoxic antimetabolites** interfere with folate metabolism by inhibiting purine ring biosynthesis. **Cytotoxic alkylating agents** inhibit mRNA transcription by cross-linking DNA strands. **Cytostatic anti-inflammatories** are the steroids (see above).

The **immunomodulator** cyclosporine blocks production of interleukin-2 (IL-2) and IL-2 receptors, inhibits proliferation of lymphocytes, and inhibits T-cell activation and recruitment. Systemically, cyclosporine is used for Mooren's ulcer, uveitis in Behçet's disease or sympathetic ophthalmia, prevention of corneal transplant rejection, ocular cicatricial pemphigoid, and thyroid-related ophthalmopathy. The topical form (Restasis) is indicated for treating dry-eye syndrome (i.e., Sjögren's syndrome) and is also used in cases of ligneous conjunctivitis, atopic keratoconjunctivitis, and necrotizing scleritis.

- **Cytotoxic antimetabolites**: methotrexate, azothioprine (Imuran).
- **Cytotoxic alkylating agents**: cyclophosphamide (Cytoxan), chlorambucil (Leukeran).
- **Cytostatic anti-inflammatories**: steroids.
- **Immunomodulator**: cyclosporine.

ANTI-INFECTIVE DRUGS

Antibiotics

Antibiotics represent one of the largest groups of drugs, but in ophthalmology their use is typically limited to topical preparations that are fewer in number than the systemic choices. It is easiest to classify the commonly prescribed ophthalmic antibiotics by their mechanism of action.

Inhibitors of intermediary metabolism are bacteriostatic. The **sulfonamides** (sulfacetamide, sulfadiazine, sulfamethoxazole) inhibit folic acid synthesis and have a broad spectrum of action (Gram-positives and negatives, toxoplasmosis, *Chlamydia*, *Actinomyces*, *Pneumocystis*). The sulfa drugs are infrequently used in ophthalmology but are commonly prescribed by the non-ophthalmologist for blepharitis and conjunctivitis. Oral forms are used for toxoplasmosis. However, resistance is a problem, as are allergy (Stevens–Johnson syndrome) and transient myopia. **Trimethoprim**, which blocks the next step in folate metabolism, is often combined with other antibiotics (polymyxin B (Polytrim), sulfamethoxazole (Bactrim)) and is used for conjunctivitis.

Inhibitors of cell wall synthesis are bactericidal and include the β-lactams (penicillins, cephalosporins, monobactams, and carbapenems), polymyxin B, bacitracin, and vancomycin.

- **β-lactams**: only cefazolin is used topically in a fortified preparation to treat bacterial keratitis (corneal ulcer) and endophthalmitis. Otherwise, the use of these drugs is limited in ophthalmology and consists of systemic administration of penicillins and cephalosporins for infections such as syphilis and preseptal cellulitis.
- **Polymyxin B** is a basic peptide that acts as a detergent and disrupts the bacterial cell membrane. It has very good Gram-negative coverage (*Haemophilus*, *Enterobacter*, *Escherichia coli*, *Klebsiella*, *Pseudomonas*) and is commonly used in combination with trimethoprim (Polytrim) for conjunctivitis.
- **Bacitracin** is a polypeptide with a spectrum against Gram-positives, *Neisseria*, *Haemophilus*, *Actinomyces*. It is often combined with neomycin or polymyxin to broaden its activity, and it is prescribed for blepharitis and conjunctivitis.
- **Vancomycin** is a glycopeptide with excellent Gram-positive activity (*Staphylococcus* (including methicillin-resistant *Staphylococcus aureus* (MRSA)), *Streptococcus* (including penicillin-resistant strains), *Bacillus*, *Propionibacterium acnes*, *Clostridium difficile*). It is used topically, usually in conjunction with cefazolin, as a fortified preparation to treat bacterial keratitis and endophthalmitis.

Inhibitors of protein synthesis are bacteriostatic except for the aminoglycosides, which are cidal. The aminoglycosides and tetracyclines inhibit the 30S ribosome, while the macrolides, chloramphenicol, and clindamycin inhibit the 50S ribosome.

- **Aminoglycosides** are used topically for conjunctivitis, keratitis, and endophthalmitis. These drugs have a good spectrum against Gram-negative bacilli and some staphylococci. Gentamicin (better for *Serratia*), tobramycin (better for *Pseudomonas*), neomycin (*Acanthamoeba*), and paromomycin (*Acanthamoeba*) are all available, but tobramycin is the least allergenic and toxic to the ocular surface.
- **Tetracyclines** are used topically as well as systemically for eye conditions. Topical tetracycline ointment is used at birth prophylactically and to treat ophthalmia neonatorum. Systemically, tetracycline, doxycycline, and minocycline are used for *Chlamydia* and also for rosacea, meibomianitis, and scleral melting due to their anti-inflammatory and anticollagenolytic properties. Patients taking oral agents must be warned about gastrointestinal upset, phototoxic dermatitis, tooth discoloration in children, teratogenicity, nephro- and hepatotoxicity, and decreased prothrombin activity (potentiates coumadin).
- **Macrolides** consist of erythromycin, azithromycin, and clarithromycin, which are active against Gram-positives, a few Gram-negatives, *Chlamydia*, *Mycoplasma*, and *Legionella*. Topical erythromycin ointment is used to treat blepharitis and conjunctivitis, while a combination of topical and oral medicine should be given for chlamydial eye infections.
- **Chloramphenicol** also has a broad spectrum of activity and is available in ophthalmic preparations, but it is rarely used any more because of its risk of causing aplastic anemia.
- **Clindamycin** is used systemically to treat toxoplasmosis, but it may cause pseudomembranous colitis (due to overgrowth of *Clostridium difficile*, which in turn is treated with vancomycin or metronidazole).

Inhibitors of genetic replication are bactericidal. These **fluoroquinolone** drugs are analogues of nalidixic acid, and they are now the most commonly used topical antibiotics in ophthalmology. Resistance has been a concern with the earlier-generation agents (ciprofloxacin (Ciloxan), ofloxacin (Ocuflox)), so the broader-spectrum newer-generation medicines (levofloxacin (Quixin), gatifloxacin (Zymar), moxifloxacin (Vigamox)) are favored. These fluoroquinolones have an extended spectrum with enhanced activitiy against Gram-positive organisms, fluoroquinolone-resistant strains, and atypical mycobacteria. They are prescribed for conjunctivitis, keratitis, surgical prophylaxis, and endophthalmitis. Oral ciprofloxacin achieves high levels in the vitreous and therefore may be useful in cases of penetrating trauma.

Antivirals

Antivirals are mostly nucleotide analogues that inhibit viral replication. They are used in ophthalmology to treat herpetic infections: HSV keratitis, herpes zoster ophthalmicus (HZO), and cytomegalovirus retinitis. Topical antivirals are only used for HSV keratitis. These eyedrops are quite toxic to the corneal epithelium. Trifluorothymidine (Viroptic) is the most commonly used because it is best tolerated. However, in cases of allergy, the other choices are idoxuridine (Stoxil), which can cause a follicular conjunctivitis, corneal epitheliopathy, and punctal stenosis, and vidarabine (Vira-A), which has less severe side-effects. Antivirals are more often used systemically. Acyclovir (Zovirax), valacyclovir (Valtrex; prodrug of acyclovir), penciclovir, or its prodrug famciclovir (Famvir) are prescribed for HSV and HZO. These pills may cause gastrointestinal upset, and high doses can cause nephro- and neurotoxicity. Cytomegalovirus retinitis is less commonly seen than it once was due to newer therapy regimens for acquired immunodeficiency syndrome (AIDS). When it does occur, this retinal infection is treated with the powerful antivirals ganciclovir (Cytovene) and foscarnet (Foscavir) either systemically or with an implant.

- **Topical antivirals**: trifluorothymidine (Viroptic), idoxuridine (Stoxil), vidarabine (Vira-A).
- **Systemic antivirals**: acyclovir (Zovirax), valacyclovir (Valtrex; prodrug of acyclovir), penciclovir, or its prodrug famciclovir (Famvir), ganciclovir (Cytovene), foscarnet (Foscavir).

Antifungals

Antifungals kill yeasts, molds, and dimorphic fungi by disrupting their cell membranes. These drugs can be compounded as eyedrops and also used orally for keratitis and endophthalmitis.

Polyenes bind to ergosterol. **Amphotericin B** is broad-spectrum and useful for ophthalmic infections caused by *Candida*, *Cryptococcus*, *Blastomyces*, *Histoplasma*, *Coccidioides*, and *Mucormycosis*. **Natamycin** is especially active against *Aspergillus* and *Fusarium*. It is only administered topically because it is too toxic for IV or intravitreal injection.

Azoles inhibit ergosterol synthesis and serve as second-line agents to amphotericin, as well as for *Acanthamoeba* keratitis. Systemic side-effects include gastrointestinal upset, headache, and rash. The **imidazoles** can be used topically or systemically: miconazole (topical, IV, intravitreal) has a broad-spectrum action against filamentous fungi and yeast, but may cause corneal erosions and anemia. Ketoconazole (topical, oral) is also broad-spectrum but can result in reversible hepatotoxicity. Clotrimazole (oral) is good for *Aspergillus* infection, but also causes hepatotoxicity. The **triazoles** (itraconazole, fluconazole) are safer oral options.

Antiamoebics

Antiamoebics kill amoeba and their cysts due to cationic surface-active properties that interfere with cell membranes and enzymes. These drugs are given topically for *Acanthamoeba* keratitis. The **biguanides** (polyhexamethylene biguanide, chlorhexadine) are the first-line agents, while the second-line **diamidines** (propamidine (Brolene), hexamidine) provide a synergistic effect but are more toxic to the cornea.

MISCELLANEOUS DRUGS

Aminocaproic acid (Amicar) is a synthetic amino acid similar to lysine with antifibrinolytic properties. It stabilizes blood clots, delays clot lysis, and decreases secondary hemorrhages. Its use in the treatment of hyphema is controversial. Contraindications include hypercoaguable states, pregnancy, renal disease, liver disease, patients at risk for myocardial infarction, pulmonary embolism, and stroke. Systemic administration may cause nausea, vomiting, diarrhea, hypotension, and rash. Topical Amicar has been used with variable success.

Botulinum toxin (Botox) is a neurotoxin that blocks the release of ACh from nerve terminals to produce temporary muscle paralysis for a period of several months. Intramuscular injections are used to treat blepharospasm, hemifacial spasm, and strabismus. Botox is also commonly given cosmetically to reduce dynamic facial wrinkles around the eyes and forehead. It is being investigated as a treatment for migraine headaches. Side-effects include ptosis, diplopia, and exposure keratopathy.

Fluorescein dye is used diagnostically. It is commonly available either as a liquid mixture with benoxinate (anesthetic) or as sterile paper strips that can be wet and applied directly to the conjunctival fornix. These topical formulations are used during the eye exam for tonometry and to help detect corneal epithelial defects. The dye is also used IV for fluorescein angiography: fluorescein is injected in a peripheral vein to allow visualization of the retinal and choroidal blood flow. Fluorescein given IV is associated with nausea, vomiting, dizziness, headache, dyspnea, hypotension, skin necrosis, phototoxic reactions, and anaphylaxis.

Indocyanine green is another dye used IV for angiography to evaluate the retinal and choroidal circulation. Side-effects are gastrointestinal upset, hypotension, urticaria, and anaphylaxis; it is contraindicated in patients who are allergic to iodine.

Toxicology

All medications have side-effects and are potentially toxic to various organs. The following is a list of common drugs that can affect the eyes (Table 3–2):

Anticholinergics (atropine, scopolamine, donnatal): dry eye, mydriasis, cycloplegia, blurry vision, angle closure.

Antihistamines (diphenhydramine): dry eye, mydriasis, cycloplegia, blurry vision.

Antibiotics:

- **Aminoglycosides**: intraocular administration may cause macular infarction.
- **Chloramphenicol**: optic neuropathy.
- **Penicillin and tetracycline**: pseudotumor cerebri.

TABLE 3–2

Ocular Toxicology

Ocular structure	Effect	Drug
Extraocular muscles	Nystagmus, diplopia	Anesthetics, sedatives, anticonvulsants, propranolol, antibiotics, phenothiazines, pentobarbital, carbamazepine, monoamine oxidase inhibitors
Lid	Edema	Chloral hydrate
	Discoloration	Phenothiazines
	Ptosis	Guanethidine, propranolol, barbiturates
Conjunctiva	Hyperemia	Reserpine, methyldopa
	Allergy	Antibiotics, sulfonamides, atropine, antivirals, glaucoma medications
	Discoloration	Phenothiazines, chlorambucil, phenylbutazone
Cornea	Keratitis	Antibiotics, phenylbutazone, barbiturates, chlorambucil, steroids
	Deposits	Chloroquine, amiodarone, tamoxifen, indomethacin, gold
	Pigmentation	Vitamin D
Increased intraocular pressure	Open-angle	Anticholinergics, caffeine, steroids
	Narrow-angle	Anticholinergics, antihistamines, phenothiazines, tricyclic antidepressants, Haldol
Lens	Opacities/cataract	Steroids, phenothiazines, ibuprofen, allopurinol, long-acting miotics
	Myopia	Sulfonamides, tetracycline, Compazine, autonomic antagonists
Retina	Edema	Chloramphenicol, indomethacin, tamoxifen, carmustine
	Hemorrhage	Anticoagulants, ethambutol
	Vascular damage	Oral contraceptives, oxygen, aminoglycosides, talc, carmustine, interferon
	Pigmentary degeneration	Phenothiazines, indomethacin, nalidixic acid, ethambutol, Accutane, chloroquine, hydroxychloroquine
Optic nerve	Neuropathy	Ethambutol, isoniazid, sulfonamides, digitalis, imipramine, streptomycin, busulfan, cisplatin, vincristine, chloramphenicol, disulfiram
	Papilledema	Steroids, vitamin A, tetracycline, phenylbutazone, amiodarone, nalidixic acid, isotretinoin

- **Sulfonamides**: conjunctivitis, transient myopia.
- **Isoniazid, rifampin, ethambutol**: optic neuropathy.

Antimalarials:

- **Chloroquine/hydroxychloroquine** (dose-related): corneal deposits, fine pigmentary macular changes (bull's-eye maculopathy).
- **Quinine**: overdose can result in acute visual loss (to no light perception).

Barbiturates (phenobarbital): nystagmus, diplopia, ptosis, conjunctivitis.

Phenothiazines (chlorpromazine, thioridazine): pigmentary retinopathy, corneal deposits, cataracts.

Tricyclic antidepressants: mydriasis, cycloplegia, dry eye, angle closure.

Dilantin: diplopia, nystagmus, papilledema.

Gold (chrysiasis): deposits in inferior corneal stroma and anterior lens capsule.

Talc: multiple tiny yellow-white glistening particles scattered through the posterior pole with macular edema, venous engorgement, hemorrhages, arterial occlusion, retinal non-perfusion, and peripheral neovascularization.

Amiodarone: corneal deposits, occasionally anterior subcapsular cataracts.

Digoxin: changes in color vision (xanthopsia (yellow vision)), scotomas.

Diuretics (hydrochlorothiazide): xanthopsia, transient myopia.

Viagra, Cialis, Levitra: decreased retinal blood flow by up to ~30%, blue vision, associated with non-arteritic anterior ischemic optic neuropathy.

Carmustine: retinal infarction, retinal pigment epithelial changes, arterial occlusions, hemorrhages, macular edema, glaucoma, optic neuritis, internuclear ophthalmoplegia.

Narcotics (opiates): miosis.

NSAIDs (indomethacin): corneal deposits, diplopia, optic neuritis, pigmentary macular changes; may have changes in vision, dark adaptation, and visual fields.

Corticosteroids: posterior subcapsular cataracts, increased IOP, delayed wound healing, infections, pseudotumor cerebri.

Oral contraceptives: dry eye, vascular occlusions, perivasculitis, optic neuritis, pseudotumor cerebri.

Tamoxifen: deposits in cornea and macula, may have macular edema.

Isotretinoin: impairment of dark adaptation.

Interferon: reversible vaso-occlusive disease.

Nicotinic acid: cystoid maculopathy.

CHAPTER FOUR

The Eye Exam

Introduction

The eye exam consists of a history and a physical examination. Often an ophthalmology consultation is ordered whenever a patient presents with an ocular complaint; however, any physician can perform the initial eye exam. In cases with significant trauma, an ominous mechanism of injury, or obvious eye findings (i.e., proptosis, restricted ocular motility, relative afferent pupillary defect, significant subconjunctival hemorrhage, or conjunctival chemosis), referral to a specialist is appropriate and usually necessary.

Ophthalmology is one of the unique medical fields in that most of the pathology is directly visible to the examiner; therefore, the eye exam alone is usually sufficient in making a diagnosis. This is a distinct advantage in certain situations when a history is difficult to elicit, insufficient, or unobtainable. However, this is not a justification for poor history-taking. As for any organ system, the ophthalmic evaluation consists of both a thorough history and physical exam.

History

A detailed history is the preliminary step in any medical encounter. The parts of the history are similar to a general medical history but are focused on the visual system:

- Chief complaint
- History of present illness
- Past ocular history
- Eye medications
- Past medical and surgical histories
- Systemic medications

- Allergies
- Family history
- Social history
- Review of systems

The patient must be questioned about specific ocular symptoms: the presence, time course, and characteristics of any change in vision, eye pain, redness, or discharge. When dealing with eye trauma, it is also necessary to ask about the mechanism of injury and any loss of consciousness. It is also important to ask specifically about the past ocular history and the use of any eye medications since the patient usually does not volunteer this information.

Physical Exam

Similar to a general physical exam, the basic eye examination consists of various parts that should be performed in a routine order. There are eight components in the eye exam: (1) vision; (2) pupils; (3) motility; (4) visual fields; (5) tonometry; (6) external; (7) anterior segment; and (8) fundus exams. A few specialized instruments are necessary to perform a comprehensive examination; however, most of the eye exam can be done without them. Specific pieces of equipment such as a slit lamp, ophthalmoscope, and tonometer are certainly available in most hospital emergency departments and are relatively easy to use.

VISION

When we check a patient's vision, only certain aspects can be quantified. These separate, discrete components of vision are measured with various tests. However, it is important to remember that our ability to measure vision is limited. The results of acuity and other tests are not a true representation of what patients actually "see" (i.e., their complete visual experience). Patients may have 20/20 vision in each eye yet notice a distinct difference in the quality of the vision. Unfortunately, we do not always have the ability to quantify this disparity.

Snellen visual acuity

Visual acuity is tested in one eye at a time and with glasses or contact lenses if the patient wears them. Distance vision is usually measured with a standard Snellen chart at 20 feet (6 meters), and is denoted with VA, Va, or V and subscript of cc or sc (i.e., V_{cc} or V_{sc}) depending on whether the acuity is measured with (cc) or without (sc) correction, respectively. The various lines of letters get progressively smaller toward the bottom of the chart. The numerator (20) is the test distance, while the denominator (20, 40, 60, etc.) is the distance at which a normal (20/20) eye can see the letters. Thus, 20/50 means that the eye sees at 20 feet (6 meters) (the numerator) what a normal eye can see at 50 feet (15 meters) (the denominator).

If a patient has decreased vision or usually wears correction but does not have his/her glasses or contact lenses, then a pinhole occluder can be used to estimate the best potential vision (Figure 4–1). Improvement of vision with pinhole testing typically indicates the presence of an uncorrected refractive error or a cataract. If the patient is unable to see the big E on the eye chart, then the vision is worse than 20/400 and is recorded as counting fingers (CF at the test distance; e.g., CF at 3 feet (1 meter)) if the patient can correctly identify the number of fingers the examiner holds up; hand motion (HM) if the patient can see the examiner's hand moving; light perception with projection (LP and the quadrants) if the patient can determine the direction from which a light is shined into the eye; light perception without projection (LP) if the patient can only identify when a bright light is shined into the eye but cannot perceive from which quadrant of the visual field the light is emanating; or no light perception (NLP) if the patient cannot determine when light from even the brightest light source is shined directly into the eye. Vision in illiterate individuals or those with a language barrier can be assessed with the tumbling E chart by having the patient indicate in which direction the open end of the E is pointing (Figure 4–2). For infants and toddlers, vision is tested by the capacity to fix and follow (F&F) objects placed in front of them or the presence of central, steady, and maintained fixation (CSM). Near vision is also tested monocularly with or without correction, and is denoted with N.

Color vision

Color vision is a sensitive indicator of optic nerve function and should be tested in any patient with a suspected optic nerve abnormality. Color vision is quickly tested monocularly with special color plates known as Ishihara pseudoisochromatic or Hardy–Rand–Ritter plates (Figure 4–3). Farnsworth tests are performed when more extensive evaluation is needed. Gross macular function is assessed by asking the patient to identify the color of a red eyedrop cap (any dilating drop bottle has a red cap). Red saturation is another test of optic nerve function that can be evaluated with the red cap by asking the patient whether it appears to be the same shade of red when the eyes are tested alternately.

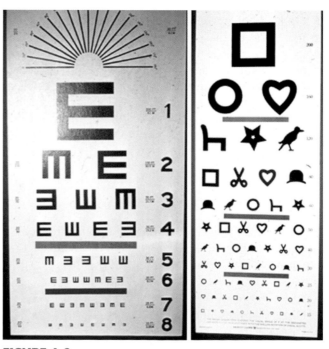

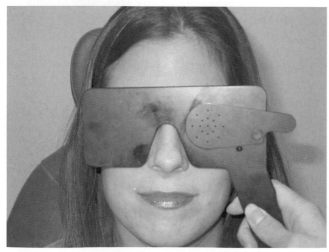

FIGURE 4–1
Patient with pinhole occluder over her left eye.

FIGURE 4–2
Eye charts for non-verbal patients or patients who cannot read English letters. Left, tumbling E chart. Right, eye chart with pictures.

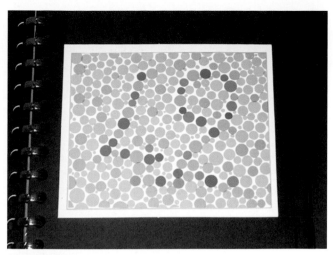

FIGURE 4–3
Ishihara color plates.

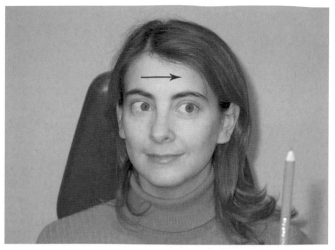

FIGURE 4–4
Patient undergoing ocular motility testing. Note: her eyes are following the pencil.

OCULAR MOTILITY

The position, alignment, and movement of the eyes are evaluated by observing the eyes in primary position (patient looking straight ahead) and while the patient looks in all directions of gaze, by following the examiner's finger or other fixation target (Figure 4–4). Normal **extraocular motility** is typically recorded as full or intact (extraocular motility intact: EOMI). When the eyes are not aligned in primary gaze, a horizontal or vertical deviation of the visual axes exists and one eye will appear to be turned inward, outward, upward, or downward. The corneal light reflex is an easy way to assess ocular alignment: a penlight is shined into the patient's eyes and the position of the light reflex is observed in each eye. The light reflexes should appear in the center of each pupil. If there is a decentration, then a misalignment exists. Similarly, if there is restriction of ocular movements in any direction or nystagmus is present, other tests are performed to differentiate and quantitate the abnormality.

PUPILS

Evaluation of the pupils (size, shape, and reaction to light) is performed while the patient fixates on a distant target. This prevents interference from the near response (accommodation, pupillary constriction, and convergence of the visual axes). The reactivity of each pupil is graded from 1+ (sluggish) to 4+ (brisk). Normal pupils are equal in size, round, and briskly reactive to light both directly and consensually. The usual abbreviation for recording this pupillary response is "pupils equal round and reactive to light" or PERRL (PERRLA if accommodation is also tested). However, ophthalmologists prefer to record the size (in millimeters) of the pupils before and after the light response (i.e., P 4 → 2 OU) since this

notation provides more information. If the reactivity to light is normal, then the pupillary response to accommodation will also be normal and does not require testing. However, there are some conditions that cause light-near dissociation. Therefore, if one or both pupils do not react to light, then the patient is asked to focus on a near object and the pupils are observed for constriction. If the pupils are unequal in size (**anisocoria**) or the reaction to light is abnormal (sluggish in one or both pupils), then the swinging flashlight test (Figure 4–5) must be performed to rule out a **relative afferent pupillary defect** or **Marcus Gunn pupil** (paradoxical dilation of the pupil in the affected eye when a light is alternately shined in the eyes). The presence of a relative afferent pupillary defect indicates optic nerve or widespread retinal damage. If anisocoria is observed, then the size of each pupil should be measured in both light and dark conditions to determine the etiology.

VISUAL FIELDS

The peripheral vision can be rapidly assessed using **confrontation visual fields**. Each eye is tested separately while the patient fixates on the examiner's opposite eye (used as a control). The patient is asked to identify correctly the number of fingers or the movement of a finger presented in each quadrant of the visual field (Figure 4–6). Normal tests are denoted as visual fields full to confrontation (VFFC or VF full). Any abnormality in the field is recorded and can be quantitated with additional tests.

EXTERNAL EXAM

The **orbit**, **eyelids**, and **lacrimal structures** (lacrimal glands and tear drainage apparatus) are inspected for any asymmetry, malposition, or other abnormalities. Palpation of the lids, globe, and orbital rim is performed for swelling, tenderness, mass, proptosis, or suspicion of orbital fracture. If **proptosis** (protruding globe) or **enophthalmos** (sunken globe) is observed, an **exophthalmometer** is used to quantify the amount (this device measures the distance the corneal apex protrudes from the lateral orbital rim). Auscultation for a bruit is

performed when a carotid cavernous sinus fistula is suspected. When indicated, facial and corneal sensation (cranial nerve (CN) V) and facial muscle function, including eyelid closure (CN VII), are tested.

SLIT-LAMP EXAM

Evaluation of the anterior segment of the eye is usually performed with a specialized biomicroscope called a **slit lamp** that allows detailed stereoscopic examination of the eye. The size, color, and orientation of the illuminating light can be controlled to enhance visualization of the ocular anatomy. A thin "slit" light beam directed through the clear media (cornea, anterior chamber, and lens) acts like a scalpel of light illuminating a cross-sectional slice of optical tissue. This feature of the instrument enables precise localization of pathology (Figure 4–7).

Anterior-segment lesions can be accurately measured by recording the height/length of the slit beam from the millimeter scale on the control knob. The technique of retroillumination (coaxial alignment of the light beam with the eyepieces) uses the red reflex from the retina to back-light the cornea and lens, making subtle abnormalities in these structures easier to visualize. Portable, hand-held versions of the slit lamp are available for bedside patient examinations. If a slit lamp is not available, a brief exam of the anterior segment can be performed with either an ophthalmoscope or a penlight and magnifying lens. Although the posterior segment can also be evaluated at the slit lamp with special hand-held or contact lenses, the slit-lamp exam typically focuses on five components of the anterior segment:

1. **Lids, lashes, and lacrimal (L/L/L):** The lids, lashes, puncta, and meibomian gland orifices at the eyelid margin are inspected with a wide slit beam. Palpation at the medial canthus or lid margin can be used to express discharge or secretions from the inferior punctum or meibomian glands, respectively.

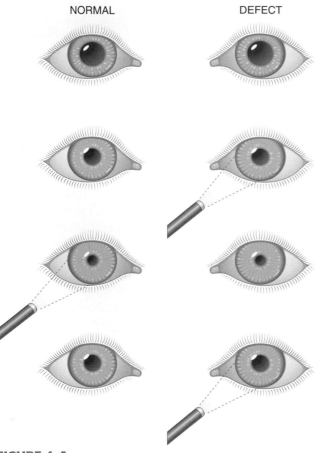

NORMAL   DEFECT

FIGURE 4–5
Swinging flashlight test.

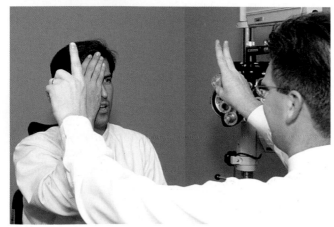

FIGURE 4–6
Patient undergoing confrontation visual field testing.

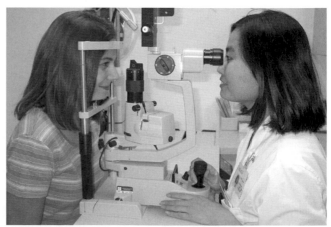

FIGURE 4–7
Patient undergoing slit-lamp examination.

2. **Conjunctiva and sclera (C/S):** The patient is asked to look in the horizontal and vertical directions so that the entire bulbar conjunctiva and anterior sclera can be inspected with a wide slit beam. In order to observe the palpebral (tarsal) conjunctival surface, the eyelids may be everted (Figure 4–8). The caruncle and plica semilunaris are also examined. The upper eyelid can be double-everted to evaluate the superior fornix, and a moistened cotton-tipped applicator can be used to sweep the fornix to remove any suspected foreign bodies. To evaluate cystic structures or masses, a thin slit beam can be utilized.

3. **Cornea (C):** All layers of the cornea are examined with a thin slit beam at an oblique angle or with retroillumination. The tear film is evaluated for break-up time as well as the height of the tear lake or meniscus. Fluorescein dye and the cobalt blue filter enable better visualization of surface irregularities and epithelial defects or abrasions.

4. **Anterior chamber (AC):** The anterior chamber is inspected for depth (graded on a scale from 1+ (shallow) to 4+ (deep)) and the presence of cell and flare with a short thin slit beam at an oblique angle and high magnification. Normally, the anterior chamber is deep and quiet (recorded as AC D&Q), indicating the absence of cells and flare.

5. **Iris and lens (I/L):** The iris and lens are evaluated both with a thin slit beam and by retroillumination. The lens is better assessed after pupillary dilation when a larger area of the lens is visible. If the eye has undergone cataract surgery and is pseudophakic, the position and centration of the intraocular lens implant are noted, and the status of the posterior capsule is recorded. The anterior vitreous can also be seen without the use of additional lenses. For aphakic eyes, the anterior hyaloid face is evaluated for its integrity and any vitreous prolapse into the anterior chamber or strands to anterior structures.

TONOMETRY

A tonometer is an instrument that measures the **intra-ocular pressure**. Various designs exist, but the most common device, the Goldmann applanation tonometer, is attached to the slit lamp, and the eye pressure reading is performed as part of the slit-lamp exam. A topical anesthetic and fluorescein dye (either individually or in a combination drop) are applied to the patient's eye, the

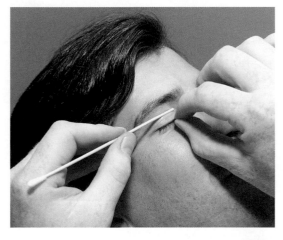
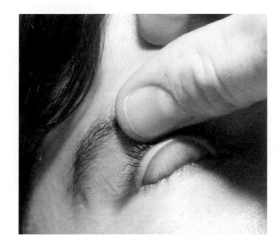
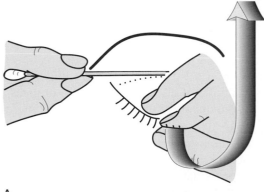
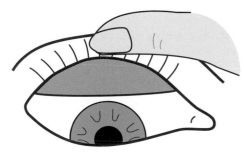

A   B

FIGURE 4–8
Technique for everting the upper eyelid.

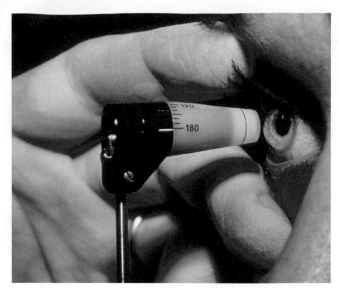

FIGURE 4–9
Goldmann applanation tonometer.

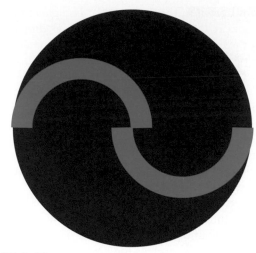

FIGURE 4–10
Applanation tonometer mires as viewed through a slit lamp. When the mires overlap, as in this figure, the intraocular pressure can be determined.

tonometer head is illuminated with a broad slit beam and cobalt blue filter, the tip is moved into gentle contact with the cornea, the tonometer dial is adjusted until the mirror-image semicircular mires slightly overlap (so that their inner margins just touch each other), and the pressure measurement in mmHg is obtained by multiplying the dial reading by 10 (i.e., "2" equals 20 mmHg)(Figures 4–9 and 4–10). It is important to record the time of the pressure measurement since there is a diurnal variation in intraocular pressure. Portable, hand-held devices like the Tono-Pen or Shiotz tonometer are easier for non-ophthalmologists to use (Figure 4–11). Estimating the intraocular pressure by digital palpation (finger tension) is sometimes helpful if the eye pressure is extremely elevated or low, but this technique is highly inaccurate and should not be relied upon.

FUNDUS EXAM

Evaluation of the **optic nerve** and **retina** can be done with or without pupillary dilation and with a variety of instruments and lenses. Direct ophthalmoscopy and indirect ophthalmoscopy are performed with either a direct or indirect ophthalmoscope, respectively (Figure 4–12–4–14). The direct ophthalmoscope is a monocular instrument that produces high magnification (15×) with a narrow field of view, whereas the indirect ophthalmoscope provides a binocular image with a wide field of view but with lower magnification (2–3×). The image obtained through the indirect ophthalmoscope (and slit-lamp fundus lenses) is flipped and inverted, a fact that must be remembered when drawing retinal diagrams. Thus, an easy way to correct for this image reversal is to turn the retinal diagram upside down and then draw the

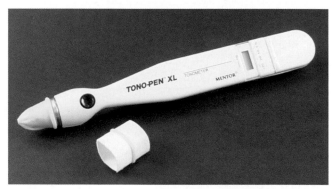

FIGURE 4–11
Hand-held tonometer (Tono-Pen).

pathology as it is seen through the lens; when the diagram is viewed right side up, the retina will be accurately depicted.

During examination of the posterior segment structures, it is important to note the appearance of the optic disc, vessels, macula, and peripheral retina. A dilated fundus exam is often denoted as DFE, and a normal exam is usually abbreviated as d/v/m/p wnl. The dimensions and location of lesions are compared to the size of the disc, so that measurements are recorded as multiples of disc diameters (DD) or areas (DA).

Components of the fundus examination include:

- **Disc**: The **optic nerve** is evaluated, with particular attention to the cup-to-disc ratio (C/D), appearance of the neural rim, and color. The normal nerve appears flat with sharp margins (i.e., no edema) and is orange-yellow in color.
- **Vessels**: The **retinal vessels** are observed as they emanate from the optic cup and branch towards the

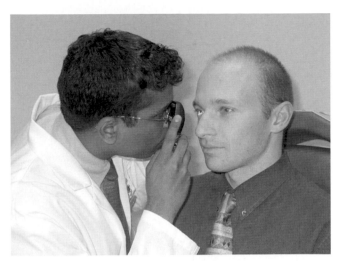

FIGURE 4–12
Patient undergoing direct ophthalmoscopic examination.

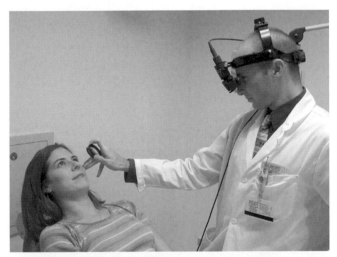

FIGURE 4–13
Patient undergoing indirect ophthalmoscopic examination.

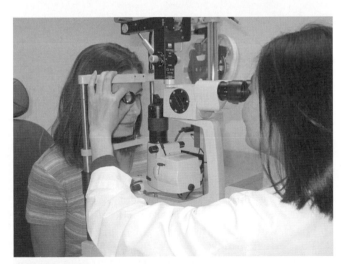

FIGURE 4–14
Patient undergoing slit-lamp fundus examination with high-magnification lens to evaluate the macula.

periphery. Spontaneous venous pulsations are sometimes appreciated at the nerve head. Any anomalous pattern or irregularity of the vasculature is noted. Any changes to the crossings between the arteries and veins should be recorded. Any changes in the vessel walls are also important to note.

- **Macula**: The center of the retina or macula, located temporal to the optic nerve and within the vascular arcades, is inspected. Often a bright light reflex is seen in the fovea at the center of the macula – the foveal reflex – particularly in younger patients.
- **Peripheral retina**: The peripheral retina is most easily viewed through a widely dilated pupil. The patient is asked to look in all directions of gaze so that the entire retina (360°) can be seen. Scleral depression, a technique used with the indirect ophthalmoscope, aids in the visualization of pathology near the ora serrata by pressing on the ora from the outside of the eye with a scleral depressor, bringing this area of the eye into view of the indirect ophthalmoscope.

Every physician should know the basic eye anatomy and examination techniques. Very few instruments are needed to perform a complete eye exam quickly and effectively. With a little practice, any doctor is able to examine the ocular structures in a knowledgeable and confident manner. If an abnormality is observed, then additional evaluation can always be obtained from an ophthalmologist.

Special Tests and Equipment

REFRACTION

Refraction is a subjective measurement of the patient's refractive error to determine the best prescription for glasses or contact lenses. Various combinations of lenses are placed in front of each eye using a phoropter or trial frame, and the patient decides which lenses are best (Figure 4–15). A manifest refraction, denoted with MR or M, is done prior to dilating the eyes, while a cycloplegic refraction, denoted with CR or C, is done after dilating the eyes with cycloplegic drops to prevent accommodation (i.e., in children and hyperopes).

LENSOMETER

A lensometer is an instrument that measures the power of spectacle lenses, and the prescription the patient is wearing is denoted with W (Figure 4–16).

POTENTIAL ACUITY METER

A potential acuity meter is an instrument that measures the visual potential of the retina by projecting an image of an eyechart directly on to the macula through corneal

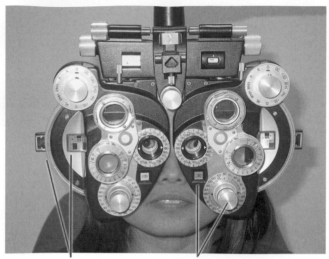

Sphere adjustment   Cylinder adjustment

FIGURE 4–15
Patient behind a phoropter undergoing manifest refraction.

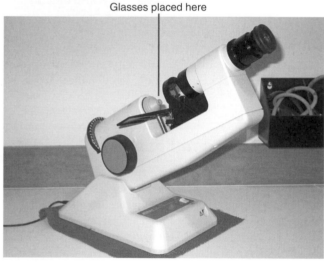

Glasses placed here

FIGURE 4–16
A lensometer measures the power of spectacle lenses placed on the middle platform.

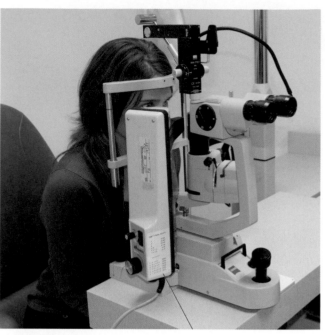

FIGURE 4–17
Patient undergoing potential acuity meter testing. The eyechart is placed on the retina by the instrument mounted on a slit lamp. The eyechart can be focused and takes into account the patient's refractive error.

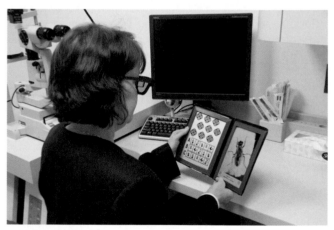

FIGURE 4–18
Patient wearing polarized glasses and performing stereo acuity test. While the patient is wearing the glasses, the fly in the picture appears three-dimensional.

or lens opacities (Figure 4–17). The potential acuity meter test is helpful in assessing visual potential prior to cataract surgery in patients with coexisting retinal pathology.

STEREOPSIS

Stereoacuity is tested binocularly, usually with **titmus** or **randot** tests. The titmus test utilizes polarized images of a fly (the patient is asked to grasp or touch the wings), animals (the patient is asked to touch the animals that are popping up), and circles (the patient is asked to touch the circles that are popping up) (Figure 4–18).

COVER TESTS

Cover tests evaluate ocular alignment by occluding one or both eyes. Measurements are made at both distance and near, with and without glasses.

The **cover–uncover test** differentiates manifest (**tropia**) from latent (**phoria**) eye turns. One eye is covered and then uncovered. If the unoccluded eye moves when the cover is in place, a tropia exists. If the

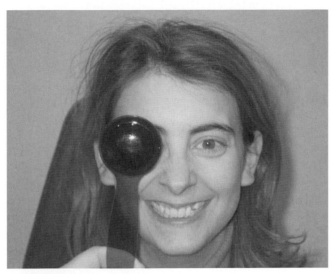

FIGURE 4–19
Patient undergoing cover–uncover test to determine if she has a tropia or phoria.

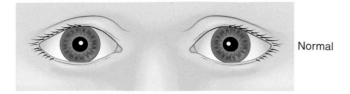

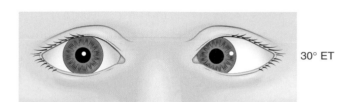

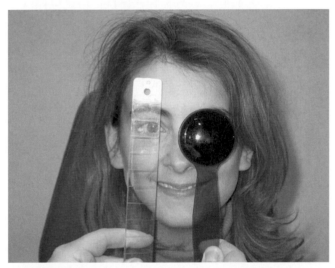

FIGURE 4–20
Patient undergoing alternate cover test where the total ocular deviation is determined by holding prisms over the eye until no movement occurs.

FIGURE 4–21
Hirschberg's method of estimating deviation. ET, esotropia.

covered eye moves when the occluder is removed, a phoria is present (Figure 4–19).

The **alternate cover test (prism and cover test)** quantifies the total ocular deviation (tropia and phoria). The eyes are dissociated by alternately holding an occluder in front of each, then prisms of increasing power are held in front of one eye until no more movement occurs (Figure 4–20).

CORNEAL LIGHT REFLEX TESTS

Corneal light reflex tests are useful in patients who cannot cooperate for the cover tests. Such tests measure ocular deviations by observing the relative position of the corneal light reflections from a light shined into the patient's eyes.

Hirschberg's method estimates the eye turn by the amount of decentration of the light reflex from the center of the cornea (1 mm of decentration corresponds to 7° or 15 prism diopters). Light reflections at the pupillary margin, mid-iris, and limbus represent decentrations of 2, 4, and 6 mm, respectively (Figure 4–21).

Modified Krimsky's method: increasing prism is held in front of the patient's fixating eye until the light reflex in the deviated eye is centered (Figure 4–22).

FORCED DUCTIONS

Forced duction testing is used to distinguish whether or not a limitation in extraocular motility is due to a restrictive etiology. Under topical anesthesia, a forceps is used to rotate the globe in the direction of abnormal movement. The eye should be grasped at the limbus on the same side in which the eye is being moved to prevent a corneal abrasion if the forceps slips.

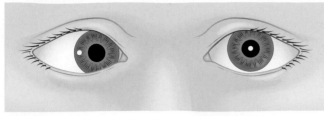

A

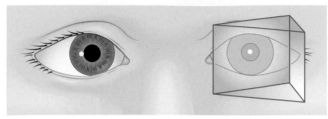

B

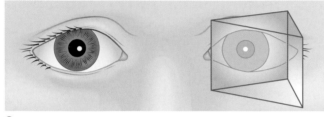

C

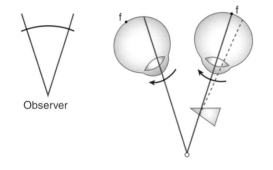

D

FIGURE 4–22
Modified Krimsky's method of estimating deviation.

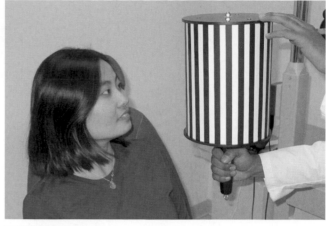

FIGURE 4–23
Patient undergoing optokinetic testing.

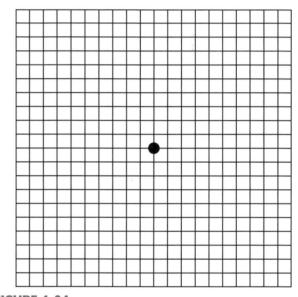

FIGURE 4–24
Amsler grid.

OPTOKINETIC TEST

Optokinetic testing uses a rotating drum with alternating black and white lines to assess nystagmus and other eye movement disorders. The test device is rotated both horizontally and vertically in front of the patient and the resulting eye movements are observed (Figure 4–23).

AMSLER GRID

The Amsler grid is a test that evaluates the central (10°) visual field and is most commonly used to assess visual changes in patients with macular degeneration. Each eye is tested monocularly by looking at a grid pattern (10 × 10 cm, composed of 5 mm squares) and any distortion or blurred areas are noted (Figure 4–24).

VISUAL FIELD TESTS

Visual field testing (**perimetry**) utilizes various devices to evaluate the peripheral vision and quantitate any field defects. Perimetry is performed one eye at a time because of the overlap of the binocular fields.

Tangent screen is a square black cloth (2 × 2 meters) over which the examiner presents round test objects of various sizes and colors to the patient seated 1 meter away.

Goldmann visual field is a manually operated machine used to perform perimetry. The patient is seated in front of a large bowl and identifies lights in the

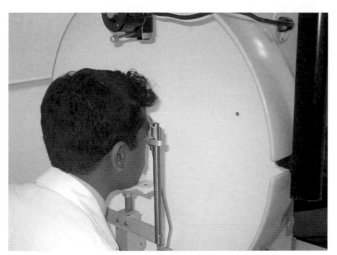

FIGURE 4–25
Patient undergoing Goldmann visual field examination.

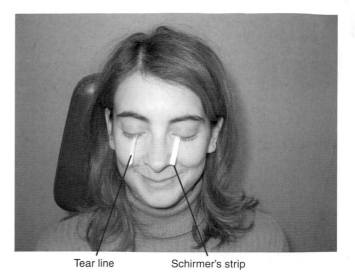

Tear line   Schirmer's strip

FIGURE 4–27
Patient undergoing Schirmer's testing for dry eyes. This patient's tears have wet the strips >10 mm, indicating that she does not have dry eyes.

visual field. The operator controls the position, size, and intensity of the light (test object) (Figure 4–25).

Humphrey visual field is a computerized perimetry test with various programs to screen for and evaluate glaucomatous, neurological, and lid-induced visual field defects (Figure 4–26).

SCHIRMER'S TEST

Schirmer's test assesses tear production in patients with dry eye. A special filter paper strip is placed over the lower eyelid into the inferior fornix to absorb tears for 5 minutes. The test, performed with or without topical anesthesia, is often unreliable because the results can be quite variable, making the reproducibility poor (Figure 4–27).

JONES' DYE TESTS

Jones' dye tests are two different tests to determine obstruction of the lacrimal drainage system. In the Jones' I test, fluorescein is instilled in the tear film and recovery from the inferior nasal meatus is attempted. The Jones' II test is performed next by attempting to recover dye after irrigating the nasolacrimal system.

ANTERIOR-SEGMENT DYES

Anterior-segment dyes include fluorescein, rose Bengal, and lissamine green, which aid in evaluating the health

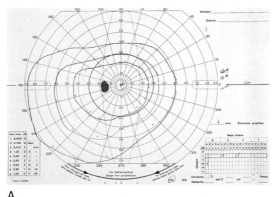

A

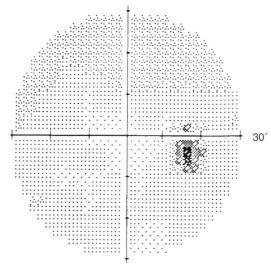

B   30°

FIGURE 4–26
Normal (**A**) Goldmann and (**B**) Humphrey visual field.

and integrity of the conjunctival and corneal epithelium. **Fluorescein**, the most common dye, stains epithelial defects and is used to check wound integrity with the **Seidel test** (the wound is painted with a moistened sterile fluorescein strip and observed for a leak which appears as a stream of diluted fluorescein emanating from the wound). **Rose Bengal** and **lissamine green** are specifically used to evaluate dry eye since they stain dry areas of conjunctiva and cornea.

GONIOSCOPY

Gonioscopy refers to examination of the angle structures with a special mirrored lens, which is placed on the cornea (Figure 4–28). This technique is the only way to ascertain whether the angle is open or closed in patients with shallow anterior chambers. Gonioscopy must be performed prior to dilating the eyes so as not to induce an angle-closure attack in patients with narrow angles.

KERATOMETRY

Keratometry can be performed with a number of devices to measure the corneal curvature and power.

A **keratometer** measures four paracentral points on the anterior corneal surface. This instrument is inaccurate in patients with altered corneal shapes.

Computerized videokeratography measures the entire corneal surface and provides more information than a keratometer. These devices generate topographic maps, and some can also measure the curvature of the posterior corneal surface as well as corneal thickness (Figure 4–29).

PACHYMETRY

Pachymetry is performed with a pachymeter, a device that uses ultrasound to measure corneal thickness. This

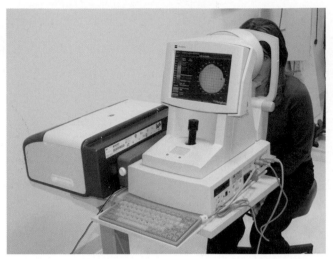

FIGURE 4–29
Patient completing a corneal topography examination.

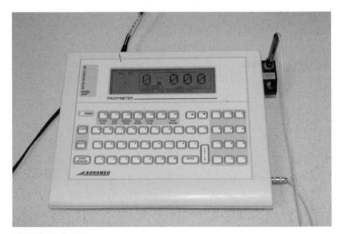

FIGURE 4–30
Pachymeter to measure corneal thickness.

information is important for patients undergoing refractive surgery and those with glaucoma (Figure 4–30).

A- AND B-SCAN ULTRASONOGRAPHY

A and B scans are types of ultrasound that measure acoustic reflectivity of interfaces to provide axial length measurements and two-dimensional images of the posterior segment, respectively (Figure 4–31). A scans are necessary to calculate the power of the intraocular lens implant for cataract surgery and are useful to differentiate ocular masses. B scans are obtained whenever the fundus cannot be directly visualized.

OCULAR COHERENCE TOMOGRAPHY

Ocular coherence tomography is an instrument that uses optical reflectivity to generate cross-sectional images of ocular structures. It is used primarily to diagnose and follow macular and optic nerve pathology (Figure 4–32).

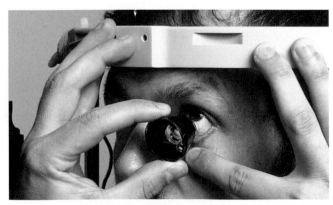

FIGURE 4–28
Goldmann gonioscopy lens.

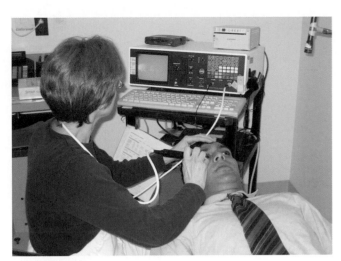

FIGURE 4–31
Patient undergoing a B-scan ultrasonography evaluation.

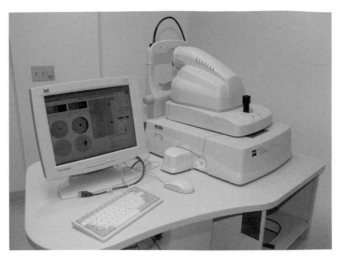

FIGURE 4–32
Optical coherence tomography scanner evaluates the retina and gives a cross-section analysis of retinal layers.

CHAPTER FIVE

Neuro-Ophthalmology

Introduction

The eye is an extension of the brain. Half of the cranial nerves (CNs) are associated with the eye, and several of these nerves as well as special gaze centers in the brain control eye movements. The retinal ganglion cells send their axons to the brain via the optic nerve. Additional connections in the brain relay the impulses transmitted by the eyes to the visual cortex where they can be interpreted into images or be "seen." Disorders affecting the eye or optic nerve cause visual loss in that eye, whereas lesions along the visual pathway to the brain disturb vision in both eyes. This chapter reviews the anatomy and pathology of the visual pathway, pupillary reflexes, gaze centers, and CNs II–VII.

Visual Pathway

ANATOMY

Images from the retina, which are upside down and inverted, travel to the brain by the visual pathway:

Optic nerve → optic chiasm → optic tract → lateral geniculate body → optic radiations → occipital lobe (visual cortex)

This mirror-image orientation (horizontally and vertically) is preserved from the retina to the visual cortex. Specifically, the information from the left half of the visual field is projected on to the right half (hemiretina) of each eye. The nasal retinal fibers in the optic nerves cross in the chiasm to the opposite optic tract so that the right occipital cortex "sees" the left field of vision of each eye, and vice versa (Figure 5–1).

Optic nerve

The optic nerve (CN II) extends from the globe to the optic chiasm to transmit information from the eye to the brain (see Ch. 1, optic nerve section). The optic nerve travels through the annulus of Zinn, the tendon ring from which the rectus muscles originate, to enter the optic canal. The vascular supply to the optic nerve varies by section with contributions from the internal carotid, anterior cerebral, anterior communicating, and ophthalmic arteries. Additional key attributes of the optic nerve include:

- The optic nerve is 1.5 mm in diameter leaving the eye.
- It widens to 3.5 mm posterior to the lamina cribrosa, where it becomes myelinated.
- It widens to 5.0 mm with the addition of the optic nerve sheath.
- The optic nerve is roughly 50 mm long and has four sections (Figure 5–2):

  1. 1 mm intraocular.
  2. 25 mm intraorbital.
  3. 9 mm canalicular.
  4. 16 mm intracranial.

- The optic nerve is surrounded by three layers of meninges:

  1. Dura mater (outer layer, merges with the sclera).
  2. Arachnoid layer.
  3. Pia mater (inner layer, fused to the surface of the nerve). The space between the arachnoid and pia contains cerebrospinal fluid.

Optic chiasm

This structure, located between the carotid arteries and 10 mm above the pituitary gland, is where 55% of the

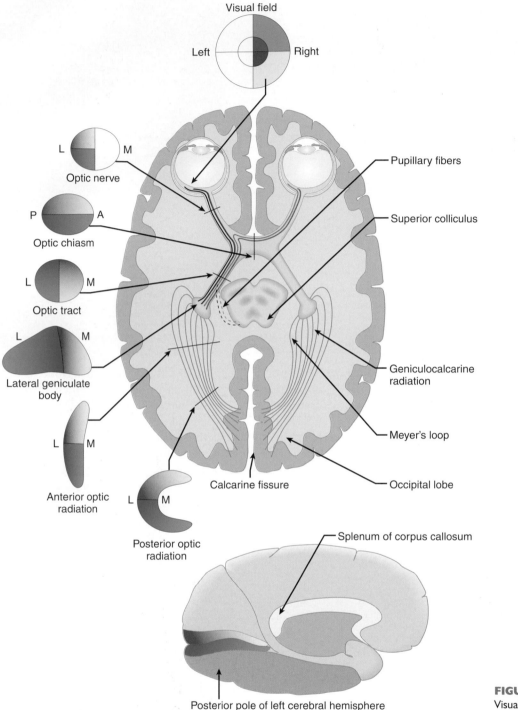

Visual field

Left   Right

L   M

Optic nerve

P   A

Optic chiasm

L   M

Optic tract

L   M

Lateral geniculate body

L   M

Anterior optic radiation

L   M

Posterior optic radiation

Pupillary fibers

Superior colliculus

Geniculocalcarine radiation

Meyer's loop

Calcarine fissure

Occipital lobe

Splenum of corpus callosum

Posterior pole of left cerebral hemisphere

FIGURE 5–1
Visual pathway.

optic nerve fibers cross to the contralateral optic tract (Figure 5–3). The fibers that cross or decussate are the nasal retinal fibers, while the temporal fibers remain uncrossed. The **knee of von Willebrand** is the name given to the inferonasal retinal fibers that cross in the chiasm and then travel anteriorly approximately 4 mm into the opposite (contralateral) optic nerve before running posteriorly to the brain. This anatomic feature gives rise to a unique binocular visual field defect (termed junctional scotoma) when a lesion of the optic nerve occurs near the chiasm. Rather than a monocular scotoma, the expected field defect of an optic nerve lesion, if the knee of von Willebrand is involved there is also a defect in the superotemporal field of the opposite eye.

Optic tract

The optic tract is the segment of the visual pathway that connects the optic chiasm to the lateral geniculate body (LGB). Fibers in the tract are rotated 90° with respect to their orientation in the optic nerve and chiasm (i.e.,

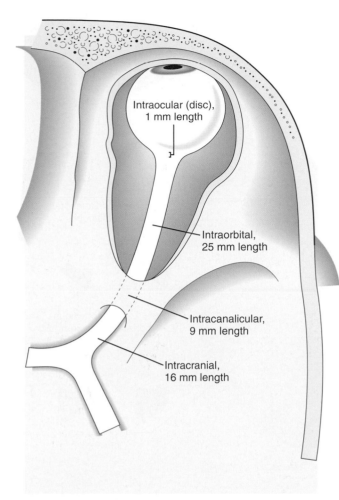

FIGURE 5–2
The four portions of the optic nerve. The lengths are given.

Labels in figure:
Intraocular (disc),
1 mm length

Intraorbital,
25 mm length

Intracanalicular,
9 mm length

Intracranial,
16 mm length

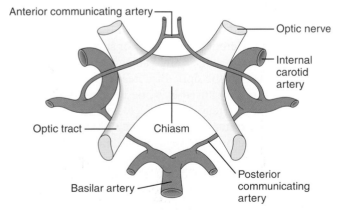

FIGURE 5–3
Relationship of the optic chiasm, optic nerves, and optic tracts to the arterial circle of Willis. The chiasm passes through the circle of Willis and receives its arterial supply from the anterior cerebral and communicating arteries from above, and the posterior communicating, posterior cerebral, and basilar arteries from below.

Labels in figure:
Anterior communicating artery
Optic nerve
Internal carotid artery
Optic tract
Chiasm
Posterior communicating artery
Basilar artery

inferior fibers lie laterally). The blood supply to the optic tract is via the anterior choroidal and posterior communicating arteries. Since the majority of retinal fibers decussate (cross) in the optic chiasm, damage to the optic tract results in a contralateral relative afferent pupillary defect (RAPD).

Lateral geniculate body

The LGB, part of the thalamus, is where the retinal ganglion cell axons that have traveled through the optic nerve, optic chiasm, and optic tract, finally synapse. The anterior communicating and choroidal arteries supply the LGB. The LGB is composed of six layers:

- Crossed fibers (from the contralateral eye) project to layers 1, 4, and 6.
- Uncrossed fibers (from the ipsilateral eye) project to layers 2, 3, and 5.

The various layers contain different types of neurons, important for different aspects of vision:

- **Magnocellular** neurons (M cells), found in layers 1 and 2, are very fast cells and function in motion detection, stereoacuity, and contrast sensitivity.
- **Parvocellular** neurons (P cells), found in layers 3–6, are slow cells, and are necessary for fine spatial resolution and color vision.

These neurons project to and synapse in the visual cortex.

Optic radiations

The optic radiations are composed of myelinated nerve fibers that extend from the LGB to the visual cortex. Signals from the superior retina (inferior visual field) travel by fibers in the parietal lobe, and those from the inferior retina (superior visual field) travel in **Meyer's loop** through the temporal lobe. Thus, temporal lobe injury may cause an incongruous homonymous superior quadrantanopia or a "pie-in-the-sky" visual field defect. Macular fibers are not affected because they travel more centrally than the inferior retinal fibers. The middle cerebral arteries provide the vascular supply to the optic radiations.

Primary visual cortex

The primary visual cortex is located on the medial face of the occipital lobe, which is divided horizontally by the calcarine fissure. This region contains a topographic map of the contralateral hemifield and receives its blood supply from the middle and posterior cerebral arteries. The central visual field from the macula has the largest representation and lies posteriorly, extending on to the lateral aspect of the occipital lobe. The peripheral visual field is located anteriorly along the calcarine fissure.

There is a temporal crescent in each visual field (from 55° to 95°) that is seen by only the nasal retina of the ipsilateral eye, and this is located most anteriorly in the

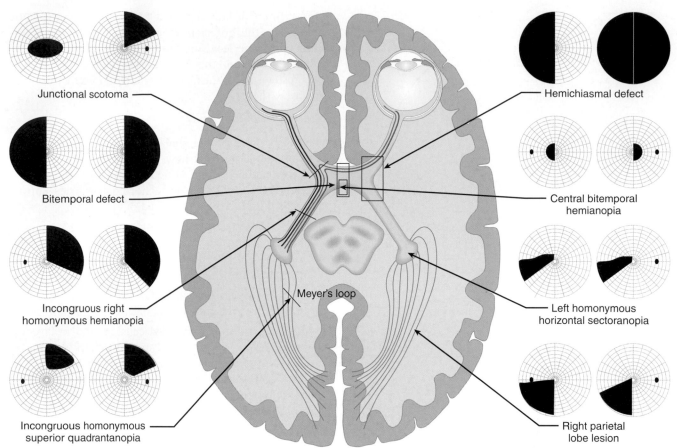

FIGURE 5–4
Visual pathway and corresponding visual field defects.

visual cortex. It is the only site posterior to the chiasm that if injured would cause a monocular visual field defect. A temporal crescent is sometimes the only portion of the visual field that is spared after occipital lobe damage.

VISUAL FIELD DEFECTS

The extent of the visual field in each eye is 60° nasally, 60° superiorly, 95° temporally, and 75° inferiorly. Damage to the retina, optic nerve, or any portion of the visual pathway may result in a visual field defect or scotoma (Figure 5–4).

There are many different types of visual field defect:

Physiologic blind spot is the naturally occurring scotoma due to the absence of retina where the optic nerve leaves the eye. It is a vertical oval-shaped area approximately 5 × 7° in size located 15° temporal to fixation and slightly below the horizontal midline. An enlarged blind spot may occur with optic disc swelling or in glaucoma (**baring of the blind spot**).

Central scotoma is a blind spot at fixation (center of vision) caused by optic nerve or macular lesions.

Cecocentral scotoma is a scotoma involving the blind spot and the macula (within 25° of fixation), and can occur in any condition that produces a central scotoma. This nerve fiber bundle defect results from damage to nerve fibers from the macula and occurs in optic neuropathies, optic neuritis, and optic pit with a serous retinal detachment.

Arcuate scotoma is a comma-shaped, macular nerve fiber bundle defect that is found in glaucoma, optic neuritis, anterior ischemic optic neuropathy (AION), branch retinal vascular occlusions (artery or vein), and optic nerve drusen.

Altitudinal defect is an inferior or superior hemifield defect that results from damage to the upper or lower pole of the optic disc, respectively. This type of scotoma is caused by optic neuritis, AION, and hemiretinal artery or vein occlusions.

Neurologic defect is a bilateral scotoma that respects (does not cross) the vertical midline.

Binasal defect is a bilateral nasal field defect that is most often associated with glaucoma (nasal defects are usually due to arcuate scotomas) but can also occur from pressure on the temporal aspect of the optic nerves and anterior angle of the chiasm (i.e., an aneurysm, pituitary adenoma, or infarct).

Pseudo-bitemporal hemianopia is not a true neurologic defect since it does not respect the vertical midline. This scotoma slopes and crosses the vertical meridian and is most commonly produced by an uncorrected refractive error, tilted optic disc, overhanging eyelid, enlarged blind spot (papilledema), or large central/cecocentral scotoma.

Constricted field or **ring scotoma** is an annular defect caused by retinitis pigmentosa, advanced glaucoma, thyroid-related ophthalmopathy, optic nerve drusen, vitamin A deficiency, occipital stroke, panretinal photocoagulation, or functional visual loss.

Spiraling visual field is an unusual pattern that suggests malingering or functional visual loss since the person taking the test cannot pinpoint the edge of the visual field defect and thus it changes every time it is tested.

Visual pathway lesions have characteristic patterns of field loss. Therefore, visual field testing is important for localizing neuro-ophthalmic pathology. The appearance of neurologic visual field defects depends upon which part of the pathway is affected:

Nerve fiber layer lesions produce arcuate, papillomacular, and temporal wedge scotomas.

Optic nerve lesions produce a monocular defect.

Optic chiasm lesions classically produce a bitemporal hemianopia. However, the chiasm is vulnerable to numerous conditions (pituitary tumor, pituitary apoplexy, craniopharyngioma, meningioma, optic nerve glioma, aneurysm, trauma, infection, metastatic tumor, multiple sclerosis (MS), sarcoidosis), and various defects occur when different areas of the chiasm are affected.

- **Anterior chiasm** lesions at the junction of the optic nerve and chiasm involve fibers in the knee of von Willebrand (the contralateral nasal retinal loop) resulting in a junctional scotoma (central scotoma in one eye and superotemporal defect in the other).
- **Body of chiasm** lesions produce a bitemporal hemianopia, which may preserve vision.
- **Posterior chiasm** lesions produce a bitemporal hemianopia (primarily involves crossing macular fibers).
- **Lateral compression** (very rare) lesions produce a binasal hemianopia (more commonly caused by bilateral optic nerve or retinal lesions).

For **retrochiasmal** lesions, the more posterior the lesion, the more congruous the defect, and a unilateral lesion does not reduce vision (macula-splitting hemianopia can have 20/20 acuity).

Optic tract lesions produce an incongruous homonymous hemianopia. The optic tracts are affected by posterior sellar or suprasellar lesions, which produce a homonymous hemianopia and a contralateral RAPD.

Retro-LGB lesions produce an isolated homonymous hemianopia and other neurologic findings.

Optic radiation lesions include those from pathology in the temporal and the parietal lobes:

- **Temporal lobe** (Meyer's loop) lesions produce a superior homonymous hemianopia ("pie-in-the-sky" defect, which is denser superiorly and spares the central region). Formed visual hallucinations and seizures can also occur.
- **Parietal lobe** lesions produce an inferior homonymous hemianopia. Hemiparesis, visual perception difficulty, agnosia, apraxia, and optokinetic (OKN) asymmetry can be present as well.

Occipital lobe lesions produce congruous defects that may have macular sparing:

- **Homonymous hemianopia with macular sparing** results from damage in the area supplied by the posterior cerebral artery. The macular region is spared since it receives dual supply from both the middle and posterior cerebral arteries.
- **Checkerboard field** is a bilateral incomplete homonymous hemianopia, that is superior on one side and inferior on the opposite side (i.e., left upper and right lower homonymous quadrant defects).
- **Bilateral homonymous altitudinal defect** is caused by infarction or trauma to both occipital lobes, above or below the calcarine fissure.
- **Monocular temporal crescent** is due to anterior occipital infarcts since the far temporal field is seen by only one eye.
- **Cortical blindness** is produced by bilateral occipital lobe destruction. Other findings include intact pupillary response, unformed visual hallucinations, the **Riddoch phenomenon** (the ability to perceive moving targets but not stationary ones), and the patient may deny blindness (**Anton's syndrome**).

Pupillary Pathways

ANATOMY

The size of the pupil is controlled by the iris sphincter and dilator muscles. The **iris dilator** has *sympathetic* innervation (Figure 5–5).

- The pathway begins in the posterior hypothalamus, where fibers travel down the spinal cord and synapse in the ciliospinal center of Budge.
- The second-order neuron ascends the sympathetic chain, goes over the apex of the lung, and synapses at the superior cervical ganglion.
- The third-order neuron travels with the internal carotid artery, joins CN VI in the cavernous sinus, enters the orbit via the long ciliary nerve, and terminates at the iris dilator and Müller's muscle.

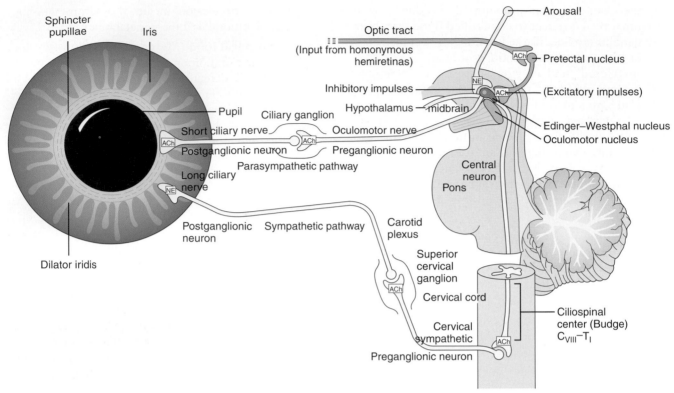

FIGURE 5–5
Parasympathetic and sympathetic innervation of the iris muscles. ACh, acetylcholine; NE, norepinephrine.

Lesions affecting the sympathetic fibers result in **Horner's syndrome**.

Iris sphincter contraction is mediated by *parasympathetic* innervation from the Edinger–Westphal nucleus (Figure 5–5). The sphincter causes pupillary constriction in response to both light and near stimulation. The pathway for the **light reflex** involves a direct connection to the midbrain.

- The afferent pupillary fibers travel with the visual fibers in the optic nerve through the chiasm into both optic tracts. They leave the tracts prior to the LGB and instead synapse in the pretectal nuclei in the midbrain.
- Fibers from the pretectal nucleus are sent to both Edinger–Westphal nuclei where they synapse again.
- The efferent (parasympathetic) fibers leave the Edinger–Westphal nucleus and travel by CN III to the ciliary ganglion.
- The postganglionic fibers reach the ciliary body and iris sphincter via the short ciliary nerves.

The anatomy of this pathway explains why the pupils react directly and consensually to light. If there is a retinal or optic nerve lesion, then an afferent pupillary defect results, whereas a CN III palsy produces an efferent defect ("blown" pupil).

The **near reflex** is a three-part response that occurs when the eyes focus on a near object:

1. Pupillary constriction.
2. Accommodation.
3. Convergence.

The exact pathway is still uncertain, but the final arm seems to be the same as for the light reflex. When checking pupillary reflexes, usually only the light response is tested. This is because if the light reflex is intact, then the near reflex will also be intact. However, the reverse is not always true. Certain disorders can result in pupillary reaction to accommodation but not to light. Such a disconnection between the two reflexes is called **light-near dissociation** (see below), and therefore, if the pupils do not react to light, then their response to near must be tested. If there is an abnormal reaction to both light and near then the cause is pharmacologic, iris damage, or a CN III palsy.

ABNORMALITIES

One or both pupils can sometimes be constricted (miotic) or dilated (mydriatic). If the pupils are not equal in size, then **anisocoria** (see below) is present.

Causes of miosis

- Horner's syndrome.
- Pharmacologic constriction (pilocarpine, brimonidine, narcotics, insecticides).
- Argyll Robertson pupil.

- Diabetes.
- Iritis.
- Spasm of the near reflex.
- Old age.

Causes of mydriasis

- CN III palsy.
- Adie's tonic pupil.
- Pharmacologic dilation (mydriatics, cycloplegics, cocaine).
- Iris damage (traumatic, ischemic, surgical).
- Hutchinson pupil.

Both Horner's and Adie's are examples of denervation hypersensitivity (sympathetic tone loss in Horner's, parasympathetic tone loss in Adie's).

RELATIVE AFFERENT PUPILLARY DEFECT (MARCUS GUNN PUPIL)

Definition

An RAPD refers to a paradoxical dilation of one pupil in response to light, due to a difference in the amount of light perceived by the two eyes, when the swinging flashlight test is performed (see below).

Etiology

An RAPD is produced when the afferent arm of the light reflex is disturbed. This occurs with asymmetric optic nerve disease (optic neuropathy and optic neuritis), retinal damage (central retinal vein or artery occlusion and retinal detachment), or chiasm lesions. Optic tract lesions can cause a contralateral RAPD because there are more nasal crossing fibers in the chiasm. Lesions posterior to the LGB *do not* produce an RAPD.

Symptoms

Patients usually have associated visual loss, often marked, and difficulty with color vision and contrast.

Signs

On examination, there is a positive RAPD. The involved pupil is often sluggish in its direct reaction to light. The consensual response is normal, as is the response to near. Other findings include decreased visual acuity and a visual field defect. Decreased color vision can usually be demonstrated as well. The optic nerve may appear swollen or pale, or there may be retinal findings suggestive of a retinal vascular occlusion or detachment.

Differential diagnosis

Other causes of **light-near dissociation** include syphilis (Argyll Robertson pupil), Adie's pupil, Parinaud's syndrome, aberrant regeneration of CN III, diabetes, myotonic dystrophy, encephalitis, alcoholism, and herpes zoster ophthalmicus.

Evaluation

- When eliciting the **history**, it is important to characterize the visual loss completely.
- The **eye exam** must include the pupillary light response with particular attention to performing the **swinging flashlight test** (a bright light is shined into one eye and then rapidly into the other in an alternating fashion; see Ch. 4). The test is positive when the pupil into which the light is shined dilates instead of constricts. If the pupil of the involved eye is non-reactive or non-functional, then observe the fellow, normal eye for a reverse afferent defect (dilation when the light is on the non-reactive eye, and constriction when the light is shined on the reactive eye). A reverse afferent pupillary defect results from a poor consensual pupillary response. Other aspects of the exam that must be noted are the visual acuity (decreased), color vision (decreased), and ophthalmoscopy (retinal or optic nerve abnormalities).
- **Neutral-density filters** can be used to grade the severity of the afferent pupillary defect.

Management

- Treat the underlying cause.

Prognosis

Depending on the etiology, the afferent pupillary defect may improve over time, but the visual loss may not.

ANISOCORIA

Definition

Anisocoria is an inequality in the size of the pupils.

Etiology

When the pupils are different sizes, it can sometimes be difficult to tell which one is abnormal, the larger or the smaller one. Observing the pupils in bright and dim lighting conditions enables the examiner to determine which one is pathologic.

If the anisocoria is *greater in dark* conditions, then the *abnormal pupil is the smaller one* since both pupils should dilate in dim light. The causes of an abnormally miotic pupil include Horner's syndrome, Argyll Robertson pupil, iritis, and pharmacologic (miotic agent, narcotic, insecticide).

If the anisocoria is *greater in bright* light, then the *abnormal pupil is the larger one* since both pupils should constrict from the light. The etiology of an abnormally mydriatic pupil is Adie's tonic pupil, CN III palsy, Hutchinson pupil (uncal herniation with CN III entrapment in a comatose patient), pharmacologic (mydriatic or cycloplegic agent, cocaine), and iris damage.

Anisocoria that is *equal in light and dark* conditions is called simple or physiologic. This is the most common cause of a relative size difference (<1 mm) between the pupils.

Epidemiology

Up to 20% of the general population has physiologic anisocoria.

Symptoms

Anisocoria rarely produces symptoms, but patients may experience glare, pain, photophobia, diplopia, or blurred vision, depending on the etiology.

Signs

The involved pupil may be larger or smaller, round or irregular, reactive or non-reactive. Other signs may coexist depending on the etiology (see below).

Evaluation

- The **history** should include information regarding associated symptoms like changes in vision (reduced acuity, difficulty reading, double vision, photophobia), or pain, medications (scopolamine patches to treat motion sickness, commonly worn behind the ear, may cause pharmacologic dilation of the ipsilateral eye), and any eyedrops that were recently administered. It is also important to inquire about past medical conditions, trauma, and surgical procedures.
- The size of the pupils must be carefully assessed in different lighting conditions. The **eye exam** should include checking the lids (for ptosis), ocular motility (for CN III palsy), anterior chamber (for cell and flare), and gonioscopy (for angle trauma) to narrow the differential diagnosis.
- **Pharmacologic pupil testing** is sometimes necessary to determine the exact etiology. Testing must be performed prior to manipulating the cornea (i.e., before any drops, applanation, or other tests have been performed) otherwise the result may be invalid.
  - *Abnormally small pupil:*
    - **Topical cocaine 4–10%** is used to detect the presence of Horner's syndrome. Two drops are administered to each eye and the pupil size is measured after 40 minutes. If there is equal dilation then the diagnosis is simple anisocoria, but if there is still asymmetry in pupil size then Horner's syndrome is present (see below).
    - **Topical hydroxyamphetamine 1% (Paredrine)** is used to distinguish the location of the Horner's lesion, but this test cannot be performed on the same day as the cocaine test. If the eyes dilate equally with Paredrine, then a central or preganglionic Horner's syndrome exists. If the pupils are still asymmetric, then the Horner's is postganglionic (see below).

- *Abnormally large pupil:*
  - **Topical pilocarpine 0.1% or methacholine 2.5%** causes constriction of an Adie's tonic pupil (see below). No constriction requires further testing with 1% pilocarpine (see below).
  - **Topical pilocarpine 1%** constricts a pupil with a CN III palsy, but does not constrict a pharmacologically dilated pupil.
- **Serology and lumbar puncture** for neurosyphilis (Venereal Disease Research Laboratory (VDRL) test, fluorescent treponemal antibody absorption (FTA-ABS) test) may be ordered in cases of suspected Argyll Robertson pupil.
- If the diagnosis is CN III palsy or Horner's syndrome, then **radiologic studies**, including head, neck, or chest computed tomography (CT) or magnetic resonance imaging (MRI) scan must be considered to rule out masses and vascular anomalies.

Management

- Treatment is directed toward the underlying cause.
- Consider a cosmetic contact lens or surgical repair of the iris for symptomatic mydriasis (usually from trauma or surgery).

Prognosis

Anisocoria is often benign, but the prognosis ultimately depends on the etiology.

HORNER'S SYNDROME

Definition

Horner's syndrome is an oculosympathetic paresis that causes a triad of findings: ptosis, miosis, and anhydrosis.

Anatomy

The sympathetic damage may occur anywhere along the three-neuron pathway:

- **First-order neuron (central):** from the hypothalamus to the ciliospinal center.
- **Second-order neuron (preganglionic):** from the ciliospinal center to the superior cervical ganglion.
- **Third-order neuron (postganglionic):** from the superior cervical ganglion to the iris dilator muscle.

Etiology

Many lesions can cause a Horner's syndrome. The etiology varies with the affected neuron.

- **First-order neuron:** cerebrovascular accident, neck trauma, tumor, demyelinating disease, polio, syringomyelia, inflammation, vertebral artery dissection, cervical disc disease, and **Foville's syndrome** (lesion of CNs V, VI, VII and Horner's syndrome). Central Horner's syndromes are rarely isolated.
- **Second-order neuron:** mediastinal mass, Pancoast tumor, cervical rib, neck trauma, abscess, thyroid

disease, neurofibroma, pneumothorax, cervical infections, upper respiratory tract tumors, and brachial plexus syndromes (congenital Horner's syndrome is usually a result of birth trauma).
- **Third-order neuron**: neck lesion, head trauma, headache syndromes (migraine, cluster headaches, **Raeder's syndrome** (middle-aged men with Horner's and daily unilateral headaches)), cavernous sinus lesion, carotid dissection, carotid cavernous fistula, internal carotid artery aneurysm, nasopharyngeal carcinoma, vascular disease, infections (complicated otitis media), trigeminal herpes zoster, and tumors of the parotid gland, nasopharynx, and sinuses.

Symptoms

Horner's syndrome is often asymptomatic. The patient may notice a droopy eyelid, blurred vision, pain (especially with a vascular postganglionic etiology), and other symptoms depending on the site and cause of the lesion (central usually has other neurologic deficits). Ipsilateral nasal stuffiness may be the initial complaint.

Sign

The hallmark of Horner's is the triad of mild (1–2 mm) ptosis, miosis, and anhydrosis. The involved pupil is smaller and dilates poorly in the dark. The presence of anhydrosis usually indicates a preganglionic lesion. There may also be a mild inverse or "upside-down" ptosis (lower-lid elevation). Initially, ipsilateral conjunctival hyperemia or reduced intraocular pressure may occur. The patient can also have facial numbness, diplopia, and vertigo. In cases of congenital or long-standing Horner's syndrome, the iris of the involved eye can be lighter in color (heterochromia iridum) (Figure 5–6).

Evaluation

- When Horner's syndrome is suspected, it is important to ask the patient specifically about any **history** of head, neck, and chest problems.
- During the examination, particular attention should be directed to the **neurologic exam** as well as the lids (ptosis), ocular motility (normal), pupils (miosis), and iris (may have heterochromia) components of the **eye exam**.
- **Pharmacologic pupil testing**:
  - **Cocaine test** determines the presence of a Horner's syndrome. Topical cocaine (4%, 10%) blocks the reuptake of norepinephrine. A functioning neuron will release norepinephrine and the pupil will dilate. The pupil does not dilate as well in Horner's syndrome.
  - **Hydroxyamphetamine (Paradrine) test** distinguishes between a preganglionic (first-order and second-order neurons) and a postganglionic (third-order neuron) lesion. Topical hydroxyamphetamine 1% releases norepinephrine from the nerve terminal.

In a preganglionic Horner's syndrome, the pupil dilates normally because the postganglionic neuron is intact and can therefore release norepinephrine. However, in a postganglionic Horner's syndrome, the pupil does not dilate because the neuron is damaged and does not have any norepinephrine to release. This test does not determine whether a preganglionic lesion affects the first-order or second-order neuron.

- Neuroblastoma must be ruled out in a young child with Horner's syndrome. This requires an **MRI of the sympathetic chain** (from the abdomen to the neck) and checking the **urine for vanillylmandelic acid and homovanillic acid**.
- For patients with suspected carotid artery dissection (i.e., Horner's syndrome associated with neck pain, shoulder pain, or an abnormal taste in the mouth) an axial **MRI of the neck** is ordered.
- Smokers should have a **chest radiograph** to rule out a Pancoast tumor.

Management

- The ptosis may be corrected with surgery to shorten Müller's muscle.

Prognosis

Lesions producing a postganglionic Horner's syndrome are usually benign, while preganglionic lesions tend to be more serious.

ARGYLL ROBERTSON PUPIL

Definition

An Argyll Robertson pupil is small, irregular, and demonstrates light-near dissociation (reacts to accommodation but not to light).

Etiology

This condition is usually caused by tertiary syphilis and affects both eyes, sometimes asymmetrically. It can also occur in sarcoidosis and MS. Herpes zoster ophthalmiscus (HZO) may cause an Argyll Robertson pupil due to involvement of the ciliary ganglion.

Symptoms

This pupillary abnormality is asymptomatic.

Signs

By definition, examination will reveal an irregular, miotic pupil with a normal near response and an absent reaction to light. These pupils respond poorly to pharmacologic dilation. Patients may also have stigmata of congenital syphilis (i.e. Hutchinson's triad (interstitial keratitis, notched teeth, and deafness), retinal changes, and skeletal deformities or sequelae of HZO (i.e., corneal scarring, glaucoma, iris atrophy).

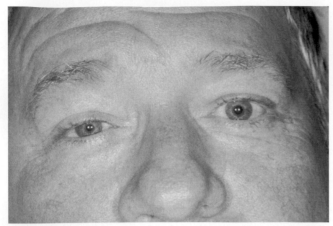

A

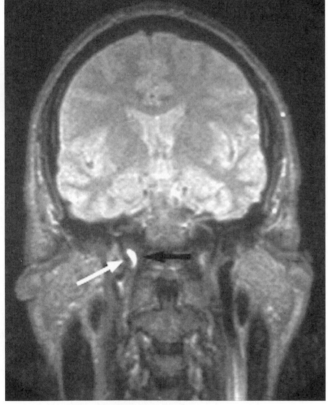

B

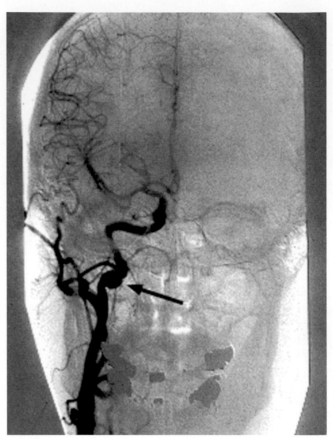

C

FIGURE 5–6
(**A**) Patient with acute right Horner syndrome illustrating miosis and ptosis of the right eye. The dissection of the internal carotid artery is shown on (**B**) the magnetic resonance imaging scan and (**C**) angiogram (arrows).

Differential diagnosis

Argyll Robertson-like pupils can also be seen in diabetes, alcoholism, and systemic lupus erythematosus.

Evaluation

- When small, irregular pupils are noted on examination, the patient should be specifically questioned about a **history** of ocular trauma or surgery, miotic eyedrop use, shingles, and systemic and sexually transmitted diseases.
- On **eye exam** the pupils must be tested carefully, and the examiner should also search for other signs of tertiary syphilis or HZO.

- **Serology and lumbar puncture** (VDRL, FTA-ABS) are necessary to rule out neurosyphilis.
- The patient should be referred to an internist for **medical consultation** and antibiotic treatment if the serologic tests are positive.

Management

- The treatment for neurosyphilis is systemic penicillin G (2.4 million U IV q4h for 10–14 days, then 2.4 million U IM once a week for 3 weeks) or tetracycline for penicillin-allergic patients.
- The serum VDRL is followed to monitor treatment efficacy.

Prognosis

The pupillary abnormality is benign; however, if the cause is untreated tertiary syphilis, then the prognosis is poor.

ADIE'S TONIC PUPIL

Definition

Adie's pupil is an idiopathic, benign form of internal ophthalmoplegia due to postganglionic parasympathetic pupillomotor damage.

Etiology

A lesion in the ciliary ganglion or short ciliary nerves with aberrant regeneration of ciliary muscle fibers to the iris sphincter causes a tonic pupil that exhibits denervation hypersensitivity.

Epidemiology

Ninety percent of Adie's pupil occurs in women, usually 20–40 years old. The lesion is unilateral 80% of the time.

Symptoms

Patients may initially experience blurred near vision and photophobia, and they often notice a slightly larger pupil in the involved eye. The condition frequently becomes asymptomatic over time.

Signs

Anisocoria is apparent. Initially the pupil is dilated and reacts poorly to light. Later the pupil becomes miotic. On slit-lamp exam, the iris exhibits segmental contraction (vermiform movements) in response to the light beam. There is poor accommodation and light-near dissociation with initial pupillary constriction and then slow (tonic) redilation to a near stimulus. Decreased deep tendon reflexes occur in 70%, and this combination is known as **Adie's syndrome** (Figure 5–7).

Differential diagnosis

The differential diagnosis of Adie's tonic pupil includes sarcoidosis, iris ischemia, botulism, giant cell arteritis, orbital and iris trauma, and any cause of light-near dissociation (see above).

Evaluation

- When gathering the **history**, it is important to ask about associated symptoms such as blurred near vision and photophobia.
- On **eye exam** attention is directed to the pupillary response. Deep tendon reflexes should be tested in all patients suspected of having Adie's pupil.
- **Pharmacologic pupil testing:**
  - **Dilute pilocarpine or methacholine** determines the presence of an Adie's pupil. Topical pilocarpine

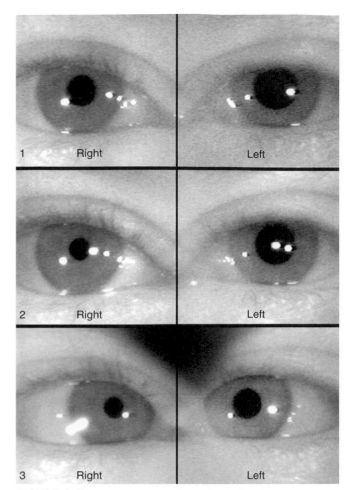

FIGURE 5–7

Adie's pupil with light-near dissociation. 1, Anisocoria is evident in room light. 2, In bright light the normal right pupil constricts, but the left pupil responds poorly. 3, On near testing, the affected pupil responds better than to light.

0.1% or methacholine 2.5% will constrict an Adie's tonic pupil (but not a normal pupil) due to cholinergic supersensitivity. False-positive tests can occur in patients with a CN III palsy.

Management

- No treatment is recommended.

Prognosis

The prognosis for Adie's pupil is good. The initial accommodative paresis is usually temporary, lasting only months.

Eye Movements

Anatomy

Eye movements are controlled by the extraocular muscles, the CNs that innervate them, and gaze centers in the brainstem. The gaze centers synchronize the eyes

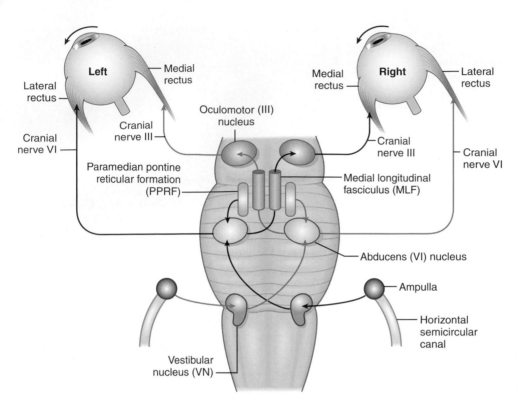

FIGURE 5–8
Horizontal eye movement pathways.

so that they move simultaneously (right, left, up, down, together, or apart). These supranuclear pathways consist of connections from the frontal cortex, occipital lobes, and semicircular canals to multiple CN nuclei (CNs III, IV, and VI).

Horizontal gaze center. The horizontal gaze center for each eye is located in the **paramedian pontine reticular formation (PPRF)** at the level of the CN VI nucleus (Figures 5–8 and 5–9). This area controls gaze to the ipsilateral side by sending projections to the ipsilateral CN VI nucleus and the contralateral CN III nucleus via the **medial longitudinal fasciculus (MLF)**. The MLF connects the CN III nuclei and the gaze centers (ipsilateral CN III and contralateral CN VI). The cortical input to each PPRF is from the cerebral cortex: contralateral frontal lobe for voluntary and ipsilateral occipital lobe for involuntary conjugate movements. There is also contralateral input from the vestibular nuclei in the pons.

Vertical gaze center. The vertical gaze center, located in the **rostral interstitial nucleus of the MLF**, receives input from the frontal eye fields, superior colliculus, and vestibular nuclei, and sends fibers to the nuclei of CN III and IV. Upgaze requires stimulation of the CN III nuclei (superior rectus and inferior oblique) while downgaze requires stimulation of the CN III (inferior rectus) and CN IV (superior oblique) nuclei (Figure 5–10).

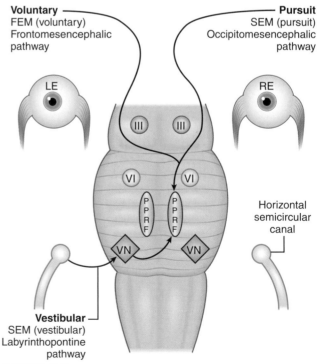

FIGURE 5–9
Fast eye movement (FEM: voluntary), slow eye movement (SEM: pursuit), and SEM (vestibular). Pathways all converge on paramedian pontine reticular formation (PPRF) for horizontal eye movements. LE, left eye; RE, right eye; VN, vestibular nuclei.

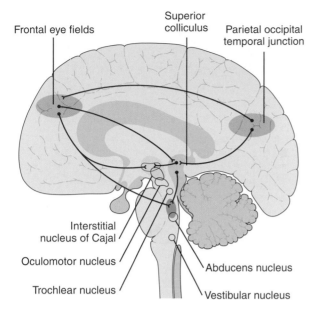

Frontal eye fields

Superior colliculus

Parietal occipital temporal junction

Interstitial nucleus of Cajal

Oculomotor nucleus

Trochlear nucleus

Abducens nucleus

Vestibular nucleus

▢ Rostral interstitial nucleus of the medial longitudinal fasciculus
▮ Paramedian pontine reticular formation

FIGURE 5–10
Supranuclear control of eye movements. The pontine horizontal gaze center (blue) and the vertical gaze center in the midbrain (yellow) receive input from the frontal eye fields to initiate saccades, and from the parietal occipital temporal junction to control pursuit. These gaze centers control ocular motility by synapsing upon the ocular motor nerve nuclei (III, IV, and VI).

GAZE PALSIES

Central eye movement (gaze) disorders are called supra-nuclear because the lesion occurs in the brain above the CN nuclei. Often there are no symptoms or complaints.

Horizontal gaze palsies

Horizontal gaze palsies may accompany many disorders. A *destructive* **frontal lobe lesion** (i.e., stroke, trauma, or infection) involving this cerebral input to the PPRF produces a tonic *deviation of the eyes toward* the side of the lesion (the patient appears to look at the lesion) due to unopposed contralateral input. However, doll's head and caloric testing can move the eyes in the contralateral direction since the vestibular pathway is intact. If the frontal lobe lesion is *irritative* (i.e., seizure), then the eyes will *deviate away* from the lesion because the increased neural activity will overpower the tonic input from the opposite hemisphere. An **occipital lobe lesion** causes an ipsilateral pursuit palsy because of ipsilateral inner-vation. A **lesion of the PPRF** results in an ipsilateral horizontal gaze palsy. Other causes of horizontal gaze palsies include Parkinson's disease, Huntington's chorea, metabolic disorders, drug-induced, and pseudo-gaze palsies such as myasthenia gravis, and chronic progressive external ophthalmoplegia (CPEO).

Internuclear ophthalmoplegia (INO) is a specific horizontal gaze palsy due to a lesion of the MLF, which produces an inability to adduct (move out) the ipsilateral eye and nystagmus of the contralateral eye. INO may be unilateral (ischemia, demyelination, tumor, infection, trauma, compression) or bilateral (most commonly demyelination or drug toxicity), and convergence may be preserved (anterior or midbrain lesion) or impaired (posterior or pons lesion) (Figure 5–11).

Vertical gaze palsies

A vertical gaze palsy is most commonly associated with **Parinaud's syndrome**. Also known as dorsal midbrain syndrome or pretectal syndrome, it is caused by lesions affecting the periaqueductal area, most commonly pineal tumors (90%), but it may also be caused by demyelination, infarction, and trauma. This syndrome is characterized by paresis of upgaze, bilateral mid-dilated pupils with light-near dissociation, convergence–retraction nystagmus on attempted upgaze (synchronous backward jerking movements of both eyes due to co-contraction of the horizontal recti), and eyelid retraction.

NYSTAGMUS

Definition

In nystagmus there are repetitive, involuntary, rhythmic oscillations of the eyes due to a disorder of the slow eye movement system. The oscillations may be horizontal, vertical, rotary, or a combination; fast or slow; symmetric or asymmetric; pendular (equal speed in both directions) or jerk (designated by the direction of the fast phase); congenital or acquired.

Etiology

Congenital nystagmus

- **Afferent**: due to sensory deprivation and associated with pediatric disorders that cause severe visual loss. A pendular nystagmus is produced.
- **Efferent**: due to an ocular motor disturbance. This condition produces a horizontal nystagmus that is present at or shortly after birth. There may be a null point (a position in which the nystagmus slows or stops) and the patient may have a head turn (to move the eyes to the null point) to counteract the nystagmus. The nystagmus decreases with convergence and stops during sleep. Other features include possible head oscillations and strabismus (33%).
- **Latent**: this is a form of nystagmus that is only present under monocular viewing conditions and is associated with certain forms of congenital strabismus. When one eye is covered the eyes jerk away from the covered eye. When the cover is removed, the nystagmus stops.

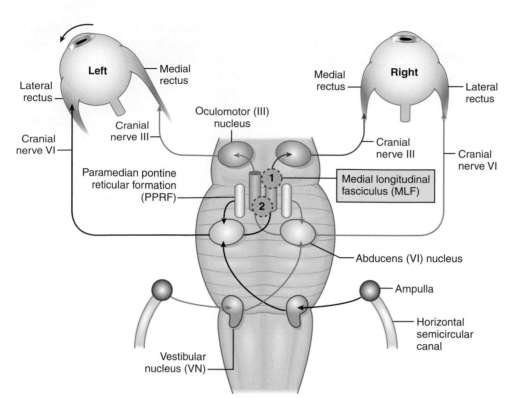

FIGURE 5–11
1. Right internuclear ophthalmoplegia (INO).
2. Bilateral INO.

- **Spasmus nutans**: this is a benign form of nystagmus consisting of fine, rapid, often monocular or asymmetric eye movements that develops during the first year of life with spontaneous resolution several years later. Characteristically, there is a triad of findings: eye movements, head nodding, and torticollis (head turning). This diagnosis is one of exclusion because similar eye movements can be seen with chiasmal gliomas and parasellar tumors. Therefore, it is important to check the pupils carefully (for an RAPD) and optic nerve (for swelling or pallor), as well as perform neuroimaging.

Acquired nystagmus. In these forms, the pattern of nystagmus often helps to localize the pathology.

- **Convergence–retraction**: due to a periaqueductal gray matter or dorsal midbrain lesion (Parinaud's syndrome, pinealoma, trauma, brainstem arteriovenous malformation, MS). Co-contraction of the lateral rectus muscles causes convergence and retraction movements of the eyes on attempted upgaze.
- **Dissociated**: due to posterior fossa disease, MS, INO. This type of nystagmus is asymmetric between the two eyes (different direction, amplitude, frequency, etc.) and is always pathologic.
- **Downbeat**: due to a lesion that affects the pathways responsible for downgaze (i.e, cervicomedullary junction lesion, spinocerebellar degeneration, drug intoxication (lithium)), but there is no identifiable cause in 50% of cases. It produces a jerk nystagmus

with rapid downbeat and slow upbeat components that worsens in downgaze and improves in upgaze. Oscillopsia (the perceived movement of one's surroundings) is present.
- **Drug-induced**: due to anticonvulsants, barbiturates, tranquilizers, and phenothiazines. Often produces gaze-evoked nystagmus that may be absent in downgaze.
- **Gaze-evoked**: due to brainstem or posterior fossa lesions, as well as certain medications (anticonvulsants, sedatives). Jerk nystagmus occurs in the direction of gaze and is absent in primary position.
- **Opsoclonus (saccadomania)**: associated with neuroblastoma or after postviral encephalopathies in children, and with visceral carcinomas in adults. It refers to rapid, unpredictable, multidirectional saccades, which are absent during sleep.
- **Periodic alternating**: due to vestibulocerebellar and cervicomedullary junction lesions. It is very rare, and is defined as horizontal jerk nystagmus that changes direction every 60–90 seconds, with 5–10 second pauses in between.
- **See-saw**: due to suprasellar lesions, cerebrovascular trauma, or may be congenital. This is a vertical and torsional nystagmus that resembles the movement of a see-saw: one eye rises and intorts while the other eye falls and extorts, then reverses.
- **Upbeat**: due to anterior vermis and lower brainstem lesions, also associated with Wernicke's syndrome or drug intoxication. The eyes drift down followed by a corrective upward saccade.

- **Vestibular**: due to an end-organ, peripheral nerve, or central lesion. Nystagmus is usually horizontal with a rotary component (fast component toward normal side, slow component toward abnormal side). Vertigo, tinnitus, and deafness may also be present.
- **Voluntary**: due to hysteria or malingering. The nystagmus is usually horizontal with rapid saccades, but cannot be sustained for more than 30 seconds. There may also be lid fluttering.

Physiologic nystagmus. These forms normally occur in certain situations:

- **End gaze**: jerk nystagmus in extreme lateral gaze with the fast component in the direction of gaze.
- **OKN**: jerk nystagmus elicited by fixating on moving targets. The slow component is in the direction of the moving target (pursuit movement), while the fast component is in the opposite direction (refixation on the next target). This is commonly tested with a rotating drum that has alternating black and white stripes. OKN nystagmus is a familiar phenomenon to all of us: the horizontal eye movements of a passenger gazing out the window of a rapidly moving train at passing objects.
- **Caloric**: water irrigated into the ear produces nystagmus. The direction of the fast component can be remembered with the mnemonic **COWS** (cold opposite, warm same) if the patient is awake. In a comatose patient, there is a tonic deviation in the opposite direction of the mnemonic. Bilateral cold water irrigation produces upbeat nystagmus in an awake patient and downward tonic deviation in a comatose patient. Bilateral warm water causes the opposite effect.
- **Rotational**: when a person is rotated, jerk nystagmus results. A special chair is used to position the patient so that the horizontal canals are aligned horizontally. Rotation will then produce nystagmus in the direction of the rotation.

Symptoms

Nystagmus itself is usually asymptomatic but acquired forms can cause oscillopsia (the perceived movement of one's surroundings). Depending on the etiology, there may be other neurologic deficits like reduced hearing, tinnitus, and vertigo.

Signs

Besides the obvious ocular movements, the visual acuity is variably decreased. There may be a head turn and other ocular or systemic pathology.

Evaluation

- The **history** should document the time of onset of nystagmus, associated symptoms, neurologic problems, and any drug or toxin ingestion.

- Complete **eye and neurologic exams** are performed with attention to visual acuity (may be decreased), head position (may have head turn), pupils (may have a positive RAPD), ocular motility (direction, type, and speed of eye movements, may have strabismus), and ophthalmoscopy (may have a retinal or optic nerve lesion).
- **Neurology or neuro-ophthalmology consultation** may be necessary.
- **Neuroimaging** with a head CT or MRI scan is used to rule out an intracranial process.

Management

- Congenital nystagmus may be amenable to treatment with prism glasses that force the eyes to converge, diminishing the nystagmus. A head posture can be corrected with extraocular muscle surgery.
- Baclofen can be used to treat periodic alternating and see-saw nystagmus.
- Clonazepam may be helpful for downbeat nystagmus.

Prognosis

Congenital nystagmus is often benign. The prognosis for acquired forms depends on the underlying etiology.

Cranial Nerve Palsies

Half of the CNs are involved with eye functions. CN II, the optic nerve, enables vision. CN III, IV, and VI innervate the extraocular muscles responsible for eye movements. CN V provides sensation to the eye and face, while CN VII controls eyelid closure and facial movements. Damage to these CNs (in isolation or combination) results in specific deficits depending on where the pathology occurs. Therefore, familiarity with the CN pathways is helpful for localizing lesions (Figures 5–12 and 5–13).

OCULOMOTOR NERVE (CN III) PALSY

Definition

Oculomotor nerve palsy is a paresis of CN III caused by a lesion anywhere along the course of the nerve from the midbrain to the orbit.

Anatomy

The CN III nucleus is located in the midbrain. The fascicle travels through the cerebral peduncle, traversing the red nucleus and corticospinal tract. The nerve enters the subarachnoid space, passes between the posterior cerebral and superior cerebellar arteries, courses lateral to the posterior communicating artery, and enters the lateral wall of the cavernous sinus. After receiving

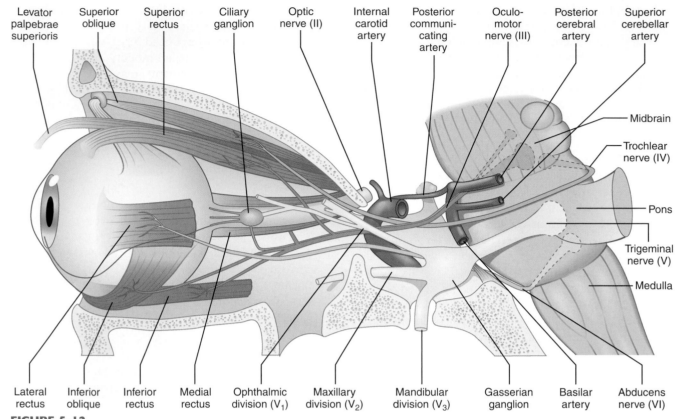

FIGURE 5–12
Cranial nerve pathways.

parasympathetic fibers from the internal carotid plexus, the nerve passes through the superior orbital fissure and divides into the superior (motor innervation to the superior rectus and levator) and inferior (motor innervation to the inferior rectus, medial rectus, inferior oblique, and parasympathetic innervation to the iris sphincter and ciliary muscle) divisions.

The CN III nucleus is actually a collection of subnuclei. Each subnucleus supplies innervation to its ipsilateral ocular muscle. Fibers from the superior rectus subnucleus, however, supply the contralateral superior rectus muscle. There is only one midline subnucleus that supplies both levator muscles, and each Edinger–Westphal nucleus supplies both pupils (Figure 5–14).

Types

CN III palsies are classified as isolated, complete, partial, and pupil-sparing.

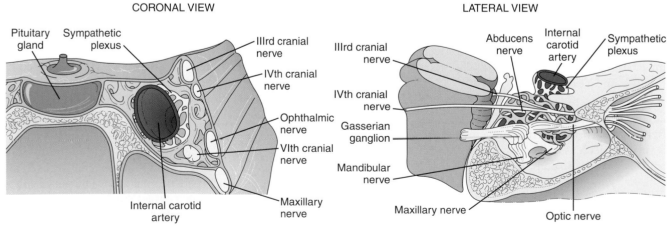

FIGURE 5–13
Anatomy of the cavernous sinus.

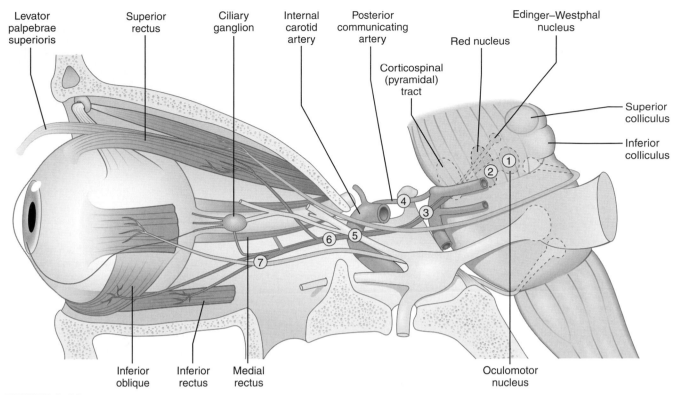

FIGURE 5-14

Seven syndromes of third cranial nerve palsy. 1, Nuclear palsy; 2, fascicular syndromes; 3, uncal herniation; 4, posterior communicating artery aneurysm; 5, cavernous sinus syndrome; 6, orbital syndrome; 7, pupil-sparing isolated palsy.

Etiology

Etiology depends on age:

- **Children**: congenital or due to postviral illness, trauma, tumor, or migraine.
- **Adults**: most commonly from ischemia or microvascular disease (hypertension or diabetes), but also due to aneurysm, trauma, and tumors. Up to 30% may be of undetermined cause.

The etiology may help localize the level of the pathology:

- **Nuclear**: very rare, usually microvascular infarctions.
- **Fascicular**: usually vascular or metastatic lesions.
- **Subarachnoid space**: usually involves the pupil and is due to aneurysm, trauma, or uncal herniation; rarely there may be microvascular disease or infection. A posterior communicating artery aneurysm is the most common cause of a non-traumatic, isolated, pupil-involving CN III palsy.
- **Cavernous sinus**: usually due to a cavernous sinus fistula, aneurysm, tumor, infection (herpes zoster), or pituitary apoplexy.
- **Orbital space**: usually due to tumor, trauma, or infection.

There are other clues to help determine etiology. **Pupil-sparing** palsies are usually seen with microvascular or ischemic (80%) disease, whereas 95% of compressive lesions involve the pupil. The explanation for this rests with the different anatomic locations of the fibers. The small-caliber parasympathetic pupillomotor fibers travel in the outer layers of CN III closer to its blood supply. These pupil fibers are more susceptible to compressive damage than are the fibers at the nerve core, which are more prone to damage by ischemia.

Another clue to determine etiology is if there is **aberrant regeneration**. This misdirection of inferior rectus and/or medial rectus nerve fibers to the levator and/or iris sphincter may occur after CN III palsies resulting from aneurysms, trauma, and tumors, but never after ischemic or microvascular injury (Figure 5–15).

Symptoms

Patients notice binocular diplopia (which disappears when one eye is closed) and an eye turn. They may also complain of pain, headache, a large pupil, or a droopy eyelid. Patients with a third-nerve palsy from an aneurysm classically present with all these symptoms and describe the headache as the worst of their life.

Signs

The characteristic findings of a CN III palsy are ptosis and a "down and out" eye (Figure 5–16). The unopposed actions of the superior oblique and lateral rectus muscles

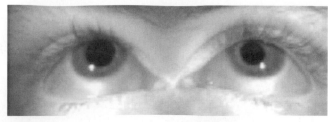

A

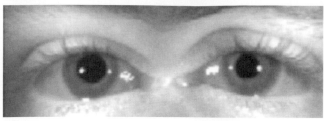

B

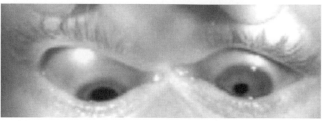

C

FIGURE 5-15
(**A–C**) Primary aberrant regeneration of the left third nerve. The left pupil constricts on downgaze because the nerves that normally supply the inferior rectus are now innervating the iris sphincter muscle.

cause this ocular misalignment (hypotropia and exotropia) in primary gaze. On ocular motility testing, the eye only abducts (moves out from CN VI innervation). The pupil may be dilated and non-reactive ("blown" pupil) due to an efferent defect.

In cases of **aberrant regeneration**, the healing nerve fibers make erroneous connections to their target muscles, resulting in anomalous lid or pupil responses with eye movements. **Lid-gaze dyskinesis,** due to inferior rectus or medial rectus fibers innervating the levator, refers to upper-lid retraction on downgaze or adduction. **Pupil-gaze dyskinesis,** that is, pupil constriction on downgaze or adduction, is caused by inferior rectus or medial rectus fibers innervating the iris sphincter.

There may be other neurologic deficits or CN palsies depending on the type and site of the lesion:

* **Nuclear**: bilateral ptosis and contralateral superior rectus involvement. Pupil involvement is bilateral or none.
* **Fascicular**: associated with various syndromes.
  * **Benedikt's syndrome**: lesion of fascicle and red nucleus causing CN III palsy with contralateral hemitremor and loss of sensation.

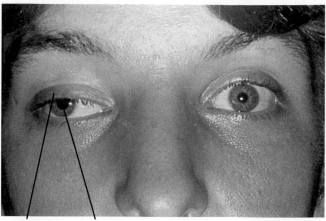

Ptosis   Dilated pupil
FIGURE 5-16
Third cranial nerve palsy with right ptosis, pupillary dilation, exotropia, and hypotropia. This is the typical appearance of the "down and out" eye with a droopy lid and large pupil.

* **Nothnagel's syndrome**: lesion of fascicle and superior cerebellar peduncle causing CN III palsy and ipsilateral cerebellar ataxia.
* **Claude's syndrome**: combination of Benedikt's and Nothnagel's syndromes.
* **Weber's syndrome**: lesion of fascicle and pyramidal tract causing CN III palsy and contralateral hemiparesis.
* **Subarachnoid space**: isolated, involving the pupil, and usually painful.
* **Cavernous sinus**: associated with multiple CN palsies (III, IV, V, VI) and Horner's syndrome. The pupil is usually spared (90%).
* **Orbital space**: associated with multiple CN palsies (II, III, IV, V$_1$, VI). Findings include proptosis (protruding globe), conjunctival chemosis (swelling), and injection (hyperemia), and the optic nerve may be normal, swollen, or atrophic. Partial palsies may be present since CN III exists in this space as separate superior and inferior divisions.

Differential diagnosis

Entities to be considered in the differential diagnosis are myasthenia gravis, thyroid-related ophthalmopathy, ophthalmoplegic migraine, and CPEO.

Evaluation

* It is critical to ask about associated neurologic symptoms in the **history**. Similarly, complete **eye and neurologic exams** must be performed with specific attention directed to the CNs (may have other palsies), pupillary response (efferent defect), lids (ptosis), ocular motility (restricted), and ophthalmoscopy (optic nerve appearance). A thorough history and physical will help to determine the type and location of the palsy.

- **Neuroimaging**, with head and orbital CT, MRI, and/or magnetic resonance angiography (MRA) scan, is warranted if: the pupil is involved, the palsy is associated with other neurologic abnormalities, there is pupil sparing in a young patient (<45 years old), signs of aberrant regeneration are present, or there is no improvement of an isolated pupil-sparing microvascular palsy after 3 months. If the pupil is involved and the MRA is inconclusive, then **cerebral angiography** is considered to rule out an aneurysm, which is a *neurosurgical emergency*.
- Certain **lab tests** should be ordered: fasting blood glucose, complete blood count (CBC), erythrocyte sedimentation rate (ESR), C-reactive protein, VDRL, FTA-ABS, and antinuclear antibody (ANA).
- The **blood pressure** is measured to check for hypertension.
- A **lumbar puncture** is performed if subarachnoid hemorrhage is suspected.
- Consider a **Tensilon test** to rule out myasthenia gravis.
- **Neurology or neurosurgery consultation** may be advisable, especially if the pupil is involved.

Management

- The treatment of a CN III palsy depends upon the etiology.
- Isolated pupil-sparing lesions must be followed closely for pupil involvement during the first week.
- Diplopia can be alleviated by occluding the paretic eye (using clear surgical tape or nail polish across one spectacle lens).
- Neurosurgery may be required for aneurysms, tumors, and trauma.

Prognosis

The prognosis depends on the etiology. Usually the prognosis is poor except for microvascular palsies, which tend to resolve within 3 months.

TROCHLEAR NERVE (CN IV) PALSY

Definition

Trochlear nerve palsy is a paresis of CN IV caused by a lesion anywhere along the course of the nerve from the midbrain to the orbit.

Anatomy

The CN IV nucleus is located in the mesencephalon at the level of the inferior colliculus. The fascicle crosses to the contralateral side as it emerges from the brainstem near the aqueduct of Sylvius, and then passes between the posterior cerebral and superior cerebellar arteries. The nerve travels in the lateral wall of the cavernous sinus, enters the orbit through the superior orbital fissure, and innervates the superior oblique muscle.

The trochlear nerve is the only CN that exits dorsally from the brainstem and that decussates (except for fibers from the CN III subnucleus that innervates the superior rectus) (Figure 5–17).

Etiology

The trochlear nerve has the longest intracranial course, making it the most frequently injured from closed-head trauma. Thus, trauma accounts for 40% of CN IV palsies. Microvascular disease (hypertension, diabetes) is responsible for 30%, and the other common etiologies are congenital and idiopathic (20%). An isolated CN IV paresis is usually congenital. Rare causes of CN IV palsies include tumor, hemorrhage, and aneurysm. Severe head trauma may produce bilateral CN IV palsies.

The etiology may help localize the level of the pathology:

- **Nuclear and fascicular**: rare, due to hemorrhage, infarction, demyelinating disease, or trauma.
- **Subarachnoid space**: due to closed-head trauma, rarely tumor or infection.
- **Cavernous sinus**: due to trauma, tumors, and inflammation.
- **Orbital space**: usually due to tumor, trauma, or infection.

Symptoms

The hallmark of an isolated CN IV palsy is acute vertical diplopia. The patient may have a head tilt toward the opposite shoulder to minimize the double vision. Other neurologic symptoms may be present.

Signs

The characteristic finding is a hypertropia due to a superior oblique palsy (Figure 5–18). Patients may present with an abnormal head posture.

There may be other neurologic deficits or CN palsies depending on the type and site of the lesion:

- **Nuclear**: contralateral superior oblique palsy.
- **Fascicular**: may have bilateral palsies or contralateral Horner's syndrome.
- **Cavernous sinus**: usually associated with multiple CN palsies (III, IV, V, VI) and Horner's syndrome.
- **Orbital space**: associated with multiple CN palsies (II, III, IV, V_1, VI). Findings include proptosis (protruding globe), conjunctival chemosis (swelling) and injection (hyperemia), and the optic nerve may be normal, swollen, or atrophic.

Differential diagnosis

A CN IV palsy can be mimicked by myasthenia gravis, thyroid-related ophthalmopathy, orbital disease, CN III palsy, skew deviation, superior oblique myokymia, and MS.

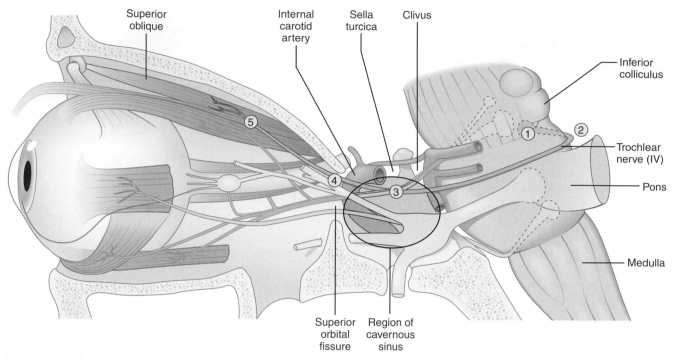

FIGURE 5-17
Five syndromes of fourth cranial nerve palsy. 1, Nuclear/fascicular syndrome; 2, subarachnoid space syndrome; 3, cavernous sinus syndrome; 4, orbital syndrome; 5, isolated palsy.

Evaluation

- The **history** should include specific questions about head posture, trauma, and associated neurologic symptoms.
- **Eye and neurologic exams** must include evaluation of the CNs (may have other palsies), ocular motility (restricted), head posture (may have head tilt), and ophthalmoscopy (optic nerve appearance). It is helpful to check old photographs for evidence of a long-standing head tilt in congenital cases.
- The **three-step test** measures the amount of ocular misalignment in various positions of gaze. This test is quickly performed by ophthalmologists to determine which muscle is paretic in cases of hypertropia due to weakness of a single muscle.
- **Lab tests** include fasting blood glucose, CBC, ESR, VDRL, FTA-ABS, and ANA.
- The **blood pressure** is measured to check for hypertension.
- **Neuroimaging**, with head and orbital CT and/or MRI/MRA scan, is obtained for: history of head trauma or cancer, signs of meningitis, young age, presence of other neurologic abnormalities, or no improvement of isolated microvascular cases after 3–4 months. Isolated and microvascular cases do not initially require neuroimaging.
- **Lumbar puncture** may be considered.
- Consider a **Tensilon test** to rule out myasthenia gravis.
- **Neurology consultation**.

Management

- The treatment of a CN IV palsy depends upon the etiology.
- Diplopia can be alleviated by occluding the paretic eye (using clear surgical tape or nail polish across one spectacle lens), or fitting the patient with prism glasses.
- Consider muscle surgery for long-standing, stable CN IV palsies.
- Neurosurgery may be required for aneurysms, tumors, and trauma.

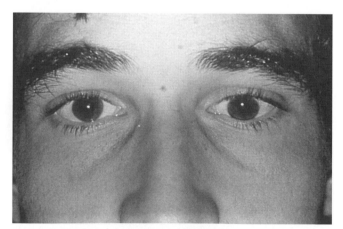

FIGURE 5-18
Fourth cranial nerve palsy with right hypertropia.

Prognosis

The prognosis depends on the etiology. Congenital palsies are well tolerated, and microvascular palsics tend to resolve within 3 months.

TRIGEMINAL NERVE (CN V) PALSY

Definition

Trigeminal neuralgia or tic douloureux is a CN V paresis due to compression of the nerve root.

Anatomy

CN V emerges from the pons, passes below the tentorium, and travels to the trigeminal ganglion where it branches into three divisions: ophthalmic (V_1), maxillary (V_2), and mandibular (V_3). These branches provide sensory innervation to the face and eye, as well as the motor supply to the muscles of mastication (Figure 5–19).

Etiology

Trigeminal neuralgia is most often caused by a superior cerebellar artery aneurysm or tumor. It may also be idiopathic or due to MS.

Symptoms

Patients with trigeminal neuralgia experience lancinating facial pain lasting seconds. The condition is unilateral in 95% and usually involves the maxillary or mandibular distribution. Pain in the ophthalmic distribution alone is rare.

Signs

There are no visible findings on exam, but testing of CN V may demonstrate altered sensation and may precipitate the pain.

Differential diagnosis

A variety of conditions may cause facial pain, so it is important to rule out sinus, ear, dental, and eye pathology. The initial symptoms of herpes zoster prior to the skin eruption may be similar, and postherpetic neuralgia can also mimic CN V palsy.

Evaluation

- The diagnosis is based on the characteristic **history** and lack of **physical** findings.
- **Neuroimaging** is obtained to identify the underlying lesion.

Management

- Medical and surgical treatment options are available. Carbamazepine may control the pain. If not, radio-frequency destruction of the trigeminal ganglion can be performed.

Prognosis

The prognosis depends on the etiology.

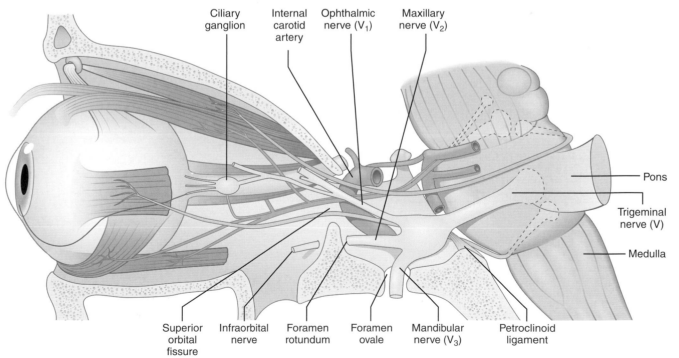

FIGURE 5–19
Fifth cranial nerve pathway.

ABDUCENS NERVE (CN VI) PALSY

Definition

Abducens nerve palsy is a paresis of CN VI caused by a lesion anywhere along the course of the nerve from the pons to the orbit.

Anatomy

From the nucleus in the pons, CN VI fibers travel to the PPRF, through the pyramidal tract, and exit at the pontomedullary groove into the subarachnoid space. The nerve climbs over the clivus and petrous ridge, runs along the base of the skull, through Dorello's canal, and enters the cavernous sinus. It enters the orbit through the superior orbital fissure and passes laterally to supply the lateral rectus muscle (Figure 5–20).

Etiology

Etiology depends on age:

- **Children** (0–15 years old): most commonly tumors (pontine glioma) or postviral, and associated with otitis media.
- **Young adults** (15–40 years old): usually miscellaneous or undetermined cause.
- **Adults** (>40 years old): usually due to trauma and microvascular disease (hypertension, diabetes), but also associated with MS, cerebrovascular accidents, increased intracranial pressure (ICP), and rarely tumors (nasopharyngeal carcinoma).

The etiology may help localize the level of the pathology:

- **Nuclear**: due to pontine infarcts, pontine gliomas, cerebellar tumors, microvascular disease, and Wernicke–Korsakoff syndrome.
- **Fascicular**: due to tumors, microvascular disease, or demyelinating disease.
- **Subarachnoid space**: due to elevated ICP (30% of patients with idiopathic intracranial hypertension have CN VI palsy); also basilar tumors (acoustic neuroma, chordomas), basilar artery aneurysm, hemorrhage, inflammation (sarcoidosis), or meningitis.
- **Petrous space**: due to trauma (basal skull fracture) and infections.
- **Cavernous sinus**: due to trauma, vascular lesion, inflammation, or tumors.
- **Orbital space**: due to trauma, tumor, idiopathic orbital inflammation, or cellulitis.

Symptoms

Patients complain of horizontal binocular diplopia, typically worse at distance than at near. They may also notice an eye turn.

Signs

On examination the involved eye appears turned inward and cannot move outward. This esotropia and inability to abduct the eye is due to the lateral rectus muscle palsy and unopposed action of the medial rectus muscle (Figure 5–21).

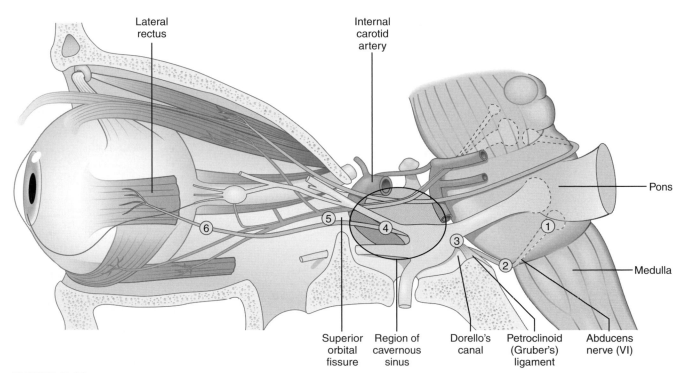

FIGURE 5–20

Six syndromes of fourth cranial nerve palsy. 1, Brainstem syndrome; 2, subarachnoid syndrome; 3, petrous apex syndrome; 4, cavernous sinus syndrome; 5, orbital syndrome; 6, isolated palsy.

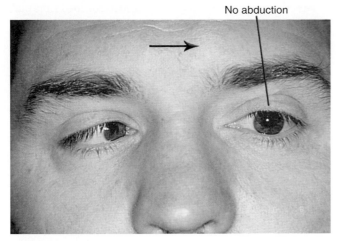

FIGURE 5–21
Sixth cranial nerve palsy demonstrating the inability to abduct the left eye on left gaze.

There may be other neurologic deficits or CN palsies depending on the type and site of the lesion:

- **Nuclear**: causes an ipsilateral, horizontal gaze palsy (cannot look to the side of the lesion).
- **Fascicular**: causes various syndromes.
  - **Millard–Gublar syndrome**: lesion of CN VI and VII fascicles and pyramidal tract causing CN VI and VII palsies with contralateral hemiparesis.
  - **Raymond's syndrome**: lesion of CN VI and pyrimidal tract causing CN VI palsy and contra-lateral hemiparesis.
  - **Foville's syndrome**: lesion of CN VI nucleus, CN V and VII fascicles, and sympathetics, causing ipsilateral V, VI, and VII palsies, horizontal conjugate gaze palsy, and ipsilateral Horner's syndrome.
  - **Mobius syndrome**: associated with CN VII lesion, supernumary digits, skeletal abnormalities, and mental retardation.
- **Petrous space**: can cause **Gradenigo's syndrome** (mastoiditis secondary to otitis media causing ipsilateral CN V, VI, and VII pareses with ipsilateral facial pain, decreased hearing, and facial paralysis in children) or **pseudo-Gradenigo's syndrome** (due to nasopharyngeal carcinoma, cerebellopontine angle tumor, petrous bone fracture, or basilar aneurysm with findings similar to those of Gradenigo's syndrome).
- **Cavernous sinus**: associated with multiple CN palsies (III, IV, V, VI), Horner's syndrome, chiasm and pituitary involvement.
- **Orbital space**: associated with multiple CN palsies (II, III, IV, V_1, VI). Findings include proptosis (protruding globe), conjunctival chemosis (swelling) and injection (hyperemia), and the optic nerve may be normal, swollen, or atrophic.

Differential diagnosis

Other conditions that should be considered are thyroid-related ophthalmopathy, myasthenia gravis, idiopathic orbital inflammation, certain forms of strabismus, orbital fracture with medial rectus muscle entrapment, and spasm of the near reflex.

Evaluation

- It is important to note any **history** of cancer, head trauma, or infections, as well as any neurologic symptoms.
- **Eye and neurologic exams** must include CNs (may have other palsies), ocular motility (restricted), and ophthalmoscopy (optic nerve appearance).
- **Lab tests** for adults include fasting blood glucose, CBC, ESR, VDRL, FTA-ABS, and ANA.
- The **blood pressure** is measured to check for hypertension.
- **Neuroimaging**, with head and orbital CT and/or MRI/MRA scan, is performed for children, a history of pain, head trauma, or cancer, signs of meningitis or other neurologic abnormalities, or no improvement of isolated microvascular cases after 3–6 months. Isolated and microvascular cases in adults > 40 years old do not initially require neuroimaging.
- Perform a **lumbar puncture** if elevated ICP is suspected.
- Consider a **Tensilon test** to rule out myasthenia gravis.
- **Neurology consultation**.

Management

- The treatment of a CN VI palsy depends upon the etiology.
- Diplopia can be alleviated by occluding the paretic eye (using clear surgical tape or nail polish across one spectacle lens).
- Consider muscle surgery in long-standing, stable cases.
- Neurosurgery may be required for aneurysms, tumors, and trauma.

Prognosis

The prognosis depends on the etiology. Microvascular palsies tend to resolve within 3 months.

FACIAL NERVE (CN VII) PALSY

Definition

Facial nerve palsy is a paresis of CN VII caused by a lesion anywhere along the course of the nerve from the pons to the orbit.

Anatomy

CN VII passes around the CN VI nucleus, exits the brainstem at the cerebellopontine angle, travels through the temporal bone, branches in the parotid gland, and innervates the muscles of voluntary facial movement. It also supplies the lacrimal and salivary glands, posterior two-thirds of the tongue, external ear sensation, and dampens the stapedius. The upper face receives bilateral supranuclear innervation, while the lower face only receives contralateral supranuclear innervation (Figure 5–22).

Etiology

The etiology may help localize the level of the pathology:

- **Supranuclear and brainstem**: due to vascular lesion or tumor.
- **Peripheral**: causes include idiopathic (**Bell's palsy**), trauma (temporal bone fracture, birth trauma, or surgical), infection (herpes zoster), inflammation, and turmor (parotid gland or facial nerve). Acute uni-

lateral facial nerve palsy is the most common cranial neuropathy.

Symptoms

Patients are aware of facial weakness and notice an asymmetric appearance and inability to move part of the face. They may complain of tearing or irritation of the eye and sometimes blurred vision. Drooling, dysarthria, and dysphagia are also common. Other neurologic symptoms may be present: hearing loss and vertigo can occur with trauma and herpes zoster. A history of pain or vesicular rash around the ear prior to the facial weakness is also indicative of herpes zoster.

Signs

The hallmark of a CN VII palsy is paralysis of facial movement. Depending on the site of the lesion, there are distinct variations in the pattern of muscle involvement that help to localize the pathology.

- **Supranuclear**: causes a contralateral paralysis of volitional facial movement involving the lower more

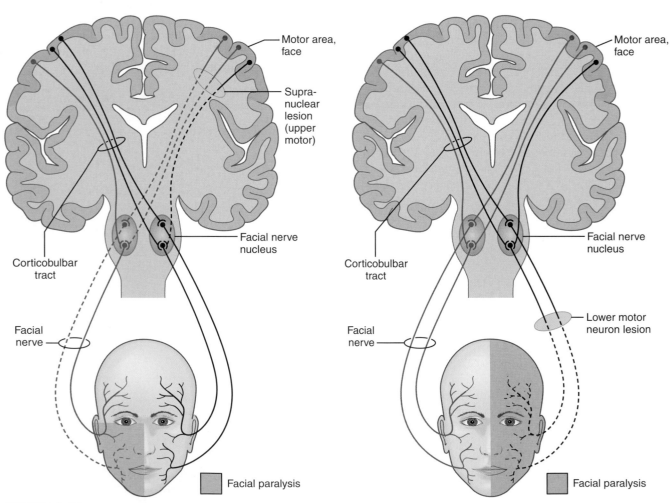

FIGURE 5–22
Facial weakness due to upper and lower motor neuron lesions.

severely than the upper face. Emotional and reflex movements like smiling and spontaneous blinking are preserved because these are extrapyramidal functions.

- **Brainstem**: causes an ipsilateral facial weakness involving both the upper and lower face. There are usually other neurologic symptoms such as CN V and VI palsies, lateral gaze palsy, cerebellar ataxia, and contralateral hemiparesis (see CN VI section above).
- **Peripheral**: causes isolated ipsilateral facial weakness.

With respect to the eyes, the patient is unable to close the lids fully due to dysfunction of the orbicularis muscle. This makes the ocular surface susceptible to dryness from exposure, which can lead to corneal erosions and infections.

Hemotympaneum, perforated tympanic membrane, and bruising over the mastoid bone may be present in traumatic cases. Associated twitching or facial spasm suggests a neoplasm. Swelling of the parotid gland or cervical lymphatics can be seen with malignant tumors and inflammatory conditions of the parotid (sarcoidosis, tuberculosis). Other findings that may occur include lacrimation (damage to the greater superficial petrosal nerve), impaired stapedius muscle reflex (damage to the stapedial nerve), and impaired taste (damage to the chorda tympani nerve). After a CN VII palsy, **aberrant regeneration** of facial innervation may be apparent with Marcus Gunn jaw winking (activation of the muscles of mastication induce orbicularis oculi contraction) or crocodile tears (lacrimation evoked by chewing).

Evaluation

- The **history** should specifically focus on the timing of the facial weakness, associated neurologic symptoms, and trauma. Acute paralysis is suggestive of Bell's palsy (isolated) while a gradually evolving paresis is more ominous. Traumatic cases of paralysis may be acute (nerve transection) or gradual (nerve contusion or swelling).
- Complete **eye and neurologic exams** must be performed with attention to the CNs (may have other palsies), lids (lagophthalmos, may have jaw winking), ocular motility (normal), and cornea (may have epithelial defects due to exposure).
- **Radiologic studies**, MRI scan of the facial nerve and CT scan of the temporal bone, are required for cases with delayed onset and progression over more than 1 week. Neuroimaging of the brainstem is performed if there is evidence of additional CN involvement.

Management

- The treatment of a CN VII palsy depends upon the etiology.
- Bell's palsy is treated initially with vigorous lubrication of the ocular surface using artificial tears (up to q1h

or more) and ointment (qhs). Sometimes it is necessary to tape the eyelids closed at night with surgical tape or a Tegaderm dressing. If this is not sufficient, then gold weight implantation or a temporary lateral tarsorrhaphy must be considered. The patient is followed each month because an absence of improvement after 4 months is ominous and requires further investigation with neuroimaging. Treatment with oral acyclovir (herpes has been linked to Bell's palsy) and prednisone may be useful. Chronic sequelae such as persistent paralysis or aberrant regeneration can be treated with surgery or botulinum toxin, respectively.
- Herpes zoster is treated with oral acyclovir and prednisone.

Prognosis

The prognosis depends on the etiology:

- Most intracranial and bone tumors that cause facial paralysis are benign, whereas parotid gland tumors are usually malignant.
- Traumatic cases tend to resolve completely.
- The prognosis is typically excellent for Bell's palsy with the majority of patients returning to nearly complete function; however, there is a 10% recurrence rate (ipsilateral or contralateral). Aberrant regeneration is common in cases with incomplete recovery.
- CN VII paresis due to herpes zoster carries a poor prognosis: only 10% of patients with complete paralysis will recover, while 66% of those with a partial paralysis recover. Patients may also develop postherpetic neuralgia.

CN VII OVERACTIVITY

There are a number of disorders that produce increased facial muscle activity.

Benign essential blepharospasm

In this condition there is frequent bilateral blinking that progresses to involuntary spasms and forceful contractions of the orbicularis muscle. The etiology of this condition is unknown, but it usually affects women over age 50 and is absent during sleep. In extreme instances, it may cause functional blindness. The treatment is botulinum toxin (Botox) injections. Surgery with orbicularis myomectomy is rarely required.

Hemifacial spasm

In hemifacial spasm there are unilateral contractions of facial muscles. This disorder is usually due to vascular compression of CN VII at the brainstem, and rarely tumor. In contrast to blepharospasm, hemifacial spasm is present during sleep. Neuroimaging is indicated.

Facial myokymia

Facial myokymia involves fasciculations of facial muscles. MS must be considered if the myokymia is multifocal and progressive.

Eyelid myokymia

In eyelid myokymia there are benign fasciculations of the eyelid. This is a very common occurrence and is self-limited. Treatment is not required.

MULTIPLE CRANIAL NERVE PALSIES

Definition

In this condition there are multiple CN abnormalities appearing simultaneously due to lesions located in the brainstem, subarachnoid space, cavernous sinus, or orbital space.

Etiology

The etiology varies with location but is generally vascular, tumor, infection, or inflammation affecting the brainstem, cavernous sinus, or superior orbital fissure. Specific entities include: arteriovenous fistula, cavernous sinus thrombosis or metastases, meningioma, mucormycosis, herpes zoster ophthalmicus, Tolosa–Hunt syndrome, mucocele, nasopharyngeal carcinoma, carcinomatous meningitis, and pituitary apoplexy.

Symptoms

Patients with multiple CN palsies usually present with pain, diplopia, droopy eyelid, and variable decreased vision.

Signs

The visual acuity is normal but may be decreased in orbital apex syndrome. Common findings include: ptosis, strabismus, limitation of ocular motility, decreased facial sensation in the CN V_1–V_2 distribution, positive RAPD, miosis (due to Horner's syndrome), and facial pain. The pupil is usually spared with CN III involvement. There may be proptosis, conjunctival injection and chemosis, increased intraocular pressure, ocular bruit, and retinopathy in cases of high-flow arteriovenous fistulas. Fever, lid edema, and signs of facial infection occur in cases of cavernous sinus thrombosis.

- **Cavernous sinus** can involve CN III, IV, V, VI and sympathetics.
- **Orbital space** can involve CN II, III, IV, V_1, and VI, with proptosis (protruding globe), conjunctival chemosis (swelling) and injection (hyperemia), and the optic nerve may be normal, swollen, or atrophic.

CN III, IV, and VI palsies occur in approximately 15% of patients with herpes zoster ophthalmicus. These individuals also suffer from facial pain and skin eruptions in the trigeminal distribution, decreased corneal sensation, and occasional pupillary involvement (tonic pupil).

Differential diagnosis

The differential diagnosis consists of thyroid-related ophthalmopathy, myasthenia gravis, giant cell arteritis, idiopathic orbital inflammation, CPEO, and Guillain–Barré syndrome.

Evaluation

- The **history** should completely characterize all the neurologic symptoms. A history of previous illness or trauma is important.
- The **eye and neurologic exams** should include CNs (which require careful examination to determine which nerves are involved), ocular auscultation (may have bruit), lids (may have ptosis or edema), pupillary response (may have a positive RAPD or miosis), ocular motility (restricted), exophthalmometry (may have proptosis), conjunctiva (may have injection and chemosis), tonometry (may have increased intra-ocular pressure), and ophthalmoscopy (retinal and optic nerve appearance).
- **Lab tests**, including fasting blood glucose, CBC, ESR, VDRL, FTA-ABS, ANA, and blood cultures, are also ordered if an infectious etiology is suspected.
- **Neuroimaging**, with head, orbital, and sinus CT and/or MRI/MRA scan, must be obtained. **Cerebral angiography** may be necessary to rule out an aneurysm or arteriovenous fistula.
- Other tests to consider are **lumbar puncture** and a **Tensilon test**.
- **Neurology, neurosurgical, and/or medical consultations** are requested as needed.

Management

- The treatment depends on the underlying etiology.
- Systemic steroids, antibiotics, or antifungals may be necessary.
- Neurosurgery may be required for aneurysms, tumors, and trauma.

Prognosis

The prognosis is usually poor.

Muscle Disorders

Extraocular muscle dysfunction can produce poor ocular motility or external ophthalmoplegia, which may be progressive or episodic. Progressive ophthalmoplegia is often caused by either a hereditary myopathy such as **oculopharyngeal dystrophy** or **myotonic dystrophy**, both of which cause **CPEO**, or an inflammatory disorder like **thyroid-related ophthalmopathy, idiopathic**

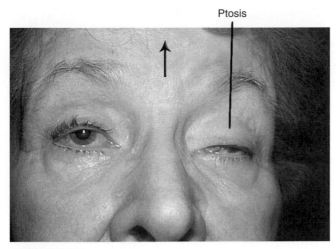

Ptosis

FIGURE 5-23
Chronic progressive external ophthalmoplegia, demonstrating ptosis and limited elevation in both eyes. The patient is attempting to look upward (note raised brows), yet the eyes remain in primary position (note the corneal light reflex centered over the pupil of the right eye) and the lids remain ptotic (markedly on the left side).

orbital inflammation, or **amyloidosis**. Episodic ophthalmoplegia is due to trauma, ischemia, vasculitis, and disorders of the neuromuscular junction such as **myasthenia gravis**, **Eaton–Lambert syndrome**, organophosphate poisoning, and botulism (Figure 5–23).

MYASTHENIA GRAVIS

Definition

Myasthenia gravis is an autoimmune disease of the neuromuscular junction that results in muscle weakness. The hallmark of this condition is variability and fatigability.

There are two types:

1. **Ocular** (20%): consists of ptosis and extraocular weakness only; does not affect pupils or ciliary muscle.
2. **Systemic** (80%): involves other skeletal muscles.

Etiology

Myasthenia gravis is caused by autoantibodies to the acetylcholine receptors in voluntary striated muscles.

Epidemiology

This disorder is more common in women than men, and usually presents between age 15 and 50 years old. Eye involvement (levator, orbicularis oculi, and extraocular muscles) occurs in 90% of patients and is the initial manifestation in 75%. There is an increased incidence of thymoma (15%) and other autoimmune disorders, including thyroid disease, rheumatoid arthritis, scleroderma, systemic lupus erythematosus, and MS.

Symptoms

Since the hallmark of myasthenia gravis is variability, symptoms can be absent or may include diplopia, droopy eyelids, dysarthria, dysphagia, and dyspnea, especially when the patient is tired.

Signs

Findings are very variable. The characteristic ocular signs are asymmetric ptosis (droopy eyelid(s) worse with fatigue, sustained upgaze, and at the end of the day), variable limitation of extraocular movements (ophthalmoplegia that can mimic any motility disturbance), strabismus, gaze-evoked nystagmus, and orbicularis oculi weakness (Figure 5–24).

Differential diagnosis

Myasthenia gravis can mimic any disorder that produces ptosis or impairment of extraocular motility: gaze palsy, MS, CN III, IV, or VI palsies, INO, thyroid-related ophthalmopathy, CPEO, idiopathic orbital inflammation, levator dehiscence, toxins (snake, arthropod, bacteria (botulism)), and Eaton–Lambert syndrome (paraneoplastic syndrome associated with small cell lung cancer due to impaired presynaptic release of acetylcholine).

Evaluation

- A key point to note in the **history** is any variability in symptoms.
- During the **eye and neurologic exams**, attention should be directed to the CNs (rule out a palsy), ocular motility (may be restricted), and lids (position and function). Specifically, the examiner should look for muscle fatigability and fluctuation in findings. Two simple tests are the rest and ice tests. The **rest test** involves having the patient relax with the eyes closed for 30 minutes to determine if there is an improvement in the ptosis (positive test). The **ice test** takes advantage of better neuromuscular transmission in the cold, therefore an ice pack is applied to the patient's eyes for 2 minutes and the test is declared positive if improvement occurs.
- A **Tensilon (edrophonium) test** can be administered in the office to help diagnose myasthenia gravis. This drug is an acetylcholinesterase inhibitor that prolongs the action of acetylcholine, resulting in stronger muscle contraction. The test involves administering a small quantity of Tensilon (2 mg IV with 1 ml saline flush), and then watching for an improvement in the diplopia and lid signs over the next minute. If there is no improvement, the test may be repeated several times (with 4 mg of Tensilon). The test is positive in 80–90% of patients, but there is a high false-negative rate. After

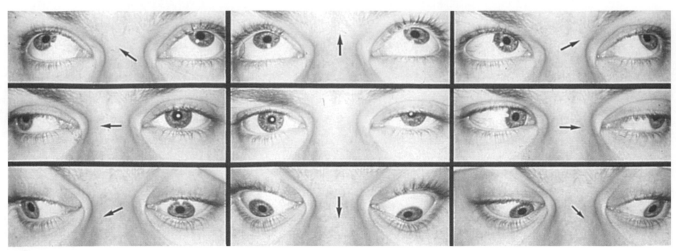

FIGURE 5–24

Myasthenia gravis with left ptosis and adduction deficit. The left ptosis is most evident in primary gaze and gaze to the left; the left adduction deficit is apparent in all right gaze positions.

three failures to respond, the test result is considered negative; however, a negative test does not rule out myasthenia gravis. It is important to perform this test with cardiac monitoring and treatment available because of the cardiovascular effects of Tensilon. If bradycardia, angina, or bronchospasm develops, then the antidote atropine (0.4 mg IV) is given immediately. Some physicians recommend pretreating patients with atropine.

- **Lab tests** may be helpful in confirming the diagnosis (acetylcholine receptor antibodies; 50% sensitive in ocular myasthenia gravis, 80% sensitive in systemic myasthenia gravis, 90% positive in myasthenia gravis with thymoma, 99% specific) or ruling out associated conditions (thyroid function tests (triiodothyronine, thyroxine, thyroid-stimulating hormone), rheumatoid factor, and ANA).
- In the event of equivocal test results, the definitive diagnosis is made by obtaining single-fiber **electromyography** of peripheral or orbicularis muscles.
- A **chest CT scan** is performed to rule out thymoma.
- **Neurology and medical consultations**.

Management

- Treatment may not be required if the symptoms are mild.
- Diplopia can be alleviated with prism spectacles, and surgery is considered for strabismus that is stable for >6–12 months.
- An oral anticholinesterase agent (pyridostigmine 60–120 mg PO qid) is prescribed for moderate symptoms.
- Other therapies that can be considered are steroids, plasmapheresis, gammaglobulin, cyclosporine, and azathioprine.
- Surgery is recommended for thymoma.

Prognosis

Myasthenia gravis is a chronic, progressive disease, but 15% of patients have spontaneous resolution. Patients with only the ocular form have a better prognosis.

Optic Nerve Problems

DISC SWELLING

Optic nerve fibers anterior to the lamina cribrosa can swell when there is obstruction of axoplasmic flow, producing disc swelling. This occurs at the level of the choroid or sclera and may result from ischemia, inflammation, increased ICP, or compression. A swollen disc has a characteristic appearance – an elevated hyperemic nerve head with blurred disc margins and loss of the physiologic cup. The optic nerve head is called the papilla, so strictly speaking there is edema of the papilla. However, the term papilledema should *not* be used since this word refers to the specific diagnosis of disc edema due to increased ICP (see below). There is also edema of the peripapillary nerve fiber layer obscuring the retinal vessels and producing chorioretinal folds. Vascular congestion causes dilated tortuous retinal veins, peripapillary flame-shaped hemorrhages, exudates, and cottonwool spots (which represent small nerve fiber layer infarcts). Chronic swelling may lead to gliosis, a pale disc, attenuated vessels, and loss of vision.

PAPILLEDEMA

Definition

Papilledema is optic disc swelling caused by increased ICP.

Etiology

Increased ICP may be caused by an intracranial mass, neoplasm, infection (meningitis, encephalitis), infiltration, hemorrhage (subdural or subarachnoid), or idiopathic intracranial hypertension (pseudotumor cerebri).

Symptoms

Papilledema may be asymptomatic, or patients may have headache, nausea, emesis, transient visual obscurations (blurred vision lasting seconds), diplopia, altered mental status, or other neurologic deficits.

Signs

Visual acuity, color vision, and pupillary responses are preserved, but visual field testing reveals enlarged blind spots. There is bilateral optic disc edema, as described above (Figure 5–25). Spontaneous venous pulsations may be absent, but this is also found in 20% of normal individuals. Unilateral or bilateral CN VI palsies occur and are usually responsible for the diplopia in these patients. In chronic papilledema, optic atrophy, visual field defects, decreased visual acuity, reduced color vision, and retinal vascular attenuation occur.

Differential diagnosis

Other causes of optic disc edema are papillitis, malignant hypertension, central retinal vein occlusion, optic neuropathy, uveitis, ocular hypotony, and optic disc drusen (**pseudopapilledema**) (Figure 5–26).

Evaluation

- The **history** should include associated neurologic symptoms.

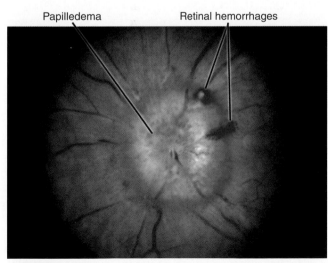

Papilledema   Retinal hemorrhages

FIGURE 5–25
Papilledema due to an intracranial tumor. There is marked edema of the nerve head with blurring of the disc margins 360° and two flame-shaped hemorrhages.

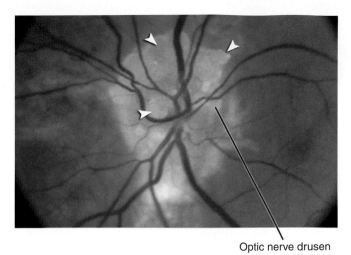

Optic nerve drusen

FIGURE 5–26
Optic nerve drusen (arrowheads). Multiple drusen are evident as elevated, chunky, refractile nodules.

- **Eye and neurologic exams** are performed with attention to color vision (normal), pupillary response (normal), ocular motility (normal), visual field testing (enlarged blind spot), and ophthalmoscopy (optic nerve appearance).
- Check the **blood pressure** to rule out malignant hypertension.
- **Emergent neuroimaging** should be carried out, with head and orbital CT or MRI scan, to rule out an intracranial process.
- **Lumbar puncture** should be performed to check the opening pressure and composition of the cerebrospinal fluid.
- Helpful **lab tests** are fasting blood sugar (to rule out diabetes), CBC, and ESR.
- **Neurology or neuro-ophthalmology consultation** is recommended.

Management

- Treat the underlying pathology.

Prognosis

The prognosis depends on the etiology.

IDIOPATHIC INTRACRANIAL HYPERTENSION (PSEUDOTUMOR CEREBRI)

Definition

Pseudotumor cerebri refers to papilledema with normal neuroimaging and cerebrospinal fluid. To be diagnosed with this disorder, the patient must meet four criteria:

1. Signs and symptoms of increased ICP (i.e., headache, vomiting, papilledema).

2. High cerebrospinal fluid pressure (>250 mm H_2O) with normal composition.
3. Normal neuroimaging studies.
4. Normal neurologic examination, with the exception that CN VI palsies may be present.

Etiology

By definition, idiopathic intracranial hypertension is a disorder of unknown etiology, but it has been linked to numerous factors. It may be related to vitamin A, tetracycline, oral contraceptive pills, nalidixic acid, lithium, or steroid use/withdrawal. It is also associated with dural sinus thrombosis, radical neck surgery, middle-ear disease, recent weight gain, chronic obstructive pulmonary disease, and pregnancy. Idiopathic intracranial hypertension is a diagnosis of exclusion.

Epidemiology

This disease typically occurs in obese 20–30-year-old women.

Symptoms

Often there are no symptoms; however, patients may present with headache, transient visual obscurations (blurred vision lasting seconds), photopsias, diplopia, tinnitus, dizziness, nausea, and emesis.

Signs

Visual acuity, color vision, and contrast sensitivity may either be normal or decreased, but bilateral optic disc edema (sometimes asymmetric) is always present (Figure 5–27). Thirty percent of patients have a CN VI palsy. Visual field defects can also occur (enlarged blind spot, constriction, or arcuate scotoma). Infants may be irritable but may not have disc swelling if their fontanelles are still open.

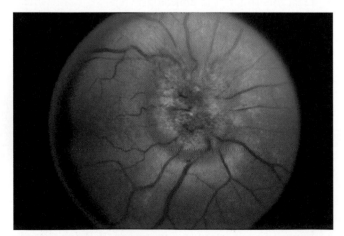

FIGURE 5–27
Idiopathic intracranial hypertension demonstrating papilledema.

Differential diagnosis

Because idiopathic intracranial hypertension is a diagnosis of exclusion, other causes of papilledema and optic disc swelling (see above) must be investigated.

Evaluation

Since idiopathic intracranial hypertension is a specific form of papilledema, the work-up is the same (see above).

Management

- If the patient is obese, a weight loss program is initiated.
- Any medication associated with idiopathic intracranial hypertension should be discontinued.
- Medical therapy is administered for progressive visual loss, visual field defects, or intractable headaches. Systemic acetazolamide (Diamox; 500–2000 mg PO qd) or diuretics (furosemide (Lasix) 60–120 mg PO divided q6h) can be initiated, and the patient's visual field, visual acuity, and color vision are monitored. Systemic steroids (prednisone 60–100 mg PO qd) are controversial.
- Surgical interventions, such as optic nerve sheath fenestration and lumboperitoneal shunt, are considered for progressive visual loss despite maximal medical therapy.

Prognosis

Idiopathic intracranial hypertension is usually self-limited, resolving over 6–12 months. However, the prognosis is variable if visual loss has occurred.

OPTIC NEURITIS

Definition

Optic neuritis is inflammation of the optic nerve. There are two types, depending on the location of the inflammation, that can be differentiated by the appearance of the optic nerve:

1. **Papillitis**: the inflammation is present in the anterior portion of the optic nerve, leading to swelling of the optic disc.
2. **Retrobulbar** (more common): the inflammation is located posteriorly (behind the globe), thus there is no optic disc swelling.

Etiology

Etiology depends on age:

- **Adults**: usually idiopathic and unilateral, but can also be associated with systemic diseases, typically demyelinating diseases (MS or, rarely, Devic's syndrome (bilateral optic neuritis with transverse myelitis)). The majority of MS patients develop optic neuritis some time during their disease, and it is the presenting diagnosis in 20% of MS cases.

- **Children**: usually bilateral, postviral, and not associated with MS.

Epidemiology

Optic neuritis is the most common optic neuropathy in people <45 years old, and it usually occurs in 15–45-year-old females.

Symptoms

Optic neuritis presents with variable visual loss that may progress for up to 7 days, then stabilizes and improves. The most characteristic feature is pain on eye movement. Patients may also notice dimmer vision, altered color perception (dyschromatopsia), and flashes of light (phosphenes) induced by eye movement or loud sounds. Although optic neuritis usually does not have any prodrome, it can occasionally be preceded by a viral (flu-like) syndrome.

Signs

Signs of optic neuritis include decreased visual acuity (ranging from minimal (e.g., 20/20–20/25) to catastrophic (no light perception (NLP), where the patient cannot even appreciate light)), color vision and contrast sensitivity, positive RAPD, visual field defects (classically, central or paracentral scotoma, but usually diffuse), and altered depth perception (known as the **Pulfrich phenomenon**: the motion of a pendulum appears elliptical due to altered depth perception from delayed conduction in the demyelinated nerve).

On clinical examination, the optic nerve usually appears normal (retrobulbar or posterior optic neuritis), and therefore optic neuritis is often described by the phrase "the patient sees nothing and the doctor sees nothing." However, in cases of anterior inflammation (papillitis), optic disc swelling is present. There may also be mild vitritis (cells in the vitreous cavity).

Differential diagnosis

Any disease that can lead to optic nerve swelling with vitritis can mimic optic neuritis, including intraocular inflammation, malignant hypertension, diabetes, cat-scratch disease, optic perineuritis, sarcoidosis, syphilis, tuberculosis, collagen vascular disease, Leber's optic neuropathy, optic nerve gliomas, orbital tumors, and AION.

Evaluation

- When taking the **history** it is important to characterize the visual loss (one versus both eyes, acute versus chronic, painful versus painless) and to ask about the presence of phosphenes and pain on eye movement. In patients without the diagnosis of MS,

eliciting other neurologic symptoms, especially if separated by space and time, should be performed. Finally, ask about any preceding viral syndromes.

- The **eye exam** should concentrate on evaluating visual acuity (decreased), color vision (decreased), pupillary response (positive RAPD), ocular motility (pain on eye movement), visual field testing (defects), and ophthalmoscopy (may have swollen optic nerve).
- The primary test that should be performed in all cases is a **head and orbital MRI scan** to evaluate for periventricular white-matter demyelinating lesions or plaques if the patient does not carry the diagnosis of MS (this is the best predictor of future development of MS). It can also rule out orbital tumors. If the MRI is positive for demyelinating lesions, then further testing to rule out other diseases is not necessary.
- **Lab tests** only need to be performed when atypical features exist and to rule out other entities in the differential diagnosis: ANA, angiotensin-converting enzyme, VDRL, FTA-ABS, ESR. Consider *Bartonella hensalae* if the optic nerve is swollen and there is an exposure to kittens.
- Consider **lumbar puncture** to rule out other intracranial processes if the previous tests are negative.
- Check **blood pressure** to rule out malignant hypertension, especially if a macular star is present on exam.

Management

- If the MRI is positive for demyelinating lesions, the primary treatment for optic neuritis is systemic intravenous steroids (methylprednisolone 250 mg IV q6h for 3 days, followed by prednisone 1 mg/kg per day for 11 days and rapid taper (20 mg/day on day 12 and 10 mg/day on days 13–15)).
- The **Optic Neuritis Treatment Trial (ONTT)** showed that this regimen led to visual recovery 2 weeks faster than other treatments, no difference in final visual acuity, and a decreased incidence of MS over the ensuing 2 years but no difference after 3 years. The trial also found that patients should not be treated with oral steroids alone, since this led to an increased risk of recurrent optic neuritis.
- The **Controlled High-risk Avonex Multiple Sclerosis Prevention Study (CHAMPS)** showed that patients receiving weekly intramuscular interferon beta-1a (Avonex) following systemic steroid therapy for their first episode of optic neuritis had a reduced incidence in the onset of clinical MS over 3 years and an improvement and/or less worsening of MRI demyelinating lesions.

Prognosis

The vision loss of optic neuritis improves over the following months after the initial inflammation, with the final acuity depending on the severity of the initial visual loss. The majority of patients (70%) recover 20/20 vision; however, permanent subtle color vision and contrast sensitivity deficits are common. After recovery, patients may experience blurred vision with increased body temperature or exercise (known as **Uhthoff's symptom**). Approximately 30% of patients have a future episode of optic neuritis in the same or fellow eye, and 30–50% of patients with isolated optic neuritis develop MS 5–10 years later.

OPTIC NEUROPATHIES

There are many types of optic neuropathies depending on the mechanism of nerve damage: ischemic, traumatic, compressive, infiltrative, toxic, or hereditary. The most common forms, due to ischemia, trauma, and compression, are discussed below. Various inflammatory diseases, infections, and malignancies can infiltrate the optic nerve (i.e., sarcoidosis, toxoplasmosis, toxocariasis, cryptococcus, coccidiomycosis, cytomegalovirus, tuberculosis, lymphoma, leukemia, plasmacytoma, and metastases). Leukemic optic nerve infiltration is a childhood *ophthalmic emergency* that requires radiation therapy to save vision. Toxicity may be caused by radiation, tobacco/alcohol amblyopia, ethambutol, isoniazid, chloramphenicol, streptomycin, arsenic, lead, methanol, digitalis, chloroquine, quinine, and various vitamin deficiencies. Regardless of the underlying etiology, the insult to the nerve results in some degree of optic atrophy and permanent visual dysfunction.

ANTERIOR ISCHEMIC OPTIC NEUROPATHY

Definition

AION is an ischemic infarction of the optic nerve head due to occlusion of the posterior ciliary arteries.

Etiology

There are two forms of AION:

1. **Arteritic**: due to giant cell arteritis (temporal arteritis), and associated with polymyalgia rheumatica.
2. **Non-arteritic (NAION)**: idiopathic, and associated with hypertension (40%), diabetes (20%), and, rarely, phosphodiesterase-5 inhibitors (i.e., Viagra, Levitra, and Cialis).

Epidemiology

The arteritic variety is more common in women and usually occurs in patients >55 years old (mostly over 70). NAION typically affects younger patients (50–75 years old).

Symptoms

Patients experience sudden, unilateral, painless visual loss and poor color perception. Other symptoms associated with giant cell arteritis and polymyalgia rheumatica may occur in the arteritic form. These include headache, fever, malaise, weight loss, scalp tenderness, jaw claudication, amaurosis fugax, diplopia, joint pain, and eye pain.

Signs

In addition to decreased visual acuity (worse for arteritic than non-arteritic) and color vision, on examination the patient also has a large visual field defect usually inferiorly, an RAPD, and a swollen optic disc (Figure 5–28). Optic nerve pallor due to atrophy develops later. The fellow nerve often appears crowded with a small or absent cup ("disc at risk"), or it may be pale from a prior episode of AION. Retinal findings such as cottonwool spots and vascular occlusions may be present. Giant cell arteritis can also cause anterior-segment ischemia, CN palsies (particularly CN VI), and a tender, swollen, ipsilateral temporal artery.

Differential diagnosis

Other disorders that need to be considered are malignant hypertension, diabetic papillitis, retinal vascular occlusion, compressive lesion, collagen vascular disease, syphilis, and herpes zoster.

Evaluation

- The **history** must document the presence or absence of giant cell arteritis and polymyalgia rheumatica symptoms. Patients also need to be questioned regarding the recent use of phosphodiesterase-5 inhibitors.

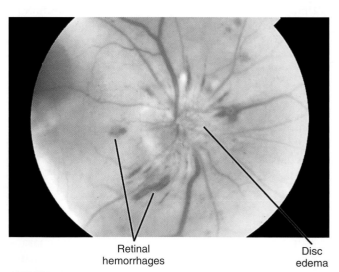

Retinal hemorrhages   Disc edema

FIGURE 5–28
Anterior ischemic optic neuropathy with disc edema and flame hemorrhages.

- The **eye exam** should concentrate on visual acuity (decreased), color vision (decreased), pupillary response (positive RAPD), visual field testing (defects), and ophthalmoscopy (swollen optic nerve).
- **Lab tests** are essential to differentiate between the two types of AION. A stat **ESR** is obtained to rule out the arteritic form. An ESR > (age/2) in men and > ((age+10)/2) in women is considered abnormal, but the ESR may be normal in 10%. Other test results indicative of arteritic AION are CBC (low hematocrit, high platelets) and C-reactive protein (>2.45 mg/dl). In addition, a VDRL, FTA-ABS, and ANA should be ordered.
- A **blood pressure** and **fasting blood glucose** level should also be obtained to rule out the non-arteritic form.
- **Temporal artery biopsy** is sometimes considered for definitive diagnosis, but a false-negative result due to skip lesions is possible.
- **Medical consultation**.

Management

NAION is not treatable; however, arteritic AION is a true *ophthalmic emergency* that requires prompt treatment to prevent involvement of the other eye.

- **Arteritic**: systemic steroids (methylprednisolone 1 g IV qd in divided doses for 3 days, then prednisone 60–100 mg PO qd with a slow-taper; decrease by no more than 2.5–5.0 mg/week) are started immediately to prevent ischemic optic neuropathy in the fellow eye. Treatment should not be delayed while awaiting temporal artery biopsy results, because these remain positive for up to 2 weeks after starting corticosteroids. Response to therapy is monitored by carefully following the patient's ESR, C-reactive protein, and symptoms.
- **Non-arteritic**: unfortunately there is no treatment, but consider starting aspirin daily.

Prognosis

Vision loss in AION is permanent. For the arteritic form, there is a 75% risk that the fellow eye will become involved within 2 weeks if treatment is not instituted. In NAION, the risk of fellow eye involvement is 25–40%.

TRAUMATIC OPTIC NEUROPATHY

Definition

Traumatic optic neuropathy involves damage to the optic nerve caused by trauma anywhere along its course from the chiasm to the globe.

Mechanism

Injury to the optic nerve can be a result of direct or indirect trauma.

- **Direct**: due to penetrating, surgical, or bone fragment injury with laceration or avulsion of the nerve.
- **Indirect**: due to compression or swelling of the nerve from a hematoma or an injury to the frontal bone or maxilla.

Epidemiology

Traumatic optic neuropathy occurs in approximately 3% of patients with severe head trauma or mid-face fractures.

Symptoms

Patients report decreased vision, altered color perception, and pain from associated injuries.

Signs

Optic nerve damage results in variable reduced visual acuity (20/20 to NLP), decreased color vision, a visual field defect, and an RAPD. Initially, the optic nerve may appear normal or show disc edema and hemorrhage (Figure 5–29). Optic atrophy with disc pallor develops later. Other signs of trauma are usually present. Hemorrhage may cause the orbit to be tense and the globe proptotic (protruding) with resistance to manual retropulsion.

Differential diagnosis

The following ocular conditions may present in a similar fashion following trauma, and need to be ruled out: open globe, retrobulbar hemorrhage, retinal detachment, macular hole, and vitreous hemorrhage.

Evaluation

- The patient must be thoroughly examined for associated **life-threatening injuries**.
- The **history** should document the exact mechanism of trauma and any other neurologic symptoms.

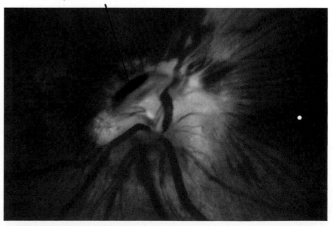

optic nerve avulsion

FIGURE 5–29
Traumatic optic nerve avulsion.

- Complete **eye and neurologic exams** are performed with attention to color vision (decreased), pupillary response (positive RAPD), ocular motility (for limitation from concomitant injury to other CNs), visual field testing (defects), tonometry (for increased intraocular pressure), anterior segment (for signs of trauma), and ophthalmoscopy (optic nerve appearance and for signs of trauma).
- **Orbital CT scan** is performed to assess the location, mechanism, and extent of injury, as well as any associated trauma.
- **Medical or neurology consultation** may be required for associated injuries.

Management

- Life-threatening injuries are treated emergently.
- A lateral canthotomy is done to drain a subperiosteal hematoma in a tense orbit.
- High-dose systemic steroid treatment (methylprednisolone 30 mg/kg IV initial dose, then starting 2 hours later 15 mg/kg every 6 hours for 1–3 days) is controversial.
- Surgical decompression is reserved for cases with an optic canal fracture or those that fail to respond to steroids.

Prognosis

The prognosis depends on the extent of optic nerve damage but is typically poor. Spontaneous improvement may occur in 20–35% of patients.

OPTIC NERVE TUMORS

Optic nerve tumors that cause a compressive optic neuropathy are optic nerve gliomas and meningiomas.

There are two types of **optic nerve glioma**:

1. **Low-grade astrocytoma (juvenile pilocytic astrocytoma)** is a rare, benign childhood tumor associated with neurofibromatosis type 1 that causes gradual, unilateral, progressive, painless proptosis, decreased vision, an RAPD, and optic disc edema. Later, optic atrophy or strabismus may develop. Half are intraorbital and half are intracranial, spreading to the chiasm and contralateral optic nerve.
2. **Malignant optic nerve glioma (glioblastoma multiforme)** is a rare, malignant tumor that produces rapid, painful visual loss in adults. Central retinal vascular occlusions may develop as the tumor interferes with the retinal blood supply. Endocrine or neurologic deficits may appear as the tumor invades other structures.

Optic nerve meningioma is a rare, histologically benign tumor that arises from the arachnoid tissue of the nerve sheath (meningothelial cells). This tumor most commonly occurs in middle-aged women (3:1) and presents with unilateral proptosis, painless, decreased visual acuity and color vision, an RAPD, and optic nerve edema. Later, optic nerve pallor and optociliary shunt vessels appear. Meningiomas may grow rapidly during pregnancy and involute after delivery.

Symptoms

Patients are initially asymptomatic, and then develop slowly progressive, sometimes painful, vision loss.

Signs

On examination, the visual acuity and color vision may be normal or decreased. There is an RAPD, proptosis, motility disturbances, increased intraocular pressure, optic disc swelling, and a visual field defect (Figure 5–30). Optic atrophy and optociliary shunt vessels (abnormal curly vessels at the disc margin, which are also commonly seen after a central retinal vein occlusion (see Figure 17–22 in Ch. 17)) are late findings.

Differential diagnosis

Other causes of compressive optic neuropathy, like thyroid-related ophthalmopathy and pituitary tumors or apoplexy, must be considered.

Evaluation

- Important elements of the **history** are the timing of the visual loss, the presence of pain, and other associated symptoms (neurologic or endocrine).
- The **eye exam** must include measurement of visual acuity (decreased), color vision (decreased), pupillary

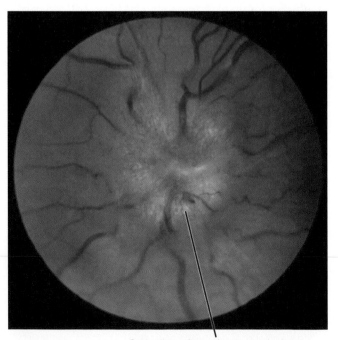

Optic disc edema due to meningioma

FIGURE 5–30
Meningioma producing optic disc edema.

response (positive RAPD), visual field testing (defects), ocular motility (restricted), exophthalmometry (proptosis), and ophthalmoscopy (optic nerve appearance).

- **Neuroimaging** may be carried out, with head and orbital CT or MRI scan, looking for optic nerve enlargement, the "railroad track" sign (meningioma; Figure 5–31), or bony erosion of the optic canal (glioblastoma).
- Consider **medical or oncology consultation**.

Management

- Surgery (resection) is controversial. Younger patients with these tumors are treated more aggressively. Meningiomas in adults are typically slow-growing and are observed, as surgical intervention may cause more morbidity.
- Treatment of increased intraocular pressure may be required (see Ch. 13).

Prognosis

Juvenile pilocytic astrocytomas, although histologically benign, cause death in 14% of patients. Glioblastoma causes fellow-eye involvement within weeks, blindness in months, and death within a year. The outcome is variable for meningiomas.

OPTIC ATROPHY

Optic atrophy represents neuronal degeneration. The nerve head becomes pale 6–8 weeks after an injury to any part of the pathway from the retinal ganglion cells to the LGB (Figure 5–32). Optic neuropathy, optic neuritis,

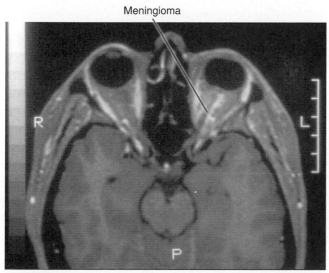

Meningioma

FIGURE 5–31
Computed tomography scan of same patient as in Figure 5–30, demonstrating tubular enlargement of the optic nerve with "railroad track" sign.

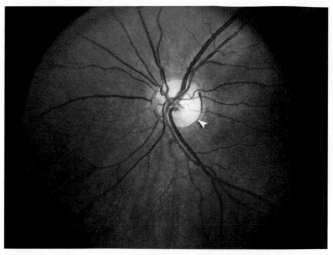

FIGURE 5–32
Optic atrophy demonstrating pale nerve. The optic nerve pallor is most striking in the inferotemporal region of the disc (arrowhead).

glaucoma, central retinal artery occlusion, tumors, and aneurysms can all produce irreversible damage to the nerve and subsequent atrophy. Patients who present with disc pallor and have not been previously diagnosed or worked up for an optic nerve lesion should undergo neuroimaging to rule out a tumor.

Chiasm and Brain Lesions

CHIASMAL SYNDROMES

Definition

Chiasmal syndromes are a variety of disorders that produce compression of the optic chiasm with resulting visual field defects.

Etiology

A mass lesion is the culprit in 95% of cases. These are typically large, since the chiasm is 10 mm above the sella turcica (i.e., pituitary microadenomas do not cause field defects). The following disorders are responsible for chiasmal syndromes: pituitary tumor, pituitary apoplexy, meningioma, aneurysm, trauma, sarcoidosis, craniopharyngioma, MS, glioma, infection, and metastasis.

Symptoms

Patients may have ophthalmic, neurologic, and/or endocrinologic symptoms such as headache, decreased vision, dyschromatopsia, visual field defects, diplopia, vague visual complaints, decreased libido, malaise, and galactorrhea.

Signs

Exam findings may be variable. There can be normal or decreased visual acuity and color vision, an RAPD, optic atrophy, a visual field defect, or signs of pituitary apoplexy (severe headache, ophthalmoplegia, and decreased visual acuity). The visual field defect may have one of several appearances: junctional scotoma, bitemporal hemianopia, or incongruous homonymous hemianopia. The reason for this is the variability in chiasm anatomy. Depending on the location of the chiasm relative to the pituitary gland, a tumor may compress different structures (optic nerves, chiasm, or optic tracts).

Evaluation

- The **history** should ask specifically about neurologic and endocrine symptoms.
- The **eye exam** must include visual acuity (may be decreased), color vision (may be decreased), pupillary response (may have a positive RAPD), visual field testing (defects that respect the vertical midline), and ophthalmoscopy (optic nerve appearance).
- **Emergent neuroimaging**, with head and orbital CT or MRI scan, should be carried out if pituitary apoplexy is suspected.
- Consider **lab tests** to check hormone levels.
- **Medical** and possibly **neurosurgery consultations**.

Management

- Treatment depends on the underlying etiology.
- Pituitary lesions requiring surgery, radiation, bromocriptine, or hormone replacement therapy should be managed by a neurosurgeon and/or internist.
- Pituitary apoplexy is treated with systemic steroids and surgical decompression.

Prognosis

Entities causing chiasmal syndromes have a generally poor prognosis.

RETROCHIASMAL DISORDERS

Retrochiasmal disorders, usually vascular lesions or tumors, cause homonymous visual field defects, which are incongruous anteriorly and become more congruous posteriorly in the visual pathway. **Cortical lesions** can produce bilateral blindness as well as disorders of visual integration. Those affecting the angular gyrus and the corpus collosum interfere with the ability to process visual information and can result in the inability to read (alexia), write (agraphia), name objects (anomia), recognize faces (prosopagnosia), and recognize objects by sight (visual agnosia). Patients may also ignore part of their visual space (visual neglect or extinction).

Headaches

Figure 5–33 shows the location of pain in common headache syndromes.

MIGRAINE

Definition

The term migraine is derived from the Greek word *hemikranos* or "half skull." Migraine is a neurologic disorder caused by changes in intracranial vasomotor control. There is often a headache, but this is not a necessary feature.

Etiology

Migraine is due to cerebral vasospasm, which produces a slow-moving concentric wave of suppressed electrical activity.

Types

There are many types of migraine:

Classic migraine (10–20%): aura or prodrome lasting approximately 10–30 minutes followed by unilateral throbbing head pain, nausea, and/or emesis. The aura usually consists of visual or other fleeting neurologic signs, including visual scintillations, dazzling zig-zag lines (fortification phenomenon), spreading scotomas, photophobia, distortion of hearing and smell, dizziness, and tinnitus. Patients may have premonitory symptoms, including hunger, thirst, mood changes, and/or a feeling of impending doom. A strong family history of migraine is common.

Common migraine (70–80%): headache with little or no prodrome and gastrointestinal disturbances (anorexia, nausea, and emesis).

Complicated migraine: headache with temporary neurologic deficits. Several types:

- **Basilar artery migraine**: mimics vertebrobasilar artery insufficiency.
- **Retinal migraine**: temporary scotoma or monocular visual loss. The headache may precede or occur within an hour.
- **Ophthalmoplegic migraine**: headache and recurrent paresis of one or more ocular motor nerves (usually CN III). Occurs in children, may last longer than 1 week.
- **Cerebral migraine**: motor or sensory defects.
- **Migraine infarction**: focal signs persist for more than 1 week. A corresponding lesion is visible on neuroimaging.
- **Status migrainosus**: an attack lasting longer than 72 hours (with or without treatment). The headache may be continuous or intermittent with interruptions of less than 4 hours.

Acephalgic migraine (migraine-equivalent): visual aura without headache. The variable visual symptoms are described as fortification phenomenon, scintillating scotoma, tunnel vision, double vision, amaurosis fugax, and altitudinal field loss.

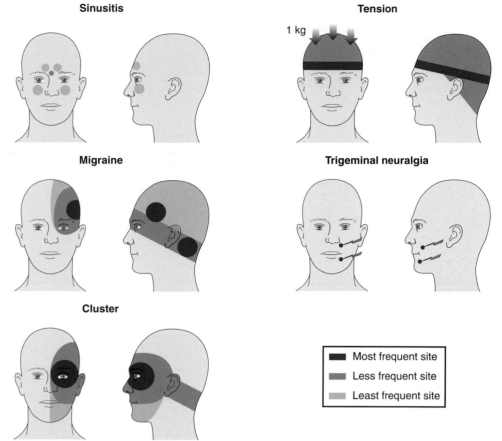

■	Most frequent site
■	Less frequent site
■	Least frequent site

FIGURE 5–33
Location of pain for the common headache syndromes.

Childhood migraine: brief attacks of nausea and vomiting, usually without headache.

Precipitating factors

Migraines may be triggered by numerous factors:

- **Diet**: tyramine (bananas, avocado, yogurt, aged cheese), phenylethylamine (chocolate, cheese, wine), sodium nitrite (preservatives, food coloring, processed meats and fish), monosodium glutamate (Chinese food, processed meats, frozen dinners, canned soup), caffeine, alcohol, artificial sweeteners.
- **Lifestyle**: excessive sleep, fasting or dieting, exertion, fatigue, stressful events, depression.
- **Hormonal**: supplemental estrogen, menses, oral contraceptives, ovulation, pregnancy.
- **Environmental**: sun exposure, loud noise, bright lights, glare, flickering lights, strong odors.

Epidemiology

Migraine affects 15% of men and 25% of women, and can begin at any age. The acephalgic variant is most common after age 40 years old. A family history of migraine is found in 60% of patients. A history of motion sickness or cyclic vomiting as a child is common.

Symptoms

Patients may suffer from an aura, photophobia, headache, nausea, and emesis.

Signs

The examination is usually unremarkable with no evident findings. Patients with complicated migraines may have a visual field defect, CN palsy, or other neurologic deficits. Venous constriction occurs acutely during a retinal migraine.

Differential diagnosis

Many diseases can present with headache and neurologic abnormalities. Serious pathology includes meningitis, subarachnoid hemorrhage, temporal arteritis, malignant hypertension, intracranial tumor, arteriovenous malformation, vertebrobasilar artery insufficiency, aneurysm, subdural hematoma, and cerebral ischemia (transient ischemic attack). Other disorders to consider are tension or cluster headaches, trigeminal neuralgia, temporomandibular joint syndrome, cervical spondylosis, sinus or dental pathology, herpes zoster ophthalmicus, uveitis, angle-closure glaucoma, post lumbar puncture, non-organic, caffeine withdrawal, carbon monoxide inhalation, and nitrite exposure.

Evaluation

- All aspects of the headache (e.g., precipitating factors, location, frequency) must be noted in the **history**, as well as any associated aura or other neurologic symptoms.
- Thorough **eye and neurologic exams** are required to rule out other causes of visual and neurologic symptoms. The exams, which should be normal, must concentrate on the CNs (for a palsy), ocular motility (for restriction), pupillary response (for a positive RAPD), visual field testing (for defects), tonometry (for increased intraocular pressure), and ophthalmoscopy (retinal and optic nerve appearance).
- Check **blood pressure** and **temperature**.
- Consider **lumbar puncture** for suspected meningitis.
- **Neuroimaging** for complicated or atypical migraines.
- **Medical or neurology consultation**.

Management

Treatment strategies are divided into abortive and prophylactic:

- **Abortive therapies**: dark, low-noise surroundings, rest, ice pack, cold shower, local scalp pressure, analgesics (non-steroidal anti-inflammatory drugs; oral narcotic medications may be necessary for severe headache), oral ergotamine (1–3 mg PO 1 tablet at onset of headache, 1 more 15–20 min later) or dihydro-ergotamine, serotonin agonist (sumatriptan (Imitrex)), and antiemetics.
- **Prophylactic measures**: avoidance of precipitating factors and systemic medications including beta-blockers (propranolol 20–40 mg PO bid to tid initially), tricyclic antidepressants (amitriptyline 25–75 mg PO qd to bid initially), calcium-channel blockers (nifedipine 10–40 mg PO tid or verapamil 80 mg PO tid), or serotonin reuptake inhibitors (fluoxetine).

Treatment should be monitored by an internist or neurologist.

Prognosis

The prognosis for migraine is good.

TENSION HEADACHES

Tension headaches are muscular, causing dull, persistent pain that feels like a tight band around the head.

CLUSTER HEADACHES

Cluster headaches consist of severe, unilateral, orbital, supraorbital and/or temporal pain lasting up to 3 hours and occurring in groups for weeks to months. Cluster headaches usually occur in men 30–40 years of age, more commonly in smokers, and can awaken the patient from sleep. Ipsilateral findings include conjunctival injection, lacrimation, nasal congestion, rhinorrhea, forehead/facial sweating, miosis, ptosis, and eyelid edema. A post-ganglionic Horner's syndrome may develop.

TEMPEROMANDIBULAR JOINT SYNDROME

Temperomandibular joint syndrome produces unilateral ear or preauricular pain radiating to the temple, jaw, or neck, and exacerbated by chewing. There is also limitation of jaw movement and an audible click when opening the mouth.

Visual Loss

FUNCTIONAL VISUAL LOSS

Definition

Functional visual loss refers to a visual abnormality not attributable to any organic disease process.

Etiology

There are two categories of non-physiologic vision loss:

1. **Malingering** is the fabrication of the existence or extent of a disorder for secondary gain. Typically the patient is involved in a legal action or compensation claim.
2. **Hysteria** is the subconscious expression of symptoms and is therefore not willful.

Symptoms

Patients often present with a chief complaint of decreased vision in one or both eyes, diplopia, metamorphopsia (distortion of vision), or oscillopsia (the perceived movement of one's surroundings). They are usually very vague about the quality of their symptoms.

Signs

The visual loss can be mild to severe (NLP). Visual field abnormalities tend to be inconsistent or have a characteristic pattern. Other possible findings include voluntary nystagmus, gaze palsy, or blepharospasm. A malingerer is often uncooperative and combative, while a hysteric is typically indifferent but cooperative.

Differential diagnosis

Functional visual loss is a diagnosis of exclusion so organic disease must be ruled out, especially amblyopia, early keratoconus, corneal dystrophy, early cataracts, central serous retinopathy, early Stargardt's disease, retinitis pigmentosa sine pigmento, rod monochromatism, cone degeneration, optic neuropathies (retrobulbar, toxic, nutritional), and cortical blindness.

Evaluation

- Vagueness and inconsistency in the **history** are suggestive.
- The **eye exam** findings may similarly be inconsistent. Attention is particularly directed toward measuring the vision and attempts are made at tricking the patient with visual tests (i.e., monocular and binocular, varying distance, fogging, prism dissociation, and stereopsis (a minimum amount of acuity is needed to distinguish different stereo images)). When the patient claims complete blindness, then the startle reflex, proprioception tests, signature, mirror tracking, and OKN response are useful for assessment. Patients may mistake proprioceptive tests and signing their name for visual tasks and be unable to perform them. Similarly, if the patient has vision, it is very difficult to suppress the startle reflex, mirror tracking, and OKN response. Visual field testing (monocular and binocular) often reveals unusual results such as tunnel vision, spiraling fields, and crossing isopters. The rest of the exam is otherwise normal (i.e., pupillary response, ocular motility, ophthalmoscopy).
- In difficult cases or if normal vision and visual fields cannot be documented, then consider **electroretinogram**, **visual evoked response**, **fluorescein angiogram**, or **neuroimaging** studies to rule out pathology.

Management

- Patients usually just require reassurance.
- Psychiatric consultation is rarely necessary.

Prognosis

There is no improvement in up to 30% of patients, and 20% may have a coexisting organic disease.

AMAUROSIS FUGAX

Definition

Amaurosis fugax is unilateral transient visual loss or temporary monocular blindness, a form of transient ischemic attack.

Etiology

Amaurosis can be caused by carotid disease, arrhythmias, cardiac valvular disease, coagulation disorders, vasospasm, migraine, orbital mass, papilledema, temporal arteritis, hypotension, and hyperviscosity syndromes.

Symptoms

Patients experience brief (2–5 minutes), reversible, monocular loss or dimming of vision.

Signs

There are no findings on exam. Rarely, emboli can be seen in retinal vessels.

Differential diagnosis

Other causes of transient visual loss include scintillating scotoma (acephalgic migraine), visual obscurations (papilledema), or vertebrobasilar artery insufficiency (bilateral amaurosis).

Evaluation

- It is essential to characterize the visual symptoms fully in the **history**. By definition, amaurosis fugax is unilateral and transient. The patient must also be asked specifically about other neurologic symptoms and cardiovascular history.
- Complete **eye and neurologic exams** should be carried out with attention to pupillary response (normal), visual field testing (normal), and ophthalmoscopy (may have emboli).
- **Medical consultation** should incorporate a complete cardiovascular evaluation including electrocardiogram, echocardiogram, and carotid Doppler studies.

Management

- Treat the underlying disease.
- Start aspirin daily (325 mg PO qd) if the etiology is embolic.

Prognosis

The prognosis depends on the etiology. The 1-year risk of a cerebrovascular accident is 2%.

VERTEBROBASILAR ARTERY INSUFFICIENCY

Definition

Vertebrobasilar artery insufficiency involves impaired vertebrobasilar circulation, producing neurologic deficits referable to the brainstem or occipital lobe.

Etiology

Vertebrobasilar artery insufficiency is due to thrombus, emboli, hypertension, arrhythmias, arterial dissection, hypercoaguable states, and subclavian steel syndrome.

Symptoms

Patients suffer from bilateral transient blurring or dimming of vision lasting seconds to minutes. Other symptoms include photopsias (flashes of light), diplopia, unilateral weakness, sensory loss, ataxia, nystagmus, dysarthria, dysphagia, hearing loss, and vertigo. Patients may report a history of drop attacks.

Signs

Neurologic findings are absent except for small, paracentral, congruous, homonymous visual field defects.

Differential diagnosis

Diseases that can mimic vertebrobasilar artery insufficiency are amaurosis fugax, migraine, papilledema, and temporal arteritis.

Evaluation

- When taking the ophthalmic **history**, it is essential to ask in detail about the visual loss (monocular versus binocular) and other neurologic symptoms.
- Complete **eye and neurologic exams** should be carried out with attention to ocular motility (for nystagmus), pupillary response (normal), visual field testing (for defects), and ophthalmoscopy (normal).
- **Lab tests** include CBC, ESR, and blood glucose (hypoglycemia).
- Check **blood pressure**.
- **Radiologic studies** include head and orbital CT or MRI scan, and cervical spine radiographs (cervical spondylosis).
- **Medical consultation** should incorporate a complete cardiovascular evaluation, including electrocardiogram, echocardiogram, and duplex and Doppler scans of the carotid and vertebral arteries.

Management

- There is no effective treatment, but a daily aspirin (325 mg PO qd) is usually prescribed.
- Long-term anticoagulation may be required.

Prognosis

Vertebrobasilar artery insufficiency has a poor outcome.

CHAPTER SIX

Pediatric Ophthalmology and Strabismus

Introduction

Certain eye diseases occur primarily during childhood, including congenital ocular defects, infections, inflammatory conditions, tumors, systemic diseases with ocular manifestations, and strabismus. Many of these conditions are vision-threatening and some are even life-threatening. Therefore, it is important to recognize and treat them promptly. Poor vision, strabismus, nystagmus, and a white pupil (leukocoria) are indications that a child has a serious eye problem that may permanently affect the vision, resulting in amblyopia or a "lazy eye."

Some of the disorders included in this chapter are also found in adults. To avoid overlap as much as possible, references to other sections of the book are provided for more detailed discussion of these topics.

Congenital Anomalies

Malformations of the eye and orbit are abnormalities that result from genetic defects or toxic insults (infection or drugs) to the fetus. The disruption of normal embryologic development may lead to a variety of problems.

COLOBOMA

Failure of the embryonic fissure to close completely produces a characteristic defect in ocular tissues called a coloboma. This absence of tissue, which may affect the optic nerve, retina, choroid, or iris, is typically located inferonasally. Eyelid colobomas can also occur (Figures 6–1–6–4).

Ocular structures or even the eye itself may be absent (aniridia, aphakia, anophthalmos) or improperly developed

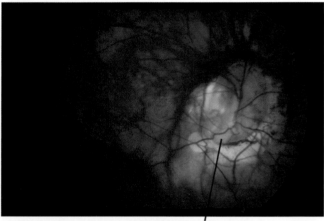

Optic nerve coloboma

FIGURE 6–1
Optic nerve coloboma demonstrating large abnormal disc that appears elongated inferiorly with irregular pattern of vessels.

(cryptophthalmos, microphthalmos, megalocornea, optic nerve hypoplasia, nasolacrimal duct obstruction (NLDO), cataracts, glaucoma, persistent hyperplastic primary vitreous).

ANIRIDIA

Aniridia refers to bilateral absence of the iris; however, sometimes a peripheral remnant or stump of tissue is present. This disorder is usually hereditary, but sporadic cases do occur and are associated with Wilms' tumor. Children with aniridia have poor vision and sensitivity to light. Common findings include nystagmus, amblyopia, strabismus, cataracts, glaucoma, foveal hypoplasia, and corneal pannus (Figures 6–5 and 6–6). Painted contact lenses may be worn for cosmesis and photophobia, and

87

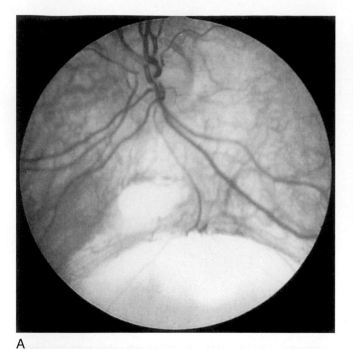

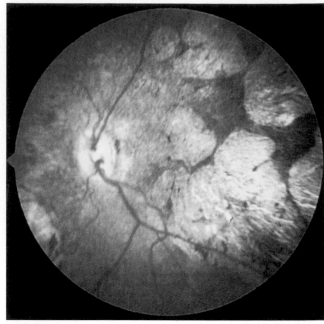

A   B

FIGURE 6–2
(**A**) Inferior choroidal coloboma and (**B**) macular coloboma due to arrested normal eye development.

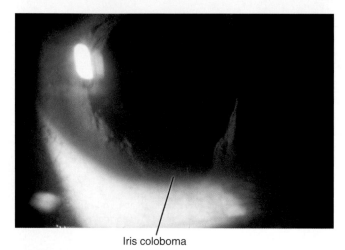

Iris coloboma

FIGURE 6–3
Coloboma of inferior iris.

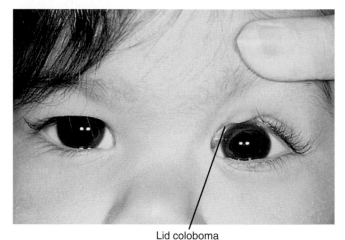

Lid coloboma

FIGURE 6–4
Superonasal coloboma of left upper eyelid in a child.

opaque implants can be inserted in conjunction with cataract surgery.

OPTIC NERVE HYPOPLASIA

Optic nerve hypoplasia results in small, underdeveloped optic nerves. The nerve head has a characteristic appearance: small with a thin ring of pigment surrounding the neural tissue (double ring sign) (Figure 6–7). Unilateral cases are usually idiopathic, while bilateral cases are associated with aniridia, midline anomalies, endocrine dysfunction, congenital intracranial tumors (optic glioma, craniopharyngioma), and maternal diabetes or drug use during pregnancy (i.e., alcohol, LSD, quinine, dilantin). Affected individuals have a variable degree of decreased vision, strabismus, nystagmus, and visual field defects. Because of the possibility of concomitant central nervous system and endocrine abnormalities, neuroimaging and lab tests must be performed.

CRANIOFACIAL CLEFT SYNDROMES

Developmental ocular defects may occur in isolation or as part of syndromes. Examples of the latter are craniofacial disorders, genetic mutations, and infections. The **craniosynostoses** and **craniofacial cleft syndromes**

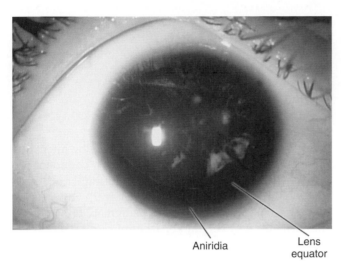

Aniridia   Lens equator

FIGURE 6–5
Aniridia with entire cataractous lens visible. The inferior edge of the lens is visible.

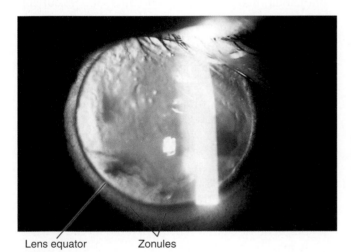

Lens equator   Zonules

FIGURE 6–6
Aniridia with the lens equator and zonules visible on retroillumination.

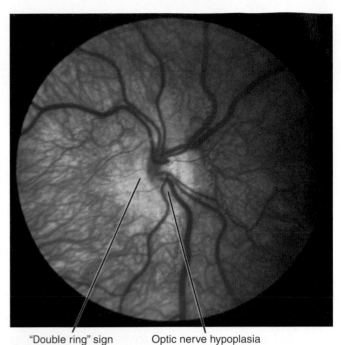

"Double ring" sign   Optic nerve hypoplasia

FIGURE 6–7
Optic nerve hypoplasia demonstrating "double ring" sign or peripapillary ring of pigmentary changes.

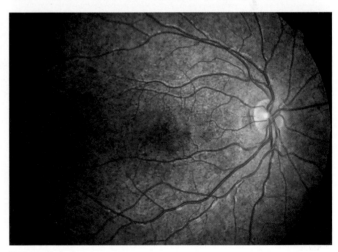

FIGURE 6–8
Rubella retinopathy demonstrating salt-and-pepper fundus appearance.

are commonly associated with shallow orbits, proptosis, and strabismus. Children with **Down syndrome** develop early cataracts. Congenital infection with **rubella** also produces cataracts as well as glaucoma, microphthalmos, and a retinopathy (Figure 6–8). **Syphilis (luetic chorioretinitis)**, the "great mimic," causes extensive uveitis with corneal involvement and retinopathy (see Figures 17–82 and 17–83). The pupil (Argyll Robertson) and nerve (optic atrophy) may also become damaged.

NASOLACRIMAL DUCT OBSTRUCTION

Definition

NLDO is a blockage of the nasolacrimal duct.

Etiology

This may be congenital or acquired (see Ch. 8). The former is usually due to a thin membrane covering the valve of Hasner.

Epidemiology

Up to 5% of infants have an obstructed nasolacrimal duct, and one-third are bilateral.

Symptoms

The infant is noted to have tearing and discharge from one or both eyes. The lashes are usually crusted nasally.

Signs

On examination, the baby's eyes are watery and discharge is often visible (Figure 6–9). Sometimes dacryocystitis or conjunctivitis is present, and the child may have a dacryocystocele (dilated lacrimal sac), or amniotic fluid or mucus trapped in the tear sac.

Differential diagnosis

Other causes of congenital tearing are glaucoma, trichiasis, conjunctivitis, nasolacrimal duct anomalies (punctal atresia), corneal abrasion, corneal trauma from forceps delivery, and an ocular surface foreign body.

Evaluation

- The **history** should note the timing and onset of symptoms as well as the lack of trauma.
- During the **eye exam**, attention is directed toward the lids (lash crusting, punctum, mass), conjunctiva (normal or injection), and cornea (normal).
- **Digital pressure** over the lacrimal sac producing mucoid reflux from the punctum indicates the nasolacrimal duct is obstructed.
- The **dye disappearance test** with fluorescein is particularly helpful in infants. A drop of fluorescein dye is instilled in each eye and the time for the dye to vanish is monitored. Prolonged or asymmetric dye clearance is found in NLDO.

Management

- Lacrimal sac massage bid–qid.
- A topical antibiotic is given acutely (Ilotycin ointment tid).
- Probing and irrigation of the lacrimal drainage system by 13 months of age (95% cure). If probing is unsuccessful, then consider silicone intubation, turbinate infracture, and ultimately dacryocystorhinostomy.

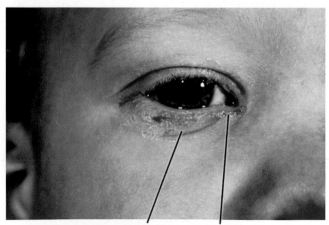

Erythema   Crusting

FIGURE 6–9
Nasolacrimal duct obstruction with tearing, crusting of eyelids, and lower-lid erythema.

Prognosis

Most congenital cases open spontaneously within 4–6 weeks of birth.

Conjunctivitis

Inflammation of the conjunctiva is caused by infectious and non-infectious etiologies. The most common eye infection, however, is not congenital but rather acquired viral conjunctivitis or "pink eye" (see Ch. 9). Other forms of conjunctivitis that only affect children are **ophthalmia neonatorum** and **vernal keratoconjunctivitis**.

OPHTHALMIA NEONATORUM

Definition

Ophthalmia neonatorum is conjunctivitis occurring within the first month of life.

Etiology

Ophthalmia neonatorum may be caused by chemical irritation or a variety of infectious organisms.

- **Chemical (silver nitrate 1% solution (Crede's prophylaxis))**-induced conjunctivitis occurs within 24 hours of birth with bulbar injection and clear watery discharge (usually bilateral), therefore erythromycin or tetracycline ointment is now used for prophylaxis. Since the conjunctivitis only lasts 24–36 hours, no treatment is required.
- *Gonococcus* presents on day 1 or 2 with copious purulent discharge, chemosis, and eyelid edema. It may be hemorrhagic, and corneal ulceration is possible. Treatment is with IV ceftriaxone for 7 days and topical bacitracin ointment. There is a high incidence of *Chlamydia* co-infection, so infected infants are also given oral erythromycin syrup and treatment is necessary for the mother and any of her sexual partners.
- **Other bacteria** produce infection on day 4–5. These are commonly due to staphylococci, streptococci, *Haemophilus* (less common now that children are vaccinated against *H. influenzae*), enterococci, and *Pseudomonas*. Broad-spectrum antibiotic ointments like bacitracin, erythromycin, gentamicin, or ciloxan are prescribed. Sometimes topical fortified antibiotics are given.
- **Herpes simplex virus** causes serous discharge, conjunctival injection, and keratitis between days 5 and 14. Vesicular lesions may be seen on the eyelids and there can be a systemic herpetic infection. The treatment is Viroptic eyedrops q2 hours for 1 week and systemic acyclovir 10 mg/kg IV tid for 10 days.

Chlamydia (**neonatal inclusion conjunctivitis**) is the most common infectious cause of neonatal conjunctivitis and also occurs between days 5 and 14 but with mucopurulent discharge. There may be an associated pneumonitis, otitis, nasopharyngitis, gastritis, or concomitant gonococcus infection. It is treated with topical erythromycin ointment and oral erythromycin syrup for 2–3 weeks (125 mg/kg per day qid) to prevent pneumonitis which begins 3–13 weeks later. Treatment is also given to the mother with doxycycline 100 mg bid for 1 week (do not use in nursing mothers).

Symptoms

Parents report tearing, discharge, and redness of one or both of the baby's eyes.

Signs

Exam reveals conjunctival hyperemia and papillae (neonates cannot produce conjunctival follicles because their immune systems are immature). Discharge and crusted eyelashes are frequently observed (Figure 6–10).

Differential diagnosis

A red, tearing eye in an infant may also be due to trauma, foreign body, corneal abrasion, glaucoma, NLDO, or dacryocystitis.

Evaluation

- Key elements of the **history** are the timing of the conjunctivitis, type of discharge, and associated symptoms.
- The **eye exam** should focus on the lids (edema, erythema, lash crusting), conjunctiva (injection, papillae, discharge), and cornea (staining). Trauma and foreign bodies must be ruled out. The lacrimal sac should be palpated to check for expressible discharge.
- **Gram stain and cultures** should be taken to identify the organism.

Management

- Treatment is tailored according to the etiologic agent (see above).
- Prophylaxis with tetracycline 1% or erythromycin 0.5% ointment is given at birth.

Prognosis

The prognosis varies depending on etiologic agent.

VERNAL KERATOCONJUNCTIVITIS

Vernal keratoconjunctivitis is a form of seasonal allergic conjunctivitis, more common in boys than girls, that presents by age 10 years old and is self-limited, lasting 2–10 years.

Vernal keratoconjunctivitis is associated with atopic dermatitis (75%) and a family history of atopy (66%). Patients suffer from intense itching, photophobia, and even pain. The eye exam is significant for large upper tarsal papillae (cobblestones), limbal follicles (gelatinous nodules at the limbus), and copious ropy mucus. Eversion of the upper eyelids is necessary to view the cobblestone papillae (Figure 6–11). There is minimal conjunctival hyperemia, and corneal changes such as peripheral scarring and vascularization or a shield-shaped ulcer may be present. Treatment is with topical allergy medication, although topical cyclosporine may

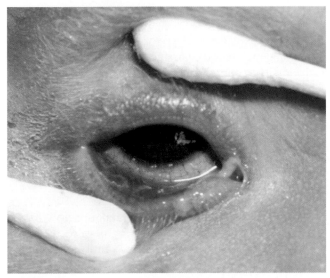

FIGURE 6–10
Hyperacute gonorrheal conjunctivitis demonstrating conjunctival injection and purulent discharge.

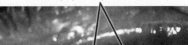
Giant papillae (cobblestones)

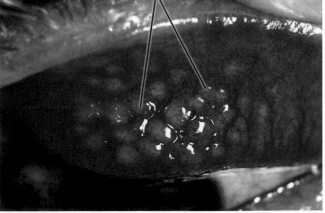

FIGURE 6–11
Vernal keratoconjunctivitis demonstrating "cobblestones" (giant papillae).

also be helpful. Since this is a chronic disease, steroid eyedrops should be used judiciously and with careful monitoring for elevated intraocular pressure (IOP) and cataract formation.

Childhood Glaucoma

Definition

There are several types of glaucoma that are classified according to the age of onset:

- **Congenital**: occurs in infants younger than 3 months old.
- **Infantile**: occurs between age 3 months and 3 years old.
- **Juvenile**: occurs between age 3 and 35 years old.

Etiology

Congenital glaucoma may be primary, secondary, or associated with a syndrome:

- **Primary**: due to developmental abnormalities of the anterior-chamber angle.
- **Secondary**: due to inflammation, trauma, tumors, steroid- or lens-induced.
- **Associated syndromes**: mesodermal dysgenesis syndromes, aniridia, persistent hyperplastic primary vitreous (PHPV), nanophthalmos, rubella, nevus of Ota, Sturge–Weber syndrome, neurofibromatosis, Marfan's syndrome, Weill–Marchesani syndrome, Lowe's syndrome, mucopolysaccharidoses.

Epidemiology

The incidence of the primary form is 1 in 12 500 births. The disease predominantly affects males bilaterally (70%). It is present at birth in 40% of cases.

Symptoms

Children with glaucoma may present with tearing, photophobia, blepharospasm, and eye rubbing. Infants less than 3 months of age are usually noted to have corneal clouding or tearing. Children older than 3 years are often asymptomatic but develop progressive myopia and insidious visual field loss.

Signs

The hallmark of glaucoma is elevated IOP (>21 mmHg) and an enlarged optic cup (cup-to-disc ratio >0.3; Figure 6–12). Cupping is reversible in childhood, so with treatment and reduction of IOP, the cup-to-disc ratio can return to normal. Other findings in congenital glaucoma include an enlarged eye (**buphthalmos** or "bull's eye"), myopia, and corneal clouding due to edema from ruptures in Descemet's membrane (**Haab's striae**) (Figure 6–13).

Differential diagnosis

Other ocular diseases that can present with similar signs and symptoms include NLDO, megalocornea, high myopia, and other causes of corneal edema (i.e., birth trauma, corneal endothelial dystrophy).

Evaluation

- The **history** should include any family history of glaucoma and the timing of symptoms.
- The **eye exam** is often difficult and therefore requires an **examination under anesthesia (EUA)** for complete evaluation with specific attention to tonometry (increased IOP), cornea (increased diameter, edema), gonioscopy (abnormal angle structures), and ophthalmoscopy (optic nerve cupping).
- **Visual field testing** is performed in older children.

Management

- Definitive treatment of congenital glaucoma is surgical, and medication is used as a temporizing measure. Therapy is conducted by a glaucoma specialist.
- Medical treatment is with hypotensive medications: topical β-blocker (timolol maleate (Timoptic) or betaxolol (Betoptic S) bid) and/or carbonic anhydrase inhibitor (dorzolamide (Trusopt), brinzolamide (Azopt) tid or acetazolamide (Diamox) 15 mg/kg per day PO). Miotics may be associated with a paradoxical increase in IOP, and brimonidine (Alphagan-P) may be associated with infant death.
- Initial surgical options include goniotomy and trabeculotomy. If these fail, then consider trabeculectomy with mitomycin C, drainage implant, or cycloablation of the ciliary body.
- The patient may require glasses for myopia and patching for amblyopia.

Prognosis

The prognosis is generally poor, but depends upon the extent of glaucomatous damage prior to treatment as well as the ability to control the IOP adequately. The outcome is best for the primary congenital form. Goniotomy and trabeculotomy have a 77% success rate.

Congenital Cataracts

Definition

A congenital cataract is a congenital opacity of the crystalline lens. Congenital cataracts are also the most frequent cause of **leukocoria** (white pupil) in children.

Etiology

The etiology depends on whether the cataracts are bilateral or unilateral:

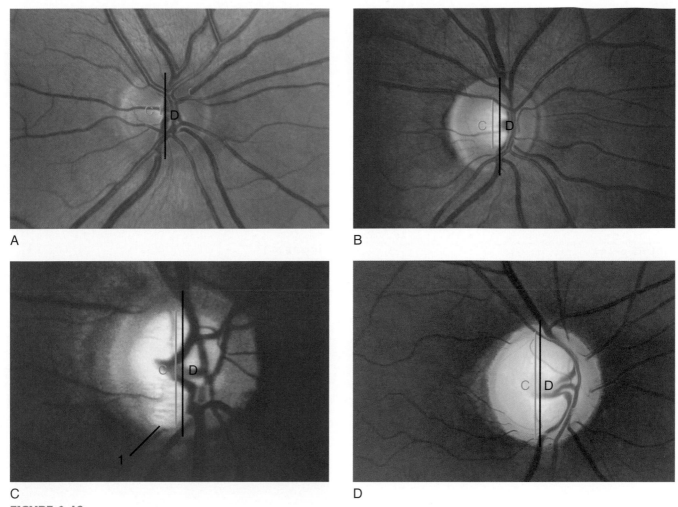

A

B

C

D

FIGURE 6–12

Different optic nerve photos showing: (**A**) normal cup-to-disc ratio of approximately 0.1. (**B**) Normal cup-to-disc ratio of approximately 0.5. (**C**) Glaucomatous optic nerve with cup-to-disc ratio of 0.8 and inferior notch (1), and (**D**) advanced glaucoma with cup-to-disc ratio of 0.9.

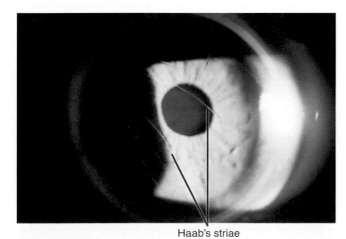

Haab's striae

FIGURE 6–13

Haab's striae appear as clear parallel lines in the cornea.

- **Bilateral cataracts**: idiopathic (60%), hereditary (30%; usually autosomal dominant, associated with or without systemic abnormalities), intrauterine infection (TORCHS syndromes (toxoplasmosis, rubella, cytomegalovirus, herpes, syphilis), mumps, vaccinia), associated with ocular disorders (Leber's congenital amaurosis, retinitis pigmentosa (RP), PHPV, retinitis of prematurity, aniridia, Peter's anomaly, ectopia lentis, posterior lenticonus, uveitis, tumors (retinoblastoma (RB), medulloepithelioma)), metabolic (diabetes, galactosemia, hypocalcemia, Lowe's syndrome, congenital hemolytic jaundice, hypoglycemia, mannosidosis, Alport's syndrome, Fabry's disease), maternal drug ingestion/malnutrition, and trauma.
- **Unilateral cataracts**: idiopathic (80%), intrauterine infection (rubella 33% unilateral), ocular abnormalities (10%), and trauma (9%).

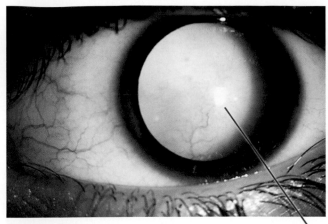

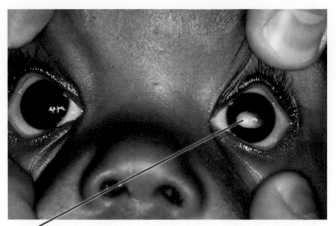

Leukocoria

FIGURE 6–14
Leukocoria in a patient with toxocariasis. The large white reflex in the dilated pupil represents the retina; a retinal vessel is visible.

Leukocoria

FIGURE 6–15
Leukocoria due to retinoblastoma in the left eye. The white pupil in the left eye is strikingly evident in comparison with the normal (black) pupil of the fellow eye.

Epidemiology

The incidence is about 1 in 2000, and approximately one-third of congenital cataracts are familial, one-third are associated with a syndrome, and one-third are isolated.

Symptoms

Parents may notice that their child has poor vision, a white pupil, an eye turn, or nystagmus.

Signs

The main findings on exam are decreased visual acuity and **leukocoria** (white pupil; Figures 6–14 and 6–15)). The child may have strabismus (especially with unilateral cataracts) and/or nystagmus (nystagmus does not usually appear until 2–3 months of age, and rarely occurs when cataracts develop after age 6 months).

   On examination, the cataract can have a variety of appearances depending on the location of the opacity within the lens (Figures 6–16 and 6–17).

Differential diagnosis

Other entities that produce leukocoria are RB, toxoplasmosis, toxocariasis, retinal detachment, retinitis of prematurity, PHPV, Coats' disease, coloboma, myelinated nerve fibers, retinal dysplasia, Norrie's disease, incontinentia pigmenti, retinoschisis, cyclitic membrane, and medulloepithelioma.

Evaluation

- When gathering the **history**, the parents must be questioned specifically about family history of cataracts, gestational and birth history, the child's general health and any eye disorders or ocular trauma. If eye findings exist, their onset and character should be noted.

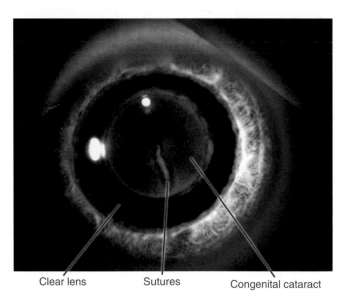

Clear lens   Sutures   Congenital cataract

FIGURE 6–16
Congenital cataract with prominent suture lines.

- A complete **eye exam** must be performed with attention to visual acuity (decreased), ocular motility (strabismus, nystagmus), lens (position, size, and density of the cataract), and ophthalmoscopy (to rule out other causes of leukocoria). An EUA may be necessary if a complete exam cannot be performed.
- **Lab tests** include TORCHS titers, and a metabolic work-up is also obtained for bilateral cataracts (i.e., fasting blood sugar (hypoglycemia), urine-reducing substances after milk feeding (galactosemia), calcium (hypocalcemia), and urine amino acids (Lowe's syndrome)).
- **B-scan ultrasonography** is obtained if the fundus cannot be adequately visualized.
- **Pediatric consultation**.

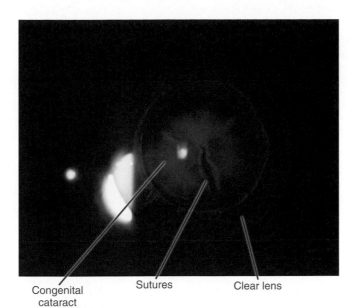

Congenital cataract   Sutures   Clear lens

FIGURE 6–17

Same patient as in Figure 6–16, demonstrating congenital sutural cataract in retroillumination.

Management

- If the cataract obscures the visual axis (opacity >3 mm) or is causing secondary ocular disease (i.e., glaucoma or uveitis), cataract surgery should be performed within days to a week after diagnosis in infants because delay may lead to amblyopia. Postoperatively, aphakic correction with a contact lens or spectacles (if bilateral) is required. Intraocular lenses are now routinely implanted in toddlers and older children. If cataracts are present in both eyes, then surgery is often done on the better-seeing eye first. Sometimes bilateral simultaneous surgery is performed.
- It is also necessary to create a primary posterior capsulotomy because children produce significant postoperative inflammation, which causes posterior capsular opacification (see Ch. 15).
- If the cataract is not causing amblyopia, glaucoma, or uveitis, then the child is observed closely for progression.
- Treatment for amblyopia may be required.
- Almost all patients with visually significant, unilateral, congenital cataracts have strabismus and may require muscle surgery after cataract extraction.

Prognosis

The visual outcome depends on whether or not amblyopia has developed. Bilateral cataracts require treatment by age 3 months, or irreversible nystagmus with poor visual acuity (≤20/200) occurs. Unilateral cataracts must be treated earlier, by 6–8 weeks of life, to prevent amblyopia.

Uveitis

Inflammation of the uvea (iris, ciliary body, and/or choroid) is classified according to location, type, and etiology (see Ch. 12). The etiology varies for adult and pediatric populations. In children, **toxoplasmosis** is the most common cause of uveitis. **Toxocariasis** is another infection that causes posterior uveitis in children, and both of these diseases may also produce leukocoria. On the other hand, pediatric anterior uveitis is most often due to **juvenile rheumatoid arthritis** (JRA).

JUVENILE RHEUMATOID ARTHRITIS

There are different types of JRA, but the one most frequently associated with ocular inflammation is pauciarticular type I, which causes chronic, bilateral uveitis with minimal symptoms (Table 6–1).

The eyes are typically white and quiet even with active inflammation, which is evident by the significant anterior-chamber flare. In addition to the standard treatment of uveitis with a topical steroid and cycloplegic, patients suffering from JRA may require systemic or subTenon's steroids, immunosuppressive agents, and treatment of complications (glaucoma (20%), cataract (40%), and band keratopathy (40%)).

TOXOPLASMOSIS

Toxoplasmosis is usually caused by congenital infection with the parasite *Toxoplasma gondii*. Eye involvement produces a necrotizing retinitis. The tachyzoites incite the inflammation, and the intraretinal cysts are responsible for recurrent disease. The classic appearance of ocular toxoplasmosis is an atrophic chorioretinal scar in the posterior pole, often in the macula (Figure 6–18). Reactivated disease is characterized by a fluffy white retinal lesion ("headlight in the fog" appearance) adjacent to an old scar, granulomatous uveitis, and vitritis (Figure 6–19). Patients present with decreased vision, photophobia, and floaters. There may be vascular sheathing, leukocoria, microphthalmia, nystagmus, and strabismus.

Systemic findings can be seen in both congenital and acquired forms of toxoplasmosis. The congenital form is associated with stillbirth, mental retardation, seizures, hydrocephalus, microcephaly, intracranial calcifications, hepatosplenomegaly, vomiting, and diarrhea, whereas the acquired form is associated with rash, meningoencephalitis, and a flu-like syndrome. The diagnosis is clinical, based on the exam, but enzyme-linked immunosorbent assay (ELISA) or indirect immunofluorescence assay for *Toxoplasma* immunoglobulin G or M is definitive. Therapy, indicated for decreased vision, moderate to severe vitritis, and lesions threatening the macula or optic nerve, is with:

TABLE 6–1

Classification of juvenile rheumatoid arthritis

Type	Polyarticular RF-negative	Polyarticular RF-positive	Pauciarticular type I	Pauciarticular type II	Systemic (Still's disease)
Age	Any	Late childhood	Early childhood	Late childhood	Any
Sex	90% girls	80% girls	80% girls	90% boys	60% boys
Rheumatoid factor (RF)	Negative	Positive	Negative	Negative	Negative
Antinuclear antibodies (ANA)	25%	75%	60%	Negative	Negative
Human leukocyte antigen (HLA) B27	N/A	N/A	N/A	75%	N/A
Joints	Any	Any	Large joints (knee, elbow, ankle)	Large joints (hip, sacroiliac joints)	Any
Uveitis	Rare	No	30% chronic	15% acute	Rare
Other findings	Low-grade fever, delayed growth, anemia, malaise	Low-grade fever, anemia, malaise, rheumatoid nodules	Few	Few	High fever, rash, organomegaly, polyserositis

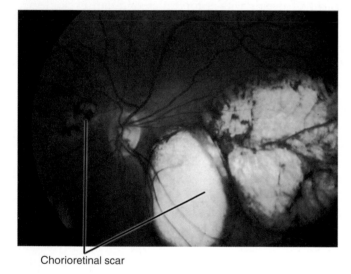

Chorioretinal scar

FIGURE 6–18
Congenital toxoplasmosis demonstrating inactive chorioretinal macular and peripheral scars.

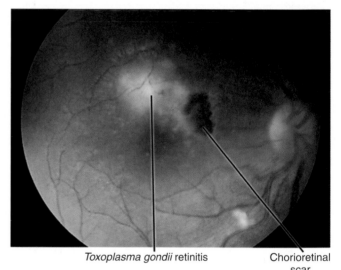

Toxoplasma gondii retinitis   Chorioretinal scar

FIGURE 6–19
Toxoplasmosis demonstrating active, fluffy white lesion adjacent to old, darkly pigmented scar.

- Clindamycin: 300 mg PO qid (risk of pseudomembranous colitis).
- Sulfadiazine: 2 grams PO loading dose, then 1 gram PO qid for maintenance.
- Pyrimethamine (Daraprim): 75–100 mg PO loading dose, then 25 mg PO qd for maintenance (bone marrow depression is prevented with coadministration of folinic acid (Leukovorin; 5 mg 2–3 times per week)).
- Steroids (prednisone): 20–80 mg PO qd for 1 week, then taper. Steroids should never be started alone, but rather 24 hours after initiating antimicrobial therapy.

Bactrim (trimethoprim–sulfamethoxazole, 1 double-strength tablet PO bid) may be used as an alternative.

Antibiotics kill the retinal tachyzoites during active infection, but do not affect the cysts. Small peripheral lesions are usually observed without treatment since they heal spontaneously.

TOXOCARIASIS

Toxocariasis, also known as ocular larva migrans, is due to infection with the dog hookworm *Toxocara canis*. The infection is acquired by ingesting contaminated soil and close contact with puppies. Usually a unilateral, solitary lesion is seen on exam; however, there are three clinical presentations depending on the patient's age (Figures 6–20 and 6–21; Table 6–2):

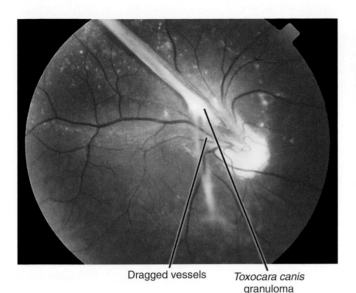

Dragged vessels   *Toxocara canis*
granuloma

FIGURE 6–20
Toxocariasis demonstrating fibrous attachment of peripheral granuloma to optic nerve with dragged retina and vessels.

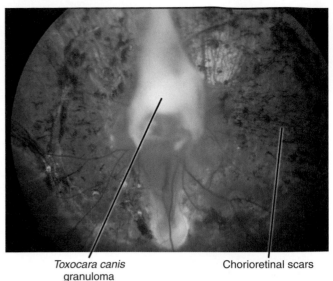

Toxocara canis   Chorioretinal scars
granuloma

FIGURE 6–21
End-stage infection with *Toxocara canis* demonstrating diffuse chorioretinal scarring, dragged vessels, and granuloma.

TABLE 6–2

Clinical Presentations of Toxocariasis

	Chronic endophthalmitis	Localized granuloma	Peripheral granuloma
Age range	2–9 years	6–14 years	6–40 years
Lesion	Exudation filling vitreous cavity, cyclitic membrane	Single localized granuloma in macula or peripapillary region	Peripheral granuloma with dense fibrotic strand, often to disk
Symptoms	Pain, photophobia, lacrimation, decreased vision, acute inflammation	Quiet eye, decreased vision, strabismus	Decreased vision, strabismus
Course	Often leads to destruction of globe	Non-progressive	Non-progressive

Other findings include leukocoria, vitreous abscess, temporal dragging of the macula and retinal vessels, and traction retinal detachments. The diagnosis is clinical based on the exam; however, certain lab tests can be helpful, such as an anterior-chamber tap for eosinophils and ELISA for *Toxocara* antibody titers. There are no ova or parasites in the stool. Treatment consists of a topical steroid and cycloplegic for active uveitis, oral and periocular steroids for severe inflammation, and surgery for retinal detachment.

Retinal Disorders

RETINOPATHY OF PREMATURITY (ROP)

Definition

ROP is a vasoproliferative retinopathy occurring almost exclusively in premature infants, especially after supplemental oxygen therapy.

Etiology

ROP is associated with a number of risk factors:

- **Low birth weight**: <1.5 kg (<750 grams: 90% develop ROP and 16% develop threshold disease; 1–1.25 kg: 45% develop ROP and 2% develop threshold disease).
- **Premature birth**: <36 weeks' gestation.
- **Supplemental oxygen**: >50 days (controversial).
- **Complicated hospital course**.

The risk of retinopathy increases exponentially the more premature and the smaller the infant.

Symptoms

This disease is asymptomatic, although the infant may be noted to have a white pupil and/or an eye turn.

Signs

The retinal findings in ROP may be acute or chronic.

- **Acute phase**: abnormal vessels develop in association with fibrous proliferation.

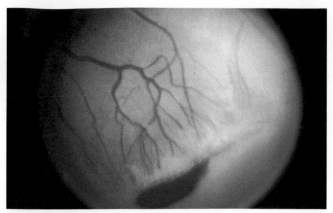

FIGURE 6–22
Stage 3 retinopathy of prematurity. Note finger-like projections of extraretinal vessels into the vitreous cavity. Hemorrhage on the ridge is not uncommon.

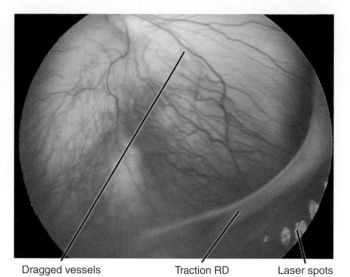

Dragged vessels   Traction RD   Laser spots

FIGURE 6–23
Retinopathy of prematurity (ROP) demonstrating dragged vessels, traction retinal detachment (RD), and laser spots anterior to the regressed fibrovascular proliferation (stage 4A ROP).

- **Chronic phase**: temporal displacement of the macula, retinal detachment, and retrolental fibroplasia.

The vasoproliferative changes are classified by stage, zone, and extent of retinal involvement. Additional terminology describes the severity of disease:

- **Plus disease**: shunted blood causes engorged, tortuous vessels in the posterior pole, vitreous haze, and iris vascular congestion, which represents a poor prognostic sign.
- **Threshold disease**: the level at which 50% will go blind without treatment; usually develops at 27 weeks postgestation.

Other findings include shallow anterior chamber, corneal edema, iris atrophy, poor pupillary dilation, posterior synechiae, ectropion uveae, leukocoria, and vitreous hemorrhage (Figures 6–22–6–24).

Differential diagnosis

Other disorders that must be considered are Coats' disease, Eales' disease, familial exudative vitreoretinopathy (FEVR), sickle-cell retinopathy, juvenile retinoschisis, PHPV, incontinentia pigmenti (Bloch–Sulzberger syndrome), and other causes of leukocoria (see cataract section above).

Evaluation

- Critical elements to note in the **history** are the gestational history, birth history and weight, and use of supplemental oxygen.
- The **eye exam** focuses on ophthalmoscopy (retinal vasculature and periphery) and must carefully document the stage, zone, and extent of disease.
- **Screen** all premature infants at 4–6 weeks of chronological age who weighed <1250–1750 grams at birth, and larger premature infants on supplemental oxygen for >50 days.
- **Pediatric consultation**.

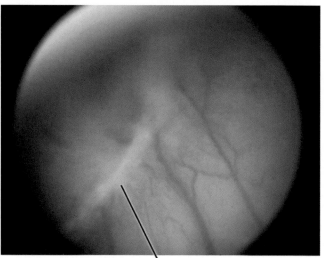

Extraretinal fibrovascular proliferation

FIGURE 6–24
Retinopathy of prematurity (ROP) demonstrating extraretinal fibrovascular proliferation along the ridge (stage 3 ROP).

Management

- Treatment consists of observation, laser, cryotherapy, and surgery. The **Cryotherapy for ROP Study (Cryo-ROP)** determined that treatment preserves visual acuity.
- Cryotherapy or laser photocoagulation of avascular retina is performed for threshold disease.
- Retinal detachment requires surgery by a retina specialist trained in pediatric retinal disease.
- Follow closely (every 1–2 weeks depending on location and severity of the disease) until the extreme retinal periphery is vascularized, then monthly.

Prognosis

The prognosis depends upon the extent of disease, but 80–90% of cases resolve spontaneously. Patients may develop high myopia, strabismus, amblyopia, macular dragging, nystagmus, glaucoma, cataracts, keratoconus, band keratopathy, retinal detachment, and phthisis bulbi.

SHAKEN-BABY SYNDROME

Shaken-baby syndrome is a form of child abuse, most commonly seen in children younger than 3 years old. Ophthalmic sequelae, which occur in 30–40% of cases, typically consist of diffuse retinal hemorrhages, papilledema, vitreous hemorrhage, and retinal tissue disruption (retinoschisis, retinal breaks, and folds) (Figure 6–25). The fundus appearance may resemble a central retinal vein occlusion, Terson's syndrome, or Purtscher's retinopathy (see Figure 17–18; Figure 6–26). Frequently, there are other associated injuries, such as subdural hematoma, subarachnoid hemorrhage, bruises, or fractures of long bones or ribs. Unfortunately, the visual outcome is usually poor due to macular scarring or retinal detachment.

RETINITIS PIGMENTOSA

RP is actually a group of rod–cone dystrophies caused by the abnormal production of photoreceptor proteins (see Ch. 17). RP, the most common hereditary retinal degeneration, can have any inheritance pattern. Many forms exist, some with atypical features and some

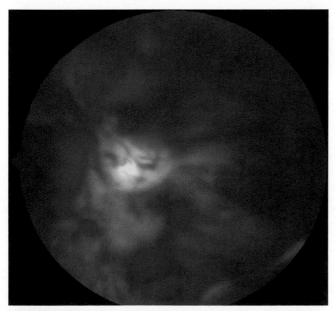

FIGURE 6–25
Retinal and viteous hemorrhage in a child with shaken-baby syndrome.

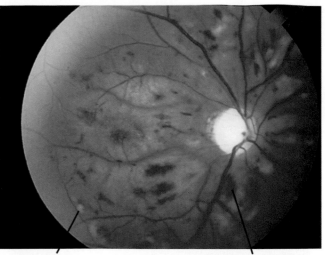

Cotton wool spot   Intraretinal hemorrhage

FIGURE 6–26
Multiple patches of retinal whitening, cotton wool spots, and intraretinal hemorrhages secondary to Purtscher's retinopathy.

with associated systemic abnormalities. The main symptoms include poor night (nyctalopia) and color (dyschromatopsia) vision, photophobia, progressive constriction of the visual fields ("tunnel vision"), and slowly, progressive, decreased central vision starting at approximately age 20 years old. The characteristic findings on retinal examination are pigmentary changes (bone spicules) in the midperiphery, attenuated vessels, and waxy pallor of the optic disc (see Figures 17–69 and 17–70). RP is also associated with macular edema, cataracts, high myopia, keratoconus, and mild hearing loss. Visual field testing shows constriction early and a ring scotoma late, and electrophysiologic tests (electro-retinogram, electro-oculogram, dark adaptation) are abnormal. Treatment is limited to a few of the forms linked to systemic disease. Otherwise, low–vision aids and dark glasses are helpful, but patients are usually legally blind by the 4th decade of life. Vitamin A therapy, which may slow the reduction of the electroretinogram, is controversial.

LEBER'S CONGENITAL AMAUROSIS

Leber's congenital amaurosis is an autosomal recessive disorder that is considered to be an infantile form of RP causing blindness or severe visual impairment in infancy or early childhood. These children have nystagmus and poorly reactive pupils. They tend to rub their eyes to stimulate the retina and elicit flashes of light (oculodigital sign). The fundus appearance ranges from normal (most common) to a variety of pigmentary changes (granular, fleck, salt and pepper, sheen, bone spicules, or atrophic; Figure 6–27). This disease is also associated with keratoconus, hyperopia, cataracts, mental retardation, deafness, seizures, renal and musculoskeletal abnormalities.

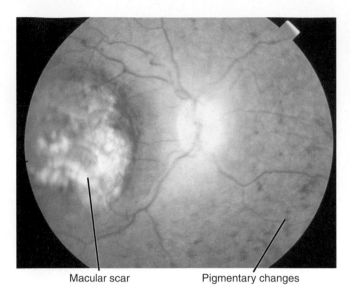

Macular scar   Pigmentary changes

FIGURE 6–27
Leber's congenital amaurosis demonstrating granular and retinitis pigmentosa-like pigmentary changes, attenuated vessels, and a macular scar.

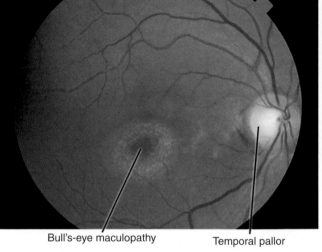

Bull's-eye maculopathy   Temporal pallor

FIGURE 6–28
Cone dystrophy with "bull's-eye" appearance and temporal optic atrophy.

COLOR BLINDNESS

Color blindness affects up to 13% of the general population. The most frequent type is red–green, which is X-linked recessive and therefore more common in men. Color vision defects do not cause decreased vision (except for rod and blue cone monochromatism) or an abnormal retinal appearance. Ninety-two percent of people are trichromats, having three types of normal cones (red (prot), green (deuter), and blue (trit)). If one or more types of cones are absent (anopia) or abnormal (anomaly), then a color vision defect results.

Anomalous trichromatism occurs when all three cones are present but in abnormal proportions:

- **Protonamaly**: abnormal level of red pigment.
- **Deuteranomaly**: abnormal level of green pigment.
- **Tritanomaly**: abnormal level of blue pigment.

Congenital dichromatism exists when there is a substantial lack of one type of color cone:

- **Protanopia**: red cones contain chlorolabe (green pigment).
- **Deuteranopia**: green cones contain erythrolabe (red pigment).
- **Tritanopia**: defect of blue cones.

Rod monochromatism (congenital achromatopsia) is the total absence of cone function with normal rod function. These children have no color vision, poor central vision, nystagmus, and photophobia from birth. The retinal exam shows granular changes and a "bull's-eye" maculopathy (Figure 6–28). Vision deteriorates to the 20/200 level by the 4th decade of life.

Tumors

Certain ocular neoplasms arise specifically in children. These are frequently orbital tumors, 90% of which are benign, but intraocular tumors also occur. It is important to be familiar with the presentation and treatment of the following pediatric neoplasms:

- **Dermoid cyst**: the most common non-inflammatory orbital mass in children.
- **Capillary hemangioma**: the most common childhood benign primary orbital tumor and most common pediatric eyelid tumor.
- **Optic nerve glioma**: benign in children, but malignant in adults (see Ch. 5).
- **Rhabdomyosarcoma**: the most common primary orbital malignancy in children.
- **Neuroblastoma**: the most common metastatic tumor to the orbit in children, followed by **Ewing's sarcoma**. **Burkitt's lymphoma** causes secondary invasion of the orbit.
- **Retinoblastoma**: the most common intraocular malignant tumor in children.
- **Leukemia**: the most common childhood malignancy.

DERMOID CYST

A dermoid cyst arises from dermal elements and is of neural crest origin. This tumor is located in the superotemporal quadrant of the orbit near the brow, often adjacent to the bony suture (Figure 6–29). Enlargement generally does not occur after age 1 year, but dermoids can rupture, causing an intense inflammatory reaction. Therefore, complete en bloc excision is required. Another type of dermoid, a **dermolipoma**, is a smooth, solid,

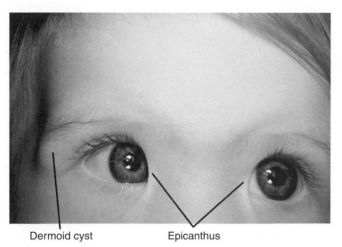

Dermoid cyst   Epicanthus

FIGURE 6–29
Dermoid cyst of the right orbit appearing as a mass at the lateral orbital rim. Also note the epicanthus causing pseudostrabismus.

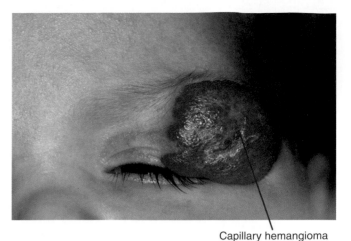

Capillary hemangioma

FIGURE 6–31
Large capillary hemangioma of the left upper eyelid in an infant, causing ptosis.

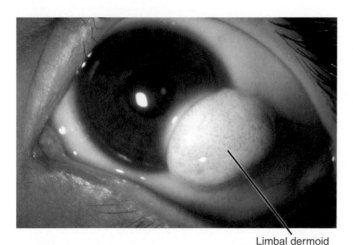

Limbal dermoid

FIGURE 6–30
Limbal dermoid at inferotemporal limbus.

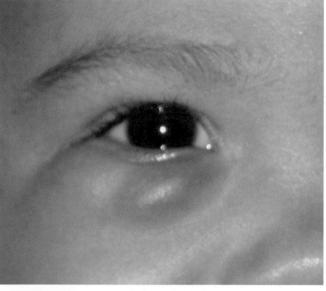

FIGURE 6–32
Capillary hemangioma demonstrating lower-eyelid swelling with bluish discoloration.

yellow-white congenital choristoma that grows at the limbus extending into the corneal stroma and may cover the visual axis or induce astigmatism (Figure 6–30).

CAPILLARY HEMANGIOMA

Definition

A diffuse high-flow mass composed of an abnormal growth of capillary blood vessels.

Epidemiology

A capillary hemangioma often manifests in the first few weeks of life and enlarges over the first 6–12 months, with complete regression by age 5–8 years old. This vascular lesion has a predilection for the superior nasal quadrant of the orbit and medial upper eyelid. It affects females slightly more frequently than males.

Signs

The classic appearance of a capillary hemangioma with skin involvement is the "strawberry nevus," which has a red, irregularly dimpled, elevated surface that blanches with direct pressure (as opposed to a port wine stain, which does not blanch). Orbital lesions can present with proptosis and a bluish appearance of the eyelids and conjunctiva (Figures 6–31 and 6–32).

Evaluation

• The **history** must characterize the growth of the mass and presence of any associated findings like ptosis, eye turn, or decreased vision.

- The **eye exam** should concentrate on the visual acuity (normal or decreased), lids (mass, ptosis), exophthalmometry (proptosis), and ocular motility (strabismus).
- **Computed tomography (CT)** or **magnetic resonance imaging (MRI) scan** shows a well-circumscribed lesion.

Management

- Treatment is required if the tumor is causing ptosis or astigmatism with resultant anisometropia, strabismus, or amblyopia. Options include observation, intralesional steroid injection, systemic steroids, laser, radiation, or excision.

Prognosis

The prognosis is generally good since 80% of cases fully regress. However, eyelid involvement may cause complications (see above).

RHABDOMYOSARCOMA

Definition

A malignant soft-tissue spindle cell tumor with a loose myxomatous matrix.

Etiology

Rhabdos originate from undifferentiated, pluripotent cells, *not* from the extraocular muscles.

Epidemiology

Besides being the most common primary orbital malignancy in children, this tumor is the most common soft-tissue malignancy of childhood. It is a unilateral tumor that tends to involve the superonasal portion of the orbit. The average age at diagnosis is 8 years old, and it is more common in males.

Symptoms

Children complain of pain, decreased vision, and a red, swollen eyelid.

Signs

The characteristic presentation of orbital rhabdomyosarcoma is rapidly progressive proptosis and reddish discoloration of the eyelid (Figure 6–33). Ptosis may occur, and tortuous retinal veins, choroidal folds, and optic nerve edema can develop later.

Evaluation

- The **history** must carefully document the age of onset and characterize any associated symptoms.
- The **eye exam** requires attention to the visual acuity (decreased), lids (ptosis, discoloration), exophthalmometry (proptosis), ocular motility (normal or

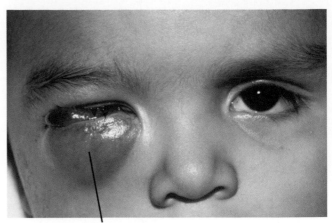
Eyelid edema/discoloration

FIGURE 6–33
Rhabdomyosarcoma of the right orbit with marked lower-eyelid edema, discoloration, and chemosis.

restriction), and ophthlamoscopy (retinal and optic nerve appearance).
- **CT scan** demonstrates a well-circumscribed orbital mass with possible extension into adjacent orbital bones or sinuses and bony destruction.
- **A-scan ultrasound** reveals an orbital mass with medium internal reflectivity.
- **Pediatric oncology consultation** should focus on a **systemic work-up**, including abdominal and thoracic CT scan, bone marrow biopsy, and lumbar puncture.

Management

- Management includes emergent diagnostic biopsy with immunohistochemical staining.
- Treatment consists of surgery for debulking, chemotherapy for microscopic metastases, and radiation therapy for local control.

Prognosis

The prognosis depends on the histologic type. Aggressive local spread through the orbital bones is possible, as well as hematogenous spread to the lungs and cervical lymph nodes. The most common location for metastasis is the chest. With chemotherapy and radiotherapy, the 3-year survival rate is 90%. The cure rate is close to 100% if the tumor is confined to the orbit, but drops to 60% if invasion of adjacent structures exists. Intrathoracic tumors have the worst prognosis, with only a 24% survival rate at 2 years.

NEUROBLASTOMA

Neuroblastoma usually originates in the adrenal gland or sympathetic ganglion chain, but also arises in the mediastinum and neck. Orbital metastases develop in 40% of patients, typically presenting at age 2 years old with sudden proptosis and periorbital ecchymosis (raccoon

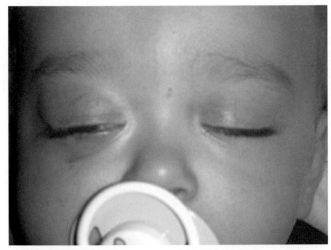

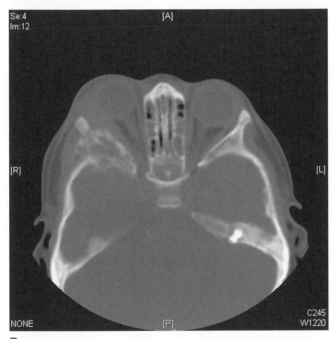

B

FIGURE 6–34
(**A**) Neuroblastoma presenting with bilateral eyelid ecchymosis and right-upper-eyelid swelling. (**B**) CT scan demonstrates the orbital metastases.

eyes; Figure 6–34). There may be an ipsilateral Horner's syndrome and opsoclonus (a paraneoplastic syndrome of random, rapid eye movements in all directions that disappear during sleep). Despite treatment with chemotherapy and local radiation treatment, the prognosis is poor if the age of onset is after 1 year old and there are bone metastases.

RETINOBLASTOMA

Definition

RB is a tumor of the retinal photoreceptors.

Etiology

The tumor originates from a genetic mutation of suppressor genes in a single retinal cell.

Epidemiology

The incidence of RB is 1 in 20 000. Ninety percent of children are diagnosed by age 5 years old. The tumor is unilateral in 70% of cases.

Genetics

The mutation that causes RB occurs on chomosome 13q14 and must involve both chromosomes. The majority are sporadic (95%); only 5% are autosomal dominant. RB is heritable 40% of the time, but only has 80% penetrance. Most tumors occur sporadically in infants with no family history, while bilateral cases are usually familial.

Signs

RB presents with leukocoria (50%), strabismus (20%), intraocular inflammation, and decreased vision (5%). The tumor appears as a white-yellow, elevated mass or masses with calcifications that may grow toward the vitreous (**endophytic**) causing vitreous seeding, toward the choroid (**exophytic**) causing retinal detachment, or diffusely infiltrating within the retina (Figures 6–35–6–37). Other findings include rubeosis (iris neovascularization), pseudohypopyon, hyphema, and angle-closure glaucoma.

Differential diagnosis

Any disease producing leukocoria must be considered: cataract, retrolental mass (PHPV, ROP, Norrie's disease, retinal detachment), tumor (choroidal metastases, retinal astrocytoma), exudates (FEVR, Coats' disease, Eales' disease), change in retinal pigment (incontinentia pigmenti, high myopia, myelinated nerve fibers, retinal

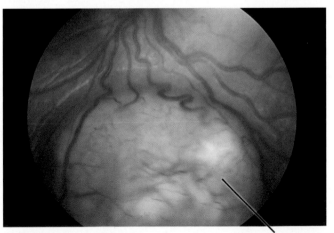

Retinoblastoma

FIGURE 6–35
Retinoblastoma demonstrating discrete round tumor.

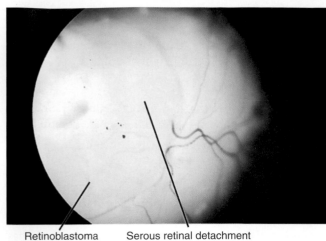

Retinoblastoma   Serous retinal detachment

FIGURE 6-36
Retinoblastoma demonstrating exophytic growth with a serous retinal detachment.

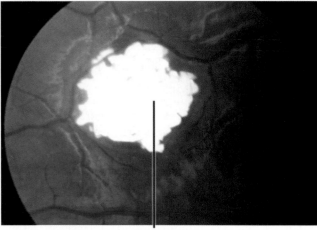

Retinoblastoma

FIGURE 6-37
Retinoblastoma appearing as a white mass.

dysplasia, choroideremia, coloboma), and infections (toxoplasmosis, toxocariasis, endophthalmitis).

Evaluation

- When gathering the **history** it is important to inquire about a family history of RB. In addition, the onset of any findings must be noted.
- The **eye exam** requires careful attention to the visual acuity (normal or decreased), pupils (leukocoria), and ocular motility (strabismus). An **EUA** is required for adequate ophthalmoscopy and treatment.
- **B-scan ultrasonography** and **CT scan** are performed to determine whether calcifications are present.
- **Head and orbital MRI scan** is ordered to evaluate for extraocular extension and trilateral RB (bilateral RB with a pinealblastoma or parasellar mass).
- **Lactate dehydrogenase levels** are helpful since increased levels are present in the aqueous, and thus

the ratio of aqueous to plasma lactate dehydrogenase is >1.0.
- A **metastatic work-up** is necessary, including bone scan, bone marrow aspirate, and lumbar puncture for cytology.
- **Oncology consultation**.

Management

Options for treating RB consist of enucleation, cryotherapy, laser photocoagulation, external beam radiation therapy, brachytherapy, and chemotherapy. Treatment should be performed by an experienced ophthalmic oncologist:

- **Enucleation**: for blind and painful eyes, the affected eye in most unilateral cases, the worst eye in most asymmetric cases, and both eyes in many symmetric cases. At least 10 mm of the optic nerve should be excised to prevent spread.
- **External beam radiation**: for salvageable eyes with vitreous seeding or large tumor, most eyes with multifocal tumors, and eyes that have failed coagulation therapy. RB is very radiosensitive.
- **Episcleral plaque radiation**: for salvageable eyes with a single medium-sized tumor that does not involve the optic nerve or macula.
- **Photocoagulation/cryotherapy**: considered for eyes with one or a few small tumors not involving the optic nerve or macula.

Prognosis

The prognosis for RB is generally good, with long-term survival approaching 85–90%. Spontaneous regression occurs in 3% of cases.

A poor prognosis is associated with optic nerve or uveal invasion, extrascleral extension, multifocal tumors (which represent seeding), and delayed diagnosis. Bilateral involvement does not worsen the prognosis, because it depends upon the status of the tumor in the worst eye. Metastases are most commonly to the central nervous system along the optic nerve, but 50% are to bone. If untreated, RB is fatal in 2–4 years.

Up to one-third of children with heritable RB may develop a secondary malignancy (often presenting around age 17 years old): osteogenic sarcoma of the femur (most common), malignant melanoma or leiomyosarcoma of the eye or orbit, lymphoma, leukemia, rhabdomyosarcoma, or medulloblastoma.

LEUKEMIA

Leukemia commonly involves the eye (80%), usually unilaterally. Patients may notice blurred vision and floaters. The most frequent ocular finding is a retinopathy due to the associated anemia, thrombocytopenia, and hyperviscosity. This is characterized by multiple hemorrhages, microaneurysms, Roth spots, cottonwool spots, dilated/

tortuous vessels, perivascular sheathing, and disc edema (see Figures 17–26 and 17–27). Infiltrative lesions of the choroid cause thickening and overlying serous retinal detachments. Direct infiltrates of the retina and optic nerve are less common. The latter causes loss of vision and papilledema, and requires emergent radiation therapy, because this situation is rapidly fatal if untreated. Orbital infiltration, which is quite rare, produces proptosis, lid swelling, and ecchymosis. The ocular disease resolves with treatment of the underlying hematologic abnormality. Nevertheless, there is a high mortality rate.

Systemic Diseases

Many systemic diseases have ocular manifestations in children. Inborn errors of metabolism result in the accumulation of abnormal substances in various tissues throughout the body, including the eye. As previously mentioned, one-third of congenital cataracts are due to systemic diseases (see section on congenital cataracts, above).

MUCOPOLYSACCHARIDOSES

The mucopolysaccharidoses are a group of disorders in which acid mucopolysaccharides accumulate, producing corneal clouding and/or pigmentary retinal changes. In the **sphingolipidoses**, accumulation of sphingolipids in the retinal ganglion cells results in a macular cherry-red spot. This is the hallmark of Tay–Sachs, Sandhoff's, Neimann–Pick, and Gaucher's diseases (Figure 6–38). Abnormal deposits in **Fabry's** disease create corneal whorls (**cornea verticillata**) (Figure 6–39).

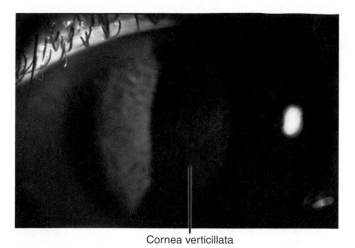
Cornea verticillata

FIGURE 6–39
Cornea verticillata demonstrating golden-brown deposits in a whorl pattern in the inferior central cornea of a Fabry's disease carrier.

ALBINISM

Albinism, another hereditary systemic disorder with ocular findings, is characterized by decreased melanin and congenitally subnormal vision. There are two forms of the disease:

1. **Ocular**: involving the eyes only.
2. **Oculocutaneous**: involving the hair, skin, and eyes.

The decreased vision is due to foveal hypoplasia and nystagmus. Ocular hypopigmentation results in iris transillumination, a pale fundus with visible choroidal vessels, and photophobia (Figures 6–40 and 6–41). These children also typically have high myopia and strabismus.

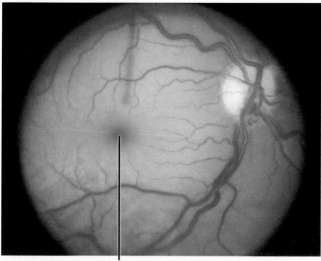
Cherry-red spot

FIGURE 6–38
Cherry-red spot in an infant with Tay–Sachs disease.

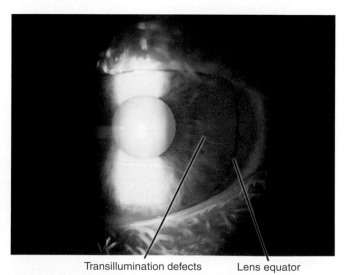
Transillumination defects   Lens equator

FIGURE 6–40
Albinism, demonstrating diffuse iris transillumination; note that the equator of the crystalline lens is visible as a dark line near the peripheral iris.

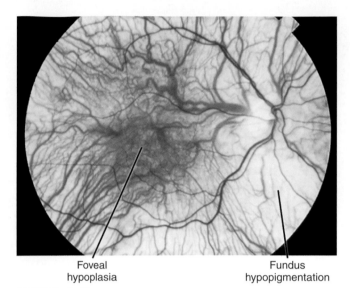

Foveal   Fundus
hypoplasia   hypopigmentation

FIGURE 6–41
Fundus hypopigmentation in a patient with albinism. The deep choroidal vasculature is clearly visible.

Amblyopia

Definition

Amblyopia, more commonly known as "lazy eye," is the unilateral or bilateral loss of best-corrected vision in an otherwise anatomically normal eye.

Etiology

In order to develop normal vision, the brain must receive clear and aligned images from the eyes. If the image from one or both eyes is blurred, then the brain learns to ignore the input from the eye(s). If this is not reversed within the first decade of life, then the subnormal vision becomes permanent. Amblyopia is classified based upon the underlying reason for the poor retinal image:

Strabismic (most common): due to a deviated eye. The visual input from the misaligned eye is ignored to prevent diplopia and visual confusion.

Refractive: due to anisometropia or high ametropia.

- **Anisometropic**: an unequal, uncorrected refractive error between the two eyes causes a constant blurred image in the eye with the higher correction. This type of refractive amblyopia usually requires a large degree of myopic anisometropia (>–6 D) but only mild degrees of hyperopic or astigmatic anisometropia (1–2 D).

- **Isometropic**: a large, but equal, uncorrected refractive error causing bilateral amblyopia. This type of refractive amblyopia usually requires myopic refractive errors >–10 D, hyperopic refractive errors >5 D, and astigmatic refractive errors >3 D.

Deprivation (uncommon): due to obstruction of vision, usually from congenital or acquired media opacities (i.e., cataracts, corneal scars) or ptosis, deprivation often results in significant loss of vision. Deprivation can also be caused by occlusion from excessive therapeutic patching during treatment of amblyopia (see below).

Epidemiology

This condition affects approximately 3% of the population.

Symptoms

Amblyopia may be asymptomatic, or the parent or child may notice decreased vision, an eye turn, droopy eyelid, or white pupil.

Signs

By definition, the visual acuity is decreased (unilateral or bilateral), and patients may have strabismus, nystagmus, ptosis, cataract, or corneal opacity.

Differential diagnosis

It is important to differentiate amblyopia from functional visual loss and optic neuropathy.

Evaluation

- The **history** should focus on the presence of decreased vision and any associated eye findings.
- On **eye exam**, particular attention must be directed to recording the vision, specifically with neutral-density filters (do not reduce acuity as much in the amblyopic eye as in the normal eye), single letters/symbols (better acuity versus a line of letters/symbols), and cycloplegic refraction, as well as pupillary response (normal), and ophthalmoscopy (rule out pathology that might be causing deprivation).

Management

- Correct any refractive error.
- Occlusion therapy with patching for children <10 years old (full-time occlusion of the better-seeing eye for no more than 1 week per year of age of child before re-examination) and continue until the vision stabilizes. Occlusion therapy is stopped if there is no improvement after 2–3 months of full-time patching. Part-time occlusion may be necessary to maintain the improved level of vision. The same effect may also be achieved pharmacologically with a cycloplegic agent (usually atropine 0.5% or 1% qd) to blur the image in the preferred eye.
- When significant amblyopia exists after age 10 years old, protective eyewear with polycarbonate lenses should be worn at all times to protect the fellow eye.
- Surgery may be required in cases of deprivation (e.g., cataract extraction, ptosis repair) and strabismus.

Prognosis

The visual prognosis depends on the extent and duration of amblyopia and the age at which appropriate corrective therapy is initiated (the earlier the better). The traditional teaching has been that treatment must be started prior to 9 years of age, but improved vision can be attained in older individuals. Deprivation amblyopia tends to have a poor outcome, whereas that for strabismus is usually good.

Strabismus

Background concepts

Strabismus is the technical term for an eye turn. This misalignment of the visual axes can be idiopathic or acquired, and the ocular deviation may cause amblyopia if left untreated. Regardless of the etiology, any child with strabismus must have a complete ophthalmic evaluation.

Eye movements are produced by the six extraocular muscles of each eye (see Ch. 1), which in turn are controlled by cranial nerves, gaze centers, and supranuclear pathways (see Ch. 5). Specific terminology is used to describe ocular motility (Table 6–3; Figure 6–42):

- **Ductions**: monocular rotations of the eye.
- **Versions**: conjugate binocular eye movements.
- **Vergence**: disconjugate binocular eye movements (i.e., convergence and divergence).
- **Agonist**: the primary muscle moving the eye in a given direction.
- **Synergist**: the secondary muscle acting with the agonist to move the eye in a given direction.
- **Antagonist**: the muscle acting to move the eye in the opposite direction as the agonist.
- **Yoke muscles**: the two muscles, one in each eye, acting to move their respective eyes into a cardinal position of gaze.

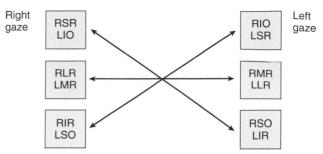

FIGURE 6–42

Cardinal positions and yoke muscles. RSR, right superior rectus; LIO, left inferior oblique; RIO, right inferior oblique; LSR, left superior rectus; RLR, right lateral rectus; LMR, left medial rectus; RMR, right medial rectus; LLR, left lateral rectus; RIR, right inferior rectus; LSO, left superior oblique; RSO, right superior oblique; LIR, left inferior rectus.

- **Cardinal positions**: the six positions of gaze in which one muscle of each eye is the prime mover.
- **Midline positions**: straight up and straight down from primary position.
- **Primary position**: the straight-ahead position of gaze. This is not a cardinal position.

Another important concept is **angle kappa** (Figure 6–43). This is the angle between the visual axis and the anatomic axis (pupillary axis) of the eye and depends on the relative position of the fovea to the pupillary axis. If the fovea is temporal to the pupillary axis (positive angle kappa), then the eyes may appear to turn outward (exotropia), while a nasal location of the fovea with respect to the pupillary axis (negative angle kappa) may produce the appearance of an inward eye turn (esotropia). Thus, angle kappa is a common cause of **pseudostrabismus**.

Definition

Strabismus is an ocular misalignment (deviation of the visual axes) that may be idiopathic or acquired; horizontal

TABLE 6–3

Agonists, Synergists, and Antagonists		
Agonist	**Synergists**	**Antagonists**
Medial rectus (MR)	SR, IR	LR, SO, IO
Lateral rectus (LR)	SO, IO	MR, SR, IR
Superior rectus (SR)	IO, MR	IR, SO
Inferior rectus (IR)	SO, MR	SR, IO
Superior oblique (SO)	IR, LR	IO, SR
Inferior oblique (IO)	SR, LR	SO, IR

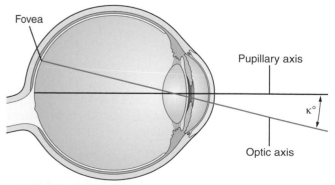

FIGURE 6–43

The angle κ. This is the displacement in degrees of the pupillary axis from the optic axis. The positive angle κ provides the illusion of exotropia in the left eye.

or vertical; comitant or incomitant; latent, manifest, or intermittent.

- **Comitant**: deviation is equal in all positions of gaze.
- **Incomitant**: deviation varies in different positions of gaze (due to paralytic or restrictive disorders).
- **Phoria**: latent deviation.
  - **Orthophoria**: normal alignment; no latent or manifest deviation exists (the eyes are straight).
- **Tropia**: manifest deviation.
  - **Esotropia**: inward deviation.
  - **Exotropia**: outward deviation.
  - **Hypertropia**: upward deviation.
  - **Hypotropia**: downward deviation (vertical deviations are usually designated by the hypertropic eye, but if the process is clearly causing one eye to turn downward, then the eye is designated hypotropic).

Etiology

Most childhood strabismus is idiopathic and numerous forms exist.

Esotropia

Esotropia is classified as follows:

- **Infantile esotropia**: develops by age 6 months with a large, constant deviation. These children usually cross-fixate and do not have a significant refractive error. A family history of strabismus is common.
- **Accommodative esotropia**: appears between age 6 months and 6 years (usually around age 2 years) with a variable angle of deviation (initially intermittent when the child is tired or sick). There are three types:
  1. **Refractive**: due to hyperopia; esotropia is equal at distance and near.
  2. **Non-refractive**: due to a high accommodative converge-to-accommodation ratio; esotropia at near is greater than at distance.
  3. **Mixed**: refractive and non-refractive components.
- **Non-accommodative esotropia**: may be due to stress, sensory deprivation, divergence insufficiency, spasm of the near reflex, consecutive (after exotropia surgery), or cranial nerve VI palsy.

Exotropia

Exotropia may be intermittent or constant. The constant type is rarely congenital, but is rather a result of esotropia surgery (consecutive), decompensated intermittent exotropia, or sensory deprivation.

- **Basic exotropia** exists when the deviation is equal at distance and near.
- **Convergence insufficiency** refers to the inability to maintain convergence as a fixation target is moved from distance to near. This type of exotropia is greater at near than at distance. Symptoms often start during the teen years with asthenopia, difficulty reading, blurred near vision, diplopia, and fatigue.
- **Divergence excess** occurs when the exotropia is larger at distance than at near.

Other causes of strabismus include cranial nerve palsy, chronic progressive external ophthalmoplegia, myasthenia gravis, thyroid-related ophthalmopathy, and orbital fractures.

Epidemiology

In children, the most common deviation is esotropia (50–75%). Exotropia, usually intermittent, accounts for 25% of childhood strabismus. Sensory deprivation typically causes esotropia in children younger than age 6 years and exotropia in older individuals.

Symptoms

Strabismus is frequently asymptomatic. The eye turn may be associated with a head turn, head tilt, decreased vision, diplopia (in older children and adults), headaches, asthenopia, and eye fatigue.

Signs

In addition to the eye turn, the other findings are normal or decreased visual acuity (amblyopia), limitation of ocular movements, and reduced stereopsis. Patients may have other ocular pathology (i.e., cataract, aphakia, retinal detachment, optic atrophy, macular scar, phthisis) causing a secondary sensory strabismus (Figures 6–44 and 6–45).

Differential diagnosis

It is important to rule out **pseudostrabismus** (Figures 6–46 and 6–47): the patient is orthophoric but appears esotropic (due to broad nasal bridge, prominent medial

Esotropia

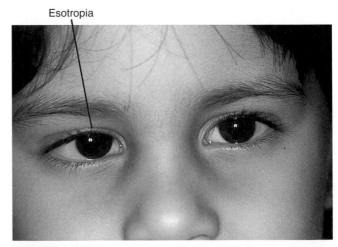

FIGURE 6–44
Esotropia (inward turn) of the right eye. The corneal light reflex in the deviated eye is at the temporal edge of the pupil rather than the center.

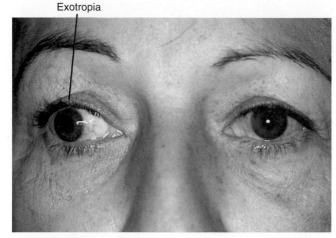

FIGURE 6–45

Exotropia (outward turn) of the right eye. The corneal light reflex in the deviated eye is at the nasal edge of the iris rather than the center of the pupil.

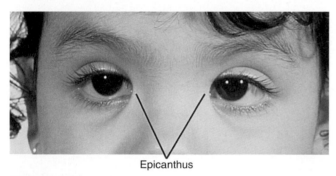

FIGURE 6–46

Epicanthus demonstrating pseudostrabismus. Note vertical skin fold over medial canthal areas.

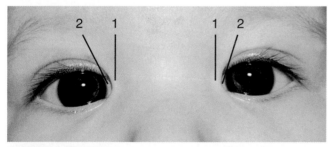

FIGURE 6–47

Pseudoesotropia gives the appearance of crossed eyes due to large epicanthal folds (1) covering the nasal sclera (2) . Notice how the corneal light reflex is centered, proving that the eyes are indeed straight.

epicanthal folds, or negative angle kappa) or exotropic (due to positive angle kappa, temporally dragged macula, or wide interpupillary distance).

Evaluation

- The critical components of the **history** include a family history of strabismus, the age of onset, charac-

teristics of the deviation (direction, timing, frequency/ duration). It is also important to inquire about trauma, associated neurologic symptoms, and systemic diseases.

- The **eye exam** must carefully assess the vision (acuity, refraction before and after cycloplegia, stereopsis, fusion), pupillary response (normal), ocular motility (identify and measure the deviation, perform forced ductions if restriction is suspected), and ophthalmoscopy (rule out pathology that might be causing deprivation).
- **Orbital CT** or **MRI scan** in cases of muscle restriction.
- **Lab tests** include thyroid function tests (triiodothyronine, thyroxine, thyrotropin) in cases of atraumatic muscle restriction, and acetylcholine receptor antibody titers if myasthenia gravis is suspected.
- Consider a **Tensilon test** to rule out myasthenia gravis.
- An **electrocardiogram** should be ordered in patients with chronic progressive external ophthalmoplegia.
- **Neurology consultation** and **brain MRI scan** if cranial nerves are involved.
- **Medical consultation** for dysthyroid and myasthenia patients.

Management

- Treatment of strabismus generally involves correction of any underlying refractive error, occlusion therapy for amblyopia, and then surgical correction of the eye deviation. Sometimes prism lenses can be helpful (Figure 6–48).
- Bifocal glasses are often useful when the child has a high accommodative converge/accommodation ratio.
- Convergence insufficiency is one of the few instances for which eye exercises are helpful. Orthoptic exercises consist of near-point pencil push-ups (fixate on a pencil, bringing it slowly toward the eyes until the breakpoint is reached, then repeat 10–15 times) or prism convergence exercises (increase the amount of base-out prism in front of the eyes until the breakpoint occurs, then repeat with lower prism power, 10–15 times). Base-out prism lenses may also be prescribed to force the eyes to converge.
- For divergence excess, consider prescribing additional minus correction in the glasses to stimulate convergence or using base-in prism lenses to help with convergence.

Prognosis

The prognosis is usually good, but depends on the etiology.

A- AND V-PATTERNS

A- and V-patterns are present when there are different amounts of horizontal strabismus in upgaze and

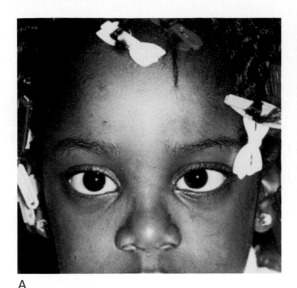

A

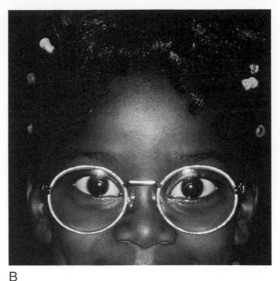

B

FIGURE 6–48
(**A**) Accommodative esotropia that improves when the child wears full hyperopic correction (**B**).

downgaze. Thus, when the child looks up and down, the eyes appear to trace the letter A or V. Muscle surgery is used to correct clinically significant patterns.

A-pattern: an esotropia that is larger in upgaze or an extropia that is larger in downgaze. This pattern is more commonly associated with exotropia and is clinically significant if the difference in horizontal deviation is 10 prism diopters (PD) or greater. The child may adopt a chin-up position to compensate.

V-pattern: an exotropia that is larger in upgaze or an esotropia that is larger in downgaze. This pattern is more commonly associated with esotropia and is clinically significant if the difference in horizontal deviation is 15 PD or greater. The child may adopt a chin-down position to compensate (Figures 6–49 and 6–50).

RESTRICTIVE STRABISMUS

Restrictive strabismus is due to various disorders that cause tethering of one or more extraocular muscles. The resulting deviation varies with different positions of gaze and is therefore incomitant. Ocular motility is restricted in the direction of action of the affected muscle, and this can be identified with forced duction testing. This form of strabismus is commonly seen in thyroid-related ophthalmopathy and orbital fractures (see Ch. 7) (Figure 6–51).

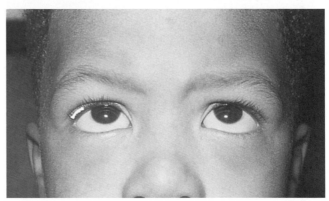

FIGURE 6–49
V-pattern esotropia demonstrating reduced esotropia in upgaze.

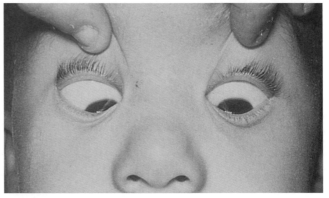

FIGURE 6–50
Same patient as shown in Figure 6–49, demonstrating increased esotropia in downgaze.

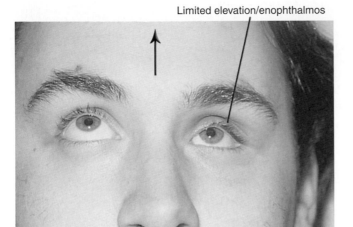

Limited elevation/enophthalmos

FIGURE 6–51
Restrictive strabismus due to an orbital fracture of the left eye with
inferior rectus entrapment, demonstrating limited elevation of the
left eye; also note enophthalmos (sunken appearance of left eye).

CHAPTER SEVEN

Orbit

Introduction

The orbit is specifically designed to protect the eye. The orbital bones surround the globe and form a strong enclosure that reduces the risk of direct ocular injury. The orbital septum serves as a barrier to prevent the spread of disease from the lids to the orbit. Finally, orbital fat cushions the globe. However, despite these protective mechanisms, various processes that affect the orbit may involve the eye.

Trauma

Orbital trauma is usually divided into blunt and penetrating injuries. The mechanism and magnitude of the trauma determine the extent of injury. Blunt trauma involving the orbit usually results in a contusion, hemorrhage, or fracture of the orbital bones rather than a rupture of the globe. This occurs because the force of the trauma blow is directed along the bones instead of being transmitted to the eye. Penetrating trauma results from projectile or lacerating injuries and is more likely to disrupt delicate ocular structures, rupture the globe, and result in intraorbital foreign bodies.

ORBITAL CONTUSION

An orbital contusion is a bruise caused by blunt trauma. An isolated contusion is confined to the eyelids (preseptal), while a more severe injury can involve the globe, paranasal sinuses, and bony socket, or cause a traumatic optic neuropathy (due to compression of the optic nerve by the bruise) or orbital hemorrhage. Examination reveals a "black eye" with lid edema, ecchymosis,

and ptosis (droopy upper eyelid). With more extensive injury, there may be signs of deeper orbital involvement (orbital signs) including a relative afferent pupillary defect (RAPD), visual field defect, restricted ocular motility, and proptosis (protruding globe). It is imperative to rule out and treat associated injuries from the trauma; therefore, a thorough examination is required. Traumatic ptosis due to contusion of the levator muscle may take up to 3 months to resolve (Figure 7–1).

- **Orbital computed tomography (CT) scan** is obtained for cases with an ominous mechanism of injury (e.g., motor vehicle accident, massive trauma, or loss of consciousness) or with orbital signs.

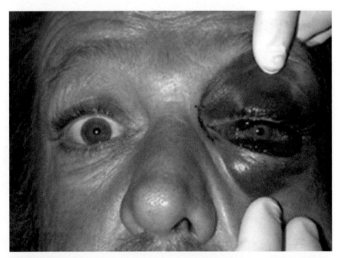

FIGURE 7–1
Orbit contusion demonstrating severe eyelid ecchymosis and edema, subconjuctival hemorrhage, and conjunctival chemosis.

- Isolated orbital contusions are treated with ice compresses every hour for 20 minutes during the first 48 hours to decrease swelling and systemic non-steroidal anti-inflammatory drugs (ibuprofen 400–600 mg PO q4h).

ORBITAL HEMORRHAGE

An orbital hemorrhage, also known as a **retrobulbar hemorrhage**, occurs when there is bleeding in the orbit behind the globe due to surgery or trauma. This condition is a *ophthalmic emergency* because blood can rapidly accumulate behind the globe and may produce a compartment syndrome, resulting in compression of the optic nerve and visual loss. Patients present with pain, decreased vision, bullous subconjunctival hemorrhage, a tense orbit, proptosis (protruding globe), and lid ecchymosis. Other findings on exam are resistance to retropulsion of the globe, restriction of ocular motility, and elevation of intraocular pressure (IOP) (Figure 7–2).

Immediate identification and treatment of this condition are required to prevent vision loss. The orbital pressure must be relieved emergently by performing a lateral canthotomy and cantholysis to free the lower eyelid, allowing the globe to proptose forward, decreasing the compartment syndrome, and the blood to drain.

- The procedure for a **lateral canthotomy** is as follows:

  1. Compress the lateral canthus with a hemostat.
  2. Make a full-thickness incision from the lateral commissure (lateral angle of the eyelids) posterolaterally to the lateral orbital rim with Stevens scissors.
  3. Transect the inferior crus of the lateral canthal tendon.

- Treatment with topical hypotensive drops (timolol (Timoptic) 0.5% bid, brimonidine (Alphagan-P) 0.15% tid, or dorzolamide (Trusopt) 2% tid) may be necessary if the IOP remains elevated (>25 mmHg) once the vision has stabilized.
- Canthoplasty to repair the eyelid can be scheduled approximately 1 week later.

ORBITAL FRACTURES

Fracture of the orbital walls and orbital rim occurs in isolation as well as with concomitant ocular, optic nerve, maxillary, mandibular, or intracranial injuries. Orbital fractures are categorized as follows:

Orbital floor (blow-out fracture)

Orbital floor (blow-out) fractures are the most common type of orbital fracture, and usually involve the maxillary bone and the posterior medial floor, which is the weakest point of the orbit. The orbital floor separates the orbit from the maxillary sinus that is situated below it. Thus, a break in the orbital floor sometimes results in the herniation or entrapment of orbital contents in the maxillary sinus.

The signs and symptoms of a blow-out fracture are diplopia on upgaze (anterior fracture) or downgaze (posterior fracture), enophthalmos (sunken globe), hypoglobus (globe ptosis), and infraorbital nerve hypesthesia (Figures 7–3 and 7–4). Orbital and lid emphysema may occur with nose blowing. Thus, patients with orbital fractures should avoid blowing their nose.

Medial wall (nasoethmoid fracture)

Medial wall (nasoethmoid) fractures can involve the lamina papricea, lacrimal, and maxillary bones. Enophthalmos

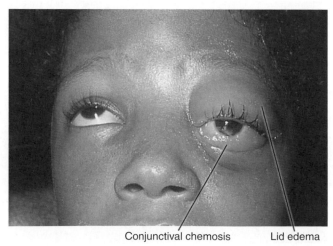

Conjunctival chemosis   Lid edema

FIGURE 7–2
Retrobulbar hemorrhage of the left eye, demonstrating proptosis, lid swelling, chemosis, and restricted extraocular motility on upgaze.

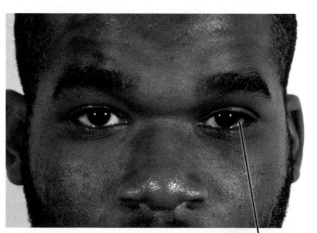

Subconjunctival hemorrhage

FIGURE 7–3
Orbital floor blow-out fracture with enophthalmos and globe dystopia of the left eye.

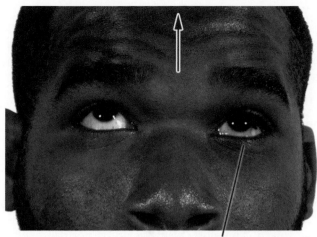

Orbital floor fracture with entrapment

FIGURE 7–4
Same patient as in Figure 7–3, demonstrating entrapment of the left inferior rectus and inability to look up.

can result from medial rectus herniation, but entrapment is rare. This injury can be associated with depressed nasal and orbital floor fractures, and complications include nasolacrimal duct injury, severe epistaxis due to anterior ethmoidal artery damage, and orbital and lid emphysema.

Orbital roof

Orbital roof fractures may involve the frontal sinus, cribriform plate, and brain. This uncommon type of fracture may present with cerebrospinal fluid rhinorrhea or pneumocephalus.

Orbital apex

Orbital apex fractures may involve the optic canal and superior orbital fissure, often with direct traumatic optic neuropathy. Such an injury is difficult to manage because of the proximity to multiple cranial nerves and vessels.

Zygomatic (tripod fracture)

Zygomatic (tripod) fractures may involve three or more fracture sites, including the inferior orbital rim (maxilla), zygomaticofrontal suture (superotemporal orbital rim), and zygomatic arch. The break usually also involves the orbit floor. Patients report pain, binocular diplopia (double vision that disappears when one eye is covered), and trismus (pain on opening mouth or chewing). On examination, there is orbital rim discontinuity or a palpable "step-off," malar flattening, enophthalmos, infraorbital nerve hypesthesia, orbital, conjunctival, or lid emphysema, restricted ocular motility, epistaxis, rhinorrhea, ecchymosis, and ptosis.

Maxillary fractures

Maxillary fractures can be classified using the classification of Le Fort:

- **Le Fort I**: low transverse fracture of the maxillary bone above the teeth that does not involve the orbit.
- **Le Fort II**: pyramidal fracture of the nasal, lacrimal, and maxillary bones that involves the medial orbital floor.
- **Le Fort III**: craniofacial dysjunction that involves the orbital floor, lateral and medial walls, and sometimes the optic canal.

Management of orbital fractures

- **Orbital CT scan** to identify the fracture and co-existing injuries is indicated for orbital signs (afferent papillary defect, diplopia, limited ocular motility, proptosis, and enophthalmos) or an ominous mechanism of injury.
- Ice compresses are used for the first 48 hours.
- Nasal decongestant (oxymetazoline HCl (Afrin nasal spray) bid for 10 days), and warn patient not to blow nose.
- Consider systemic steroids and oral antibiotics (amoxicillin/clavulanate (Augmentin) 250–500 mg PO tid for 10 days).
- Surgical repair depends on the type and extent of the fracture and associated findings.
- Orbital surgery consultation for fractures associated with diplopia, muscle entrapment, enophthalmos, and facial asymmetry. Surgery, when indicated, is usually delayed for 1 week to allow for reduction of swelling. However, for children with entrapment due to a "trapdoor" phenomenon, surgery is performed urgently (within 24 hours).
- Neurosurgery and otolaryngology consultations for cerebrospinal fluid rhinorrhea or pneumocephalus.
- Treatment of traumatic optic neuropathy may be required (see Ch. 5).

INTRAORBITAL FOREIGN BODY

An intraorbital foreign body can be associated with penetrating trauma due to projectiles. Depending upon the extent of injury and ocular involvement, patients may be asymptomatic or may have pain or decreased vision. The entry wound is often apparent as an eyelid or conjunctival laceration, and other findings include lid ecchymosis and edema, bullous subconjunctival hemorrhage, or chemosis. Proptosis and restricted ocular motility occur when there is retrobulbar hemorrhage associated with the penetrating trauma. Penetration of the globe and optic nerve involvement must be ruled out with a thorough eye exam.

- Emergent **orbital CT scan** should be carried out to localize and characterize the foreign body (Figure 7–5). If a metallic object is suspected, then a magnetic resonance imaging (MRI) scan is *contraindicated*.
- Initial treatment consists of culturing the entry wound, starting broad-spectrum oral antibiotics (e.g.,

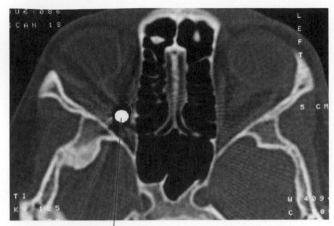

Intraorbital foreign body

FIGURE 7–5
Orbital computed tomography scan demonstrating intraorbital foreign body.

Augmentin or Keflex), and administering a tetanus booster if necessary.

- A small piece of inert material such as glass, lead, or plastic is generally well tolerated, so, depending on the location in the orbit, it may be best to observe rather than attempt removal and possible damage to delicate ocular structures.
- Surgical removal by an orbital surgeon is indicated for fistula formation, infection, optic nerve compression, large or intolerable foreign bodies, or those that are easily removed (i.e., anterior to the equator of the globe). Foreign bodies composed of iron and copper are poorly tolerated, as is organic material, which has a significant risk for infection. These types of foreign bodies require prompt removal.
- The prognosis is favorable if the eye and optic nerve are not affected.

Infections

Orbital infections can be benign or devastating. Thus, it is vital that physicians be able to differentiate preseptal (usually benign) from orbital cellulitis (which can be devastating). The former is a superficial infection, which, if not recognized and treated appropriately, can quickly become the latter. Orbital cellulitis is a grave condition which requires emergent treatment to prevent vision loss and even death.

PRESEPTAL CELLULITIS

Definition

Preseptal cellulitis is infection and inflammation anterior to the orbital septum and limited to the superficial periorbital tissues and eyelids. There is no involvement of the globe and orbit.

Etiology

Preseptal cellulitis usually results from periorbital trauma (even minor) or dermal infection. The most common organism is *Staphylococcus aureus*.

Symptoms

Patients present with eyelid swelling, redness, ptosis, and pain, sometimes with a low-grade fever.

Signs

The hallmark of preseptal cellulitis is that the findings are confined to the eyelid, which demonstrates erythema, edema, ptosis, and warmth (Figure 7–6). The eye is *not* involved. Therefore, visual acuity is normal, ocular motility is full, the conjunctiva and sclera are not injected, and there is no proptosis or RAPD.

Differential diagnosis

It is important to rule out the more severe conditions of orbital cellulitis, idiopathic orbital inflammation, eyelid abscess, dacryoadenitis, dacryocystitis, trauma, and rhabdomyosarcoma (in children).

Evaluation

- When gathering the **history**, the patient must be asked about even minor trauma, sinus disease, recent dental work or infections, and a history of diabetes or immunosuppression. The patient should be questioned specifically about visual and constitutional symptoms.
- A complete **eye exam** is necessary to rule out ocular involvement. Attention is directed to the vision (normal acuity and color vision), pupillary response (normal), ocular motility (normal), exophthalmometry (no proptosis), lids (red and swollen, often ptotic), and conjunctiva and sclera (normal).
- It is also important to check **vital signs, head and neck lymph nodes, meningeal signs** (rule out nuchal

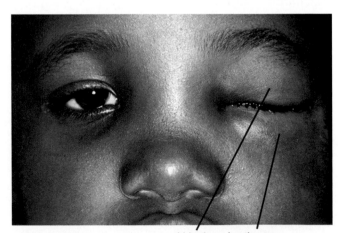

Lid edema/erythema

FIGURE 7–6
Moderate preseptal cellulitis with left-eyelid edema and erythema.

rigidity), and **mental status** to rule out more wide-spread involvement.

- **Orbital and sinus CT scan** should be considered in the absence of trauma or in the presence of orbital signs to check for paranasal sinus opacification.
- **Lab tests** include complete blood count (CBC) with differential, blood cultures, and wound culture if relevant.

Management

- Systemic antibiotics are prescribed to prevent spread of infection:
  - **Oral** for mild cases: amoxicillin/clavulanate (Augmentin) 250–500 mg PO tid or cefaclor (Ceclor) 250–500 mg PO tid or trimethoprim/sulfamethoxazole (Bactrim) 1 double-strength tablet PO bid for penicillin-allergic patients.
  - **Intravenous** for moderate to severe cases, septic patients, non-compliant patients, children younger than 5 years old, and patients who do not respond to oral antibiotic treatment after 48 hours: cefuroxime 1 g IV q8h or ampicillin/sulbactam (Unasyn) 1.5–3 g IV q6h.
- Warm compresses tid.
- Daily follow-up until improvement occurs.
- Consider surgical drainage if an abscess exists.

Prognosis

The prognosis is good when treatment is initiated early, otherwise orbital involvement may develop.

ORBITAL CELLULITIS

Definition

Orbital cellulitis is infection and inflammation posterior to the orbital septum within the orbit. There may also be involvement of the eyelids.

Etiology

Infection within the orbit is usually secondary to sinusitis, typically ethmoid, but other causes include dacryocystitis, dental caries, intracranial infection, orbital trauma, and surgery. The most common organisms are streptococci and staphylococci. Fungal infections from *Phycomycetes* (i.e., *Mucor*) are extremely aggressive and occur more frequently in sick patients with malignancy, immunosuppression, diabetes mellitus, or renal disease.

Symptoms

Orbital cellulitis presents with a red, painful eye, blurred vision, headache, and fever.

Signs

At a glance, orbital and preseptal cellulitis look similar, with lid edema, erythema, and tenderness. However, the

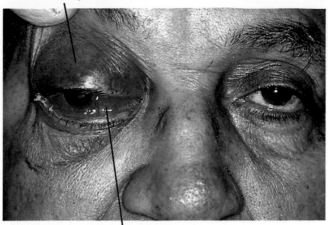
Lid edema/erythema

Conjunctival chemosis/injection

FIGURE 7–7
Orbital cellulitis with right-sided proptosis, lid edema and erythema, conjunctival injection and chemosis, and right exotropia (note decentered right corneal light reflex at the limbus).

hallmark of an orbital infection is the presence of orbital findings. These may include decreased visual acuity, restriction of and/or painful ocular movements, proptosis (protruding globe), a positive RAPD, conjunctival hyperemia and swelling (chemosis), and even optic disc edema (Figure 7–7). Fungal infections classically present with proptosis and orbital apex syndrome (see Ch. 5). There may also be a black eschar in the nose or palate.

Differential diagnosis

Other entities that may present with similar findings are thyroid-related ophthalmopathy, idiopathic orbital inflammation, subperiosteal abscess, orbital tumors, lacrimal gland tumors, orbital vasculitis, trauma, carotid cavernous fistula, cavernous sinus thrombosis, and cranial nerve palsies.

Evaluation

- During the **history**, it is important to document any trauma, sinus disease, recent dental work or infections, and history of diabetes mellitus or immunosuppression. The patient should be questioned specifically about visual and constitutional symptoms.
- A complete **eye exam** is performed focusing particularly on the vision (reduced acuity and/or abnormal color vision), pupillary response (positive RAPD), ocular motility (restricted, painful), exophthalmometry (proptosis), lids (red and swollen), conjunctiva (injection, chemosis), cornea (exposure keratopathy), and ophthalmoscopy (optic disc edema).
- It is also important to check **vital signs**, **head and neck lymph nodes**, **meningeal signs** (rule out nuchal rigidity), **cranial nerves**, and **mental status**.
- **Orbital and sinus CT scan** should be carried out to check for paranasal sinus opacification.

- **Lab tests** include CBC with differential, blood cultures (usually negative in phycomycosis), and wound culture if relevant.
- **Otolaryngology consultation** is necessary for sinusitis.

Management

- Orbital cellulitis is a true *ophthalmic emergency* that requires immediate diagnosis and treatment to prevent complications.
- Emergent treatment with systemic antibiotics (intravenous then oral) and surgical drainage of the abscess by an orbital surgeon is required:
  - **Intravenous** (1-week course): nafcillin 1–2 g IV q4h and ceftriaxone 1–2 g IV q12–24h, or ampillicin/sulbactam (Unasyn) 1.5–3 g IV q6h.
  - **Oral** (10-day course) only after improvement is noted: amoxicillin/clavulanate (Augmentin) 250–500 mg PO tid or cefaclor (Ceclor) 250–500 mg PO tid or trimethoprim/sulfamethoxazole (Bactrim) 1 double-strength tablet PO bid for penicillin-allergic patients.
- Topical antibiotics (bacitracin or erythromycin ointment qid) are used to treat conjunctivitis and corneal exposure.
- Daily follow-up is required to monitor the ocular signs.
- Mucormycosis has a high mortality rate and therefore requires emergent debridement, biopsy, antifungal therapy (amphotericin B 0.25–1.0 mg/kg IV divided equally q6h), and treatment of the underlying medical condition.

Prognosis

The prognosis depends on the causative organism and the extent of infection. Complications such as orbital apex syndrome, cavernous sinus thrombosis, and meningitis can produce permanent neurologic deficits. Mucormycosis has the worst outcome and may be fatal due to intracranial spread.

Inflammation

The two major inflammatory diseases affecting the orbit are thyroid-related and idiopathic. These can mimic infections, tumors, and vascular processes.

THYROID-RELATED OPHTHALMOPATHY (TRO)

Definition

TRO is an autoimmune disease associated with thyroid gland dysfunction. It is also referred to as dysthyroid orbitopathy or ophthalmopathy, and Graves' ophthalmopathy.

Epidemiology

TRO is the most common cause of unilateral or bilateral proptosis in adults, affecting women more often than men (8:1). Abnormal thyroid function tests are found in 80% of cases, usually hyperthyroidism (particularly Graves' disease), although patients may be hypothyroid or even euthyroid (25%). TRO is also associated with myasthenia gravis.

Symptoms

Patients are usually asymptomatic, but they may experience foreign-body sensation, tearing, decreased vision, dyschromatopsia, diplopia, prominent ("bulging") eyes, red eyes, or retracted eyelids.

Signs

The ocular manifestations of this disease can be divided into four clinical categories: (1) eyelid disorders; (2) eye surface disorders; (3) ocular motility disorders; and (4) optic neuropathy.

The classic signs of TRO are eyelid retraction (90%) and proptosis (protruding globe). The palpebral fissure is wider, especially laterally. Other findings on exam include lagophthalmos (incomplete eyelid closure), lid lag on downgaze, corneal exposure (from a combination of eyelid retraction, proptosis, and lagophthalmos), dry eye (due to corneal exposure and infiltration of the lacrimal glands), conjunctival injection and chemosis, restricted ocular movements (most commonly upgaze), increased IOP on upgaze, resistance to retropulsion of the globe, choroidal folds, optic disc hyperemia, and compressive optic neuropathy (<5%) with decreased acuity and color vision, positive RAPD, and visual field defects (Figures 7–8 and 7–9; Box 7–1).

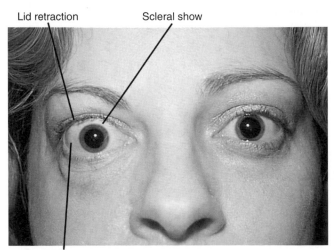

Lid retraction   Scleral show

Proptosis

FIGURE 7–8
Thyroid ophthalmopathy with proptosis, lid retraction, and superior and inferior scleral show of the right eye.

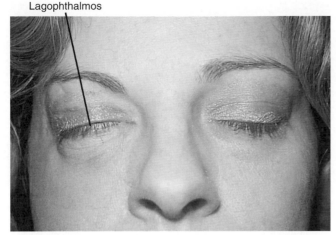

Lagophthalmos

FIGURE 7–9
Same patient as shown in Figure 7–8, demonstrating lagophthalmos on the right side with eyelid closure (note the small incomplete closure of the right eyelid).

BOX 7–1

Werner Classification of Eye Findings in Graves' Disease (NO SPECS)

N No signs or symptoms
O Only signs

S Soft-tissue involvement (signs and symptoms)
P Proptosis
E Extraocular muscle involvement
C Corneal involvement
S Sight loss (optic nerve compression)

Differential diagnosis

Other conditions that may resemble TRO are idiopathic orbital inflammation, orbital and lacrimal gland tumors, orbital vasculitis, trauma, cellulitis, arteriovenous fistula, cavernous sinus thrombosis, gaze palsies, and aberrant regeneration of cranial nerve III.

Evaluation

- It is important to record a complete medical **history** trying to elicit a history of thyroid disease, auto-immune disease, or cancer. The patient should be questioned specifically about hyperthyroid symptoms such as heat intolerance, weight loss, palpitations, sweating, and irritability.
- The **eye exam** should pay particular attention to the cranial nerves (rule out a palsy), visual acuity (may be decreased), color vision (may be decreased), pupillary response (may have a positive RAPD), ocular motility (restricted, forced duction testing), lids (position), exophthalmometry (proptosis), conjunctiva (injection and chemosis), cornea (may have staining or ulceration from exposure), tonometry (increased IOP on upgaze), and ophthalmoscopy (retina and optic nerve appearance).
- Automated **visual field testing** should be obtained as a baseline study in early cases and to rule out optic neuropathy in advanced cases.
- **Lab tests** include thyroid function tests (thyroid-stimulating hormone, thyroxine (total and free), and triiodothyronine).
- **Orbital CT scan** demonstrates extraocular muscle enlargement *sparing* the tendons (inferior rectus is most commonly involved, followed by the medial, superior, and lateral).
- **Endocrinology consultation**.

Management

- As a general principle, the disease should be stable for at least 6 months before performing any surgical interventions, except in cases of optic neuropathy and severe proptosis, which require *emergent* decompression. Surgery should proceed in a stepwise fashion, with orbital decompression first, then strabismus surgery, and finally eyelid reconstruction as indicated.
- Specific treatment recommendations are as follows:
  - **Exposure keratopathy**, depending on the degree, is treated with topical lubrication (artificial tears up to q1h while awake and ointment qhs), taping the eyelids shut or wearing humidifying goggles at bedtime, punctal occlusion, and/or lateral tarsorrhaphy.
  - **Eyelid retraction** may require surgical eyelid lengthening.
  - **Diplopia** is treated acutely with systemic steroids (prednisone 80–100 mg PO qd for 1–2 weeks, then taper over 1 month), and then prism glasses may be prescribed or strabismus surgery is considered when the condition is stable.
  - **Optic neuropathy** is immediately treated with systemic steroids (prednisone 100 mg PO qd for 2–7 days) and orbital decompression. External-beam radiation (15–30 Gy) may also be considered.
- Treatment of any underlying thyroid disease by an endocrinologist should be performed concurrently, but this may not affect the acute orbital process.

Prognosis

The prognosis depends on the severity of ocular involvement and the presence of a compressive optic neuropathy; however, most patients do well. Multiple surgeries may be required.

IDIOPATHIC ORBITAL INFLAMMATION

Definition

Orbital pseudotumor or idiopathic orbital inflammation is an idiopathic inflammatory disorder of the orbital tissues. It may be acute or chronic and involve the lacrimal gland (dacryoadenitis), extraocular muscles (myositis), sclera (scleritis), optic nerve sheath (optic perineuritis), orbital fat, and/or orbital apex (**Tolosa–Hunt syndrome**). A sclerosing type may also occur.

Epidemiology

Idiopathic orbital inflammation affects patients of all ages. Children commonly have bilateral disease, while adults usually have unilateral disease. Adults require an evaluation for systemic vasculitis (e.g., Wegener's granulomatosis, polyarteritis nodosa) or lymphoproliferative disorders.

Symptoms

Idiopathic orbital inflammation presents with orbital pain, decreased vision, binocular diplopia, red eye, headaches, and constitutional symptoms (present in 50% of children).

Signs

The examination is notable for tenderness of the involved region, lid edema and erythema, ptosis, lacrimal gland enlargement, restricted and painful ocular movements, proptosis (protruding globe), resistance to retropulsion of the globe, induced hyperopia, conjunctival injection and chemosis, reduced corneal sensation (due to cranial nerve V_1 involvement), and increased IOP (Figures 7–10 and 7–11). Children may also have papillitis or iritis. Patients with Tolosa–Hunt syndrome present with painful ophthalmoplegia and decreased vision.

Differential diagnosis

Idiopathic orbital inflammation is essentially a diagnosis of exclusion, so it is important to rule out thyroid-related ophthalmopathy, orbital cellulitis, orbital tumors, lacrimal

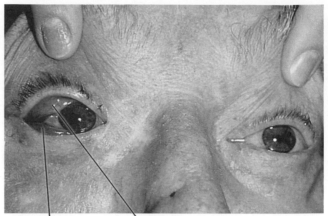

Conjunctival   Lacrimal gland
chemosis   enlargement

FIGURE 7–11
Idiopathic orbital inflammation of the right orbit with lacrimal gland involvement. Note the swollen, prolapsed lacrimal gland superiorly.

gland tumors, orbital vasculitis, trauma, arteriovenous fistula, cavernous sinus thrombosis, gaze palsies, and herpes zoster ophthalmicus.

Evaluation

- It is important to obtain a **history** of previous episodes, cancer, or other systemic disease.
- The **eye exam** must include examination of the cranial nerves (rule out a palsy), visual acuity (decreased), pupillary response (may have a positive RAPD), ocular motility (restricted, forced duction testing), lid and orbital palpation (lacrimal gland mass, resistance to retropulsion), exophthalmometry (proptosis), conjunctiva (injection and chemosis), cornea (staining from exposure), tonometry (increased IOP), and ophthalmoscopy (retina and optic nerve appearance).
- **Orbital CT scan** shows extraocular muscle enlargement *involving* the tendons (as opposed to TRO, which spares the tendons), scleral thickening and enhancement, and diffuse inflammation with orbital fat streaking. Lacrimal gland involvement can also be seen.
- **Lab tests** are ordered for bilateral or unusual cases to rule out vasculitis: CBC with differential, erythrocyte sedimentation rate, antinuclear antibodies, blood urea nitrogen, creatinine, fasting blood glucose, antineutrophil cytoplasmic antibodies, and urinalysis.
- Consider **orbital biopsy** for cases that are unusual or unresponsive to steroids.

Management

- Idiopathic orbital inflammation is treated with systemic steroids (prednisone 80–100 mg PO qd for 1 week, then taper slowly over 6 weeks). A dramatic response should be seen within 24–48 hours; if not, another diagnosis must be considered.

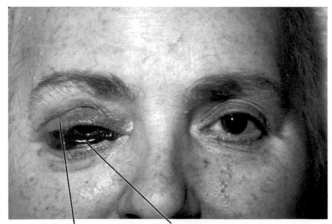

Lid erythema   Conjunctival chemosis

FIGURE 7–10
Idiopathic orbital inflammation of the right orbit with lid edema, ptosis, and chemosis.

- Orbital decompression for compressive optic neuropathy.

Prognosis

Although recurrences are common, the prognosis is generally good for acute disease. The sclerosing form of idiopathic orbital inflammation has a more insidious onset and is often less responsive to treatment.

Tumors

Many tumors involve the orbit. Most orbital masses produce proptosis with or without pain as well as displacement of the eye (globe dystopia). Sometimes the medical history is suggestive of the specific type of tumor, but more commonly, the diagnosis is made based upon the lesion's appearance on imaging studies. The childhood tumors are discussed in Chapter 6, while those that occur in adults are reviewed below.

CAVERNOUS HEMANGIOMA

Cavernous hemangioma is the most common adult orbital tumor. This venous malformation typically presents in the 4th to 6th decades, more often in women. Patients usually notice painless decreased vision or diplopia. They develop slowly progressive proptosis and a compressive optic neuropathy. Other findings include induced hyperopia, strabismus, increased IOP, and chorioretinal folds. The tumor may enlarge during pregnancy.

- **Orbital CT scan** reveals a well-circumscribed intraconal (within the extraocular muscles) or extraconal lesion *without* bony erosion.
- **B-scan ultrasonography** demonstrates a smooth lesion. **A-scan ultrasonography** shows high internal reflectivity within the lesion.
- Complete surgical excision by an oculoplastic surgeon is indicated for compressive optic neuropathy, intractable diplopia, or proptosis.

MUCOCELE

Mucocele represents a cystic sinus mass caused by obstructed excretory ducts. This lesion may produce bony erosion and invade the orbit, most commonly in the superonasal quadrant. There is usually a history of chronic sinusitis (frontal and ethmoid), but a mucocele can also be associated with cystic fibrosis (Figures 7–12 and 7–13).

- **Head and orbital CT scan** is performed to rule out encephalocele and meningocele. A mucocele appears as an orbital lesion and orbital wall defect with sinus opacification.

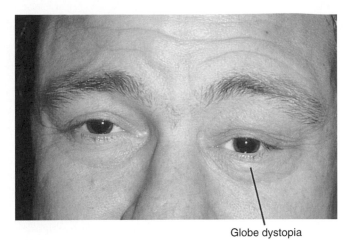

Globe dystopia

FIGURE 7–12
Mucocele of the orbit with left globe dystopia.

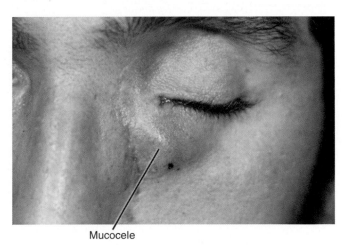

Mucocele

FIGURE 7–13
Mucocele of the left eye.

- Complete surgical excision should be performed by an oculoplastic surgeon, and the patient is placed on systemic antibiotics (ampillicin/sulbactam (Unasyn) 1.5–3 g IV q6h).

NEURILEMMOMA (SCHWANNOMA)

Neurilemmoma (schwannoma) is a rare, benign tumor composed of Schwann cells. It is usually located in the superior orbit of middle-aged individuals and rarely is associated with neurofibromatosis. These tumors can grow along any peripheral or cranial nerve, most commonly cranial nerve VIII (acoustic neuroma). Patients experience gradual, painless proptosis and globe displacement; however, pain may occur from perineural spread and nerve compression (Figure 7–14).

- **Orbital CT scan** demonstrates a well-circumscribed lesion similar in appearance to a cavernous hemangioma.

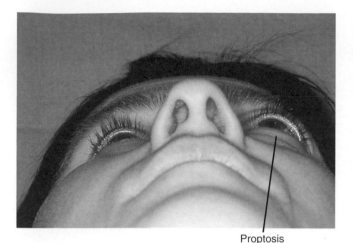

Proptosis

FIGURE 7–14
Neurilemmoma (schwannoma) producing proptosis of the left eye.

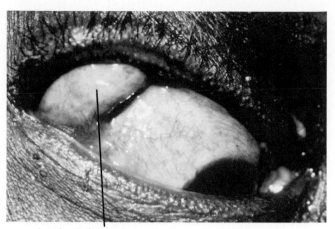

Lacrimal gland enlargement

FIGURE 7–15
Lacrimal gland enlargement due to reactive lymphoid hyperplasia.

- **B-scan ultrasonography** demonstrates a smooth lesion. **A-scan ultrasonography** shows low internal reflectivity, which differentiates this tumor from a cavernous hemangioma.
- Complete surgical excision should be performed by an oculoplastic surgeon.

MENINGIOMA

Meningioma (see Ch. 5) may arise from the optic nerve (primary orbital meningioma) or sphenoid bone with expansion into the orbit.

LYMPHOID TUMORS

Lymphoid tumors represent a spectrum of disorders characterized by the abnormal proliferation of lymphoid tissue. Lymphoid infiltrates, which account for approximately 10% of all orbital tumors, are classified as benign reactive lymphoid hyperplasia, atypical lymphoid hyperplasia, and malignant lymphoma. These lesions usually occur in patients 50–70 years old, more commonly in women, and are extremely rare in children (invasion by Burkitt's lymphoma). Patients present with painless proptosis, diplopia, and visual disturbances, and may have conjunctival salmon patches or lacrimal gland enlargement (Figures 7–15 and 7–16).

Lymphoid tumors are clinically indistinguishable, and therefore tissue biopsy and immunohistochemical studies are required for diagnosis. Lymphoma is nearly always extranodal, B-cell, non-Hodgkin's type, and more than 50% are mucosa-associated lymphoid tissue (MALT)-type lymphomas. Orbital lymphoma carries a 50% risk of systemic involvement. The location of the ocular tumor appears more important than the histopathology in determining systemic involvement: eyelids (67% will have systemic involvement) > orbit (35%) > conjunctiva

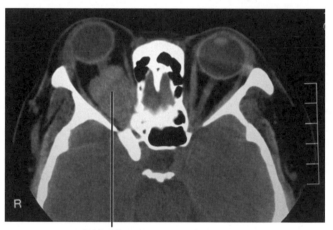

Orbital tumor

FIGURE 7–16
Orbital computed tomography scan showing right orbital lymphoid tumor and proptosis.

(20%). Forty percent of patients with atypical lymphoid hyperplasia develop systemic disease within 5 years. The 5-year survival rate of orbital lymphoma is 90%.

- **Orbital CT scan** reveals a solid tumor with molding to surrounding structures.
- A **systemic evaluation** by an internist or oncologist must be performed in the presence of biopsy-proven orbital lymphoma. This should be done every 6 months for 2 years and includes a thoracic, abdominal, and pelvic CT scan, CBC with differential, serum protein electrophoresis, erythrocyte sedimentation rate, bone marrow biopsy, and possibly a bone scan.
- Localized orbital disease is controlled with low-dose, fractionated radiotherapy (15–20 Gy for benign lesions, and 20–30 Gy for malignancy).
- Systemic disease is treated with radiation to the orbit and chemotherapy.

METASTATIC TUMORS

Metastatic tumors are the most common orbital malignancy, comprising 10% of all orbital tumors. The primary sources are most frequently the breast, lung, prostate, and gastrointestinal tract. Patients with metastatic tumors present with rapid-onset, painful proptosis, restricted ocular motility, and diplopia. A notable exception is scirrhous breast cancer, which characteristically causes enophthalmos due to orbital fibrosis.

- **Orbital CT scan** demonstrates bony erosion and destruction of adjacent structures.
- An immediate **hematology and oncology consultation** is indicated for treatment of the underlying malignancy.
- Palliation with local radiotherapy should be performed by a radiation oncologist experienced in orbital processes.

Atrophia Bulbi/Phthisis Bulbi

Progressive ocular degeneration and decompensation may occur after severe eye trauma or even surgery. There are three stages of ocular atrophy:

1. **Atrophia bulbi without shrinkage**: the size and shape of the globe are normal, but intraocular findings may include cataract, retinal detachment, synechiae, and/or cyclitic membranes.
2. **Atrophia bulbi with shrinkage**: the globe is softer and smaller than normal, with decreased IOP, flat anterior chamber, and an edematous cornea with vascularization, fibrosis, and opacification.
3. **Atrophia bulbi with disorganization (phthisis bulbi)**: the globe is approximately two-thirds normal size with thickened sclera, intraocular disorganization, and calcification of the cornea, lens, and retina. There may be spontaneous hemorrhages, inflammation, or bone formation in uveal tissue. These eyes have an increased risk of intraocular malignancies and usually have no vision (Figure 7–17).
   - **B-scan ultrasonography** is recommended annually to rule out intraocular malignancy.
   - Painful phthisical eyes are initially treated with a topical steroid (prednisolone acetate 1% qid) and cycloplegic (atropine 1% tid). Retrobulbar alcohol or chlorpromazine (Thorazine) injections are alternatives for severe ocular pain in eyes with no vision.
   - A cosmetic shell may be worn over the atrophic globe to improve the appearance and support the eyelid.
   - Enucleation usually cures the pain as well as improves cosmesis. Modern techniques involve the insertion of porous orbital implants to which the extraocular muscles are attached, allowing for natural-appearing movement of the prosthesis.

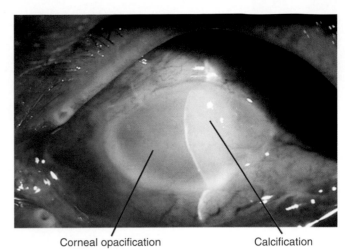

Corneal opacification   Calcification

FIGURE 7–17
Phthisis bulbi demonstrating shrunken globe. The cornea is opaque, edematous, and thickened, and the anterior chamber is shallow.

Anophthalmia

Anophthalmia refers to absence of the eye. This condition is rarely congenital but rather results from enucleation or evisceration of the globe. After removal of an eye due to malignancy, severe trauma, or pain and blindness, the patient commonly receives an integrated or separate orbital implant and cosmetic shell (Figures 7–18 and 7–19). These are generally well tolerated; however, there is a risk that the socket may become infected or the implant may erode through the remaining conjunctiva.

- In the event of such an occurrence, the patient may present with mucopurulent discharge, pain in one direction of gaze, or serosanguineous tears. Prompt examination is necessary to inspect the eyelids, conjunctiva, and socket. In particular, it is important to look for cellulitis, ptosis, eyelid retraction, superior

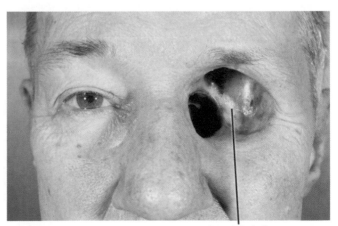

Anophthalmia

FIGURE 7–18
Acquired anophthalmia of the left eye secondary to evisceration for orbital tumor.

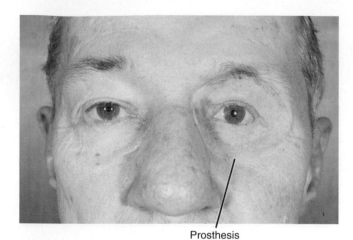

Prosthesis

FIGURE 7–19
Same patient as in Figure 7–18 with prosthesis in place.

tarsal giant papillae, and conjunctival inflammation, dehiscence, or erosion with exposure of the implant. If there is no conjunctival defect or lesion, then treatment with a broad-spectrum antibiotic drop (polytrim 1 gtt qid) is sufficient. However, if a conjunctival defect is observed, then the patient must be referred to an orbital surgeon for exploration and wound closure.

- An exposed implant is at risk for orbital cellulitis, and therefore treatment with systemic oral antibiotics (cephalexin 250–500 mg PO qid or amoxicillin/clavulanate (Augmentin) 250–500 mg PO tid) must be instituted.

- The orbital prosthesis is replaced with a conformer for the duration of the infection since the absence of a prosthesis or conformer in the socket for greater than 24 hours is a risk for conjunctival scarring (cicatrization), forniceal foreshortening, and socket contracture.

CHAPTER EIGHT

Lids and Adnexa

EYELIDS

Introduction

The eyelids protect the eye by serving as a physical barrier as well as a lubricating system. Proper lid function contributes to a healthy tear film and ocular surface, which are important for clear vision. Therefore, various processes that affect the eyelids can interfere with sight. These include trauma, infections, inflammation, malpositions, and tumors.

Trauma

Trauma involving the eyelid requires a thorough evaluation because apparently minor injuries may actually be vision-threatening. Blunt and penetrating trauma can result in either open or closed soft-tissue injury. An orbital computed tomography (CT) scan should be ordered if the trauma is associated with an ominous mechanism of injury, orbital signs, or massive periocular injury. Retained foreign matter, improper wound repair, or canalicular damage may produce undesirable complications such as infection, chronic discomfort, lid deformities, and tearing (epiphora).

CONTUSION

An eyelid contusion or bruise usually occurs after blunt trauma. A diffuse hematoma forms within the lid, producing ecchymosis and edema (Figure 8–1). Ptosis, from a mass effect or direct injury to the levator muscle, may also occur and can last for up to 6 months. Frequently, there is concomitant ocular injury, so it is important to

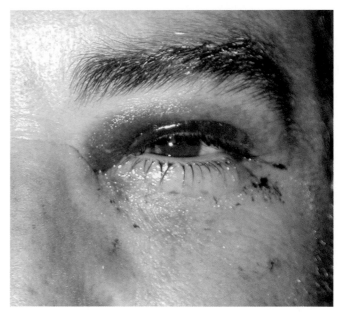

FIGURE 8–1
Eyelid contusion with prominent ecchymosis of the upper lid and eyelid swelling nasally.

assess the eye carefully. A lid contusion is treated with cold compresses (10–15 minutes qid for 24–48 hours) to reduce the bleeding and swelling. In contrast to a retrobulbar hemorrhage, an orbital compartment syndrome does not result from a preseptal hematoma so a canthotomy is not necessary. The prognosis is excellent in the absence of ocular or bony injuries.

LACERATION

A lid laceration is a partial or full-thickness cut in the eyelid involving superficial (skin) and deep structures

125

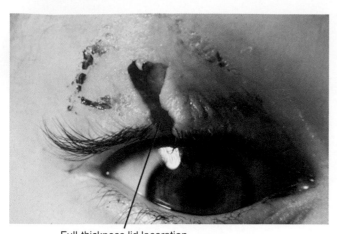

Full-thickness lid laceration

FIGURE 8–2
Full-thickness upper-eyelid laceration.

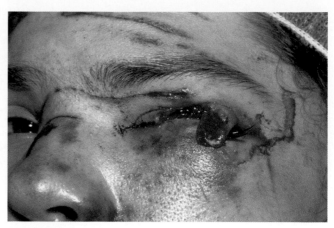

FIGURE 8–3
Severe eyelid laceration with large-tissue defect and fragment of upper lid dangling.

(muscle and fat). Fat prolapsing into the wound indicates violation of the orbital septum. Lacerations are most commonly due to penetrating trauma and are categorized according to whether or not the lid margin, canthus, or canaliculus (tear duct) is involved (Figure 8–2). Lacerations involving the nasal lid margin between the punctum and the medial canthus of either eyelid require probing of the lacrimal system to diagnose involvement of the canaliculus. Sometimes it is identified on inspection as a pouting gray structure.

All wounds must be inspected for foreign bodies and probed to evaluate for penetration of the septum and involvement of the canaliculus. As much tissue as possible must be preserved, and the wound may require two-layer closure. The lid margin is reapproximated with three interrupted sutures carefully placed at the muco-cutaneous junction, posterior lid margin, and lash line to minimize the risk of lid notching. Sutures are removed 7–10 days later. Canalicular lacerations require naso-lacrimal duct intubation with a silicone stent for 3 months. Depending on the mechanism of injury, a prophylactic tetanus booster and rabies shot (for animal bites) may be necessary. Dirty wounds require systemic antibiotics (dicloxacillin 250–500 mg PO qid for 7–10 days, consider penicillin V 500 mg PO qid for animal or human bites). Early wound repair is usually successful, but complications such as lid notching, entropion, ectropion, cicatrix, epiphora, and infection, may develop.

AVULSION

A special type of laceration, an eyelid avulsion, refers to a tearing injury causing part of the lid or the entire lid to be severed. The resulting tissue defect requires surgical repair, and the technique used depends upon the degree and location of the injury. The procedure may be complicated if there is tissue loss, so care must be taken to preserve any avulsed portion. Defects are classified by size

(small (<25%), moderate (25–50%), and large (>50%)) and location (upper versus lower eyelid; Figure 8–3). Small defects are amenable to direct closure, while moderate or large ones require flap advancements, reconstructions with grafts, and sometimes lid-sharing procedures. The latter should be avoided in young children to prevent deprivation amblyopia (see Ch. 6).

Infections

Eyelid infections are caused by a variety of organisms. The most serious lid infection is cellulitis since it can quickly spread to the orbit without proper treatment (see section on preseptal cellulitis in Ch. 7). Superficial infections of the eyelid skin are due to bacteria, viruses, and lice. Herpetic infections, which are very common in ophthalmology, initially occur on the eyelids, while recurrences affect the eye itself.

BLEPHARITIS/MEIBOMITIS

Definition

Inflammation of the eyelid margins (**blepharitis**) and clogging of the eyelid oil glands (**meibomitis**) often occur together.

Etiology

Blepharitis and meibomitis are very common conditions caused by chronic *Staphylococcus* or *Demodex* infection, seborrhea, and eczema. Seborrheic or staphylococcal blepharitis affects the anterior lid margin, while meibomitis affects the posterior lid margin. Another type of blepharitis that affects the lateral canthal angles, angular blepharitis, is due to *Moraxella* infection. Anterior and posterior lid margin disease is associated with dry eyes, acne rosacea, and chalazia.

Symptoms

The severity of symptoms varies, but patients usually complain of itching, burning, tearing, mild pain, foreign-body sensation, and redness, which is often worse in the morning and late in the day.

Signs

On examination, the lid margins appear thickened and erythematous with telangiectatic blood vessels. Crusting of the eyelashes ("scurf" and "collarettes") is found in blepharitis. Swollen, blocked meibomian glands are the hallmark of meibomitis, and often gentle pressure on the lids expresses columns of thick, white sebaceous material ("toothpaste sign") (Figures 8–4 and 8–5). Eye findings may include conjunctival injection and corneal staining.

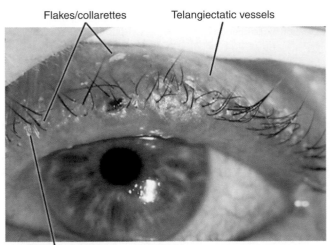

Flakes/collarettes   Telangiectatic vessels

Thickened lid margin

FIGURE 8–4
Blepharitis with thickened eyelid margins, flakes, and collarettes.

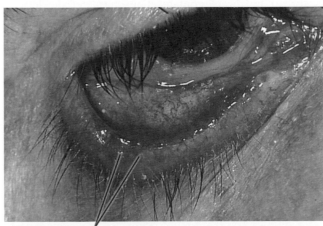

Blocked meibomian glands

FIGURE 8–5
Meibomitis demonstrating inspissated right lower-eyelid meibomian glands with obstructed, pouting orifices.

Differential diagnosis

Other conditions that present in a similar manner are dry-eye syndrome, herpes simplex virus (HSV), corneal foreign body, allergic or infectious conjunctivitis, sebaceous cell carcinoma, squamous or basal cell carcinoma, discoid lupus, medicamentosa, and ocular cicatricial pemphigoid.

Evaluation

- When gathering the **history**, it is important to ask about a history of skin cancer, acne rosacea, allergies, eye medications, and chronic, recurrent eyelid disease. Unilateral, chronic, refractory symptoms suggest malignancy.
- The **eye exam** must focus on the appearance of the lids (lid margins, meibomian gland orifices, and lashes), conjunctiva (injection), and cornea (inferior staining with fluorescein).
- **Biopsy** lesions that are suspicious for malignancy (ulcerated, chronic, scarred, or unilateral lid lesions).

Management

- There is no cure for the lid inflammation, but rather, treatment is aimed at minimizing the inflammation to resolve the symptoms.
- The mainstay of therapy is daily lid hygiene with warm compresses (applied to closed lids for 10 minutes) followed by lid scrubs (commercial preparations or a warm solution of baby shampoo and water applied rigorously to the lids and lashes using cotton, a face cloth, or cotton-tipped applicator).
- Apply topical antibiotic ointment (bacitracin or erythromycin) at bedtime for 2–4 weeks.
- Consider oral doxycycline (50–100 mg qd), oral flaxseed oil and omega-3 fatty acids (TheraTears Nutrition gel capsules, 2 bid), and/or topical Restasis eyedrops bid for recalcitrant cases. A short (1–2-week) course of topical steroids may be useful but should be used with caution.
- Treatment may also be required for associated rosacea or dry eye.

Prognosis

Recurrence is common and maintenance treatment is often required indefinitely.

HERPES SIMPLEX VIRUS

Primary infection with HSV causes a vesicular dermatitis, which is usually mild and easily overlooked. When HSV is mentioned in relation to the eye, our initial response is to imagine the classic corneal dendrite. However, this characteristic lesion actually represents a secondary or recurrent lesion (see Ch. 11). The primary infection affects the skin and therefore is seen on the

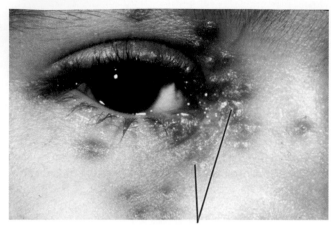

FIGURE 8–6
Primary herpes simplex virus with eyelid vesicles.

Seropurulent vesicles

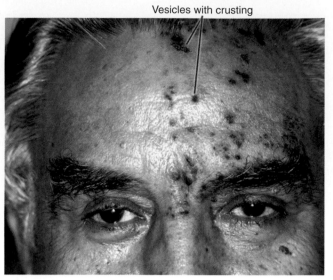

Vesicles with crusting

FIGURE 8–7
Herpes zoster virus demonstrating unilateral cranial nerve V_1 dermatomal distribution (trigeminal nerve ophthalmic branch).

eyelids, usually in children, who may have pain, itching, and redness. The dermatitis appears as small crops of seropurulent vesicles that rupture and then form scabs (Figure 8–6). Lesions on the lid margin may produce ulcerative blepharitis, follicular conjunctivitis, and punctate or dendritic keratitis. There may also be preauricular lymphadenopathy. Treatment of primary HSV consists of applying cool compresses (bid to qid) and topical antibiotic ointment to the affected skin area. Topical antiviral medications (trifluridine 0.1% 9 times a day or vidarabine 3% 5 times a day for 14 days) are reserved for concomitant blepharoconjunctivitis or corneal involvement. Patients are given a systemic antiviral (acyclovir (Zovirax) 400 mg PO 5 times a day for 10 days or famciclovir (Famvir) 500 mg PO tid for 7 days) if constitutional symptoms are present.

HERPES ZOSTER VIRUS/VARICELLA ZOSTER VIRUS

Reactivation of latent varicella zoster virus causes the classic unilateral dermatomal skin eruption known as shingles. Facial involvement is along the distribution of cranial nerve V, most commonly V_1, with a maculopapular rash followed by vesicular ulceration and crusting (Figure 8–7).

Patients may have constitutional symptoms, including fever, lymphadenopathy, headache, malaise, nausea, and altered sensation (i.e., tingling, paresthesias, burning) over the affected dermatome. Herpes zoster ophthalmicus refers to the potentially severe and recurrent keratouveitis resulting from nasociliary nerve involvement (see Chs 11 and 12). Thus, a skin lesion on the tip of the patient's nose (**Hutchinson's sign**) is a clue that the eye may be affected. Even if herpes zoster ophthalmicus is not present, eyelid involvement alone may be complicated by scarring with entropion, ectropion, lash loss, canalicular and punctal

stenosis, and lid retraction with exposure keratitis. Management of the eyelid infection is similar to that for HSV: cool compresses and topical antibiotic ointment (erythromycin or bacitracin) bid to tid to the affected skin, and systemic antivirals (acyclovir (Zovirax) 800 mg PO 5 times a day for 10 days or famciclovir (Famvir) 500 mg PO tid for 7 days). Immunocompromised patients are placed on acyclovir 10–12 mg/kg/day IV in divided doses q8h for 10–14 days. Postherpetic neuralgia can be treated with Zostrix (capsaicin 0.025% tid to qid) cream to the affected area or amitriptyline (25 mg PO tid).

MOLLUSCUM CONTAGIOSUM

Molluscum contagiosum is another viral infection usually seen in children. This infection, caused by the poxvirus, is spread by direct contact. The characteristic lesions are usually asymptomatic and appear as shiny dome-shaped papules with central umbilication on the lid or lid margin, although they may be present anywhere on the body (Figure 8–8). Lid involvement can cause a chronic follicular conjunctivitis and punctate keratitis. The disease is self-limited, but may take years to resolve. Treatment of one or more lesions with curettage, cryotherapy, or cautery may stimulate the immune system to eliminate the others.

PHTHIRIASIS PALPEBRUM

Phthiriasis palpebrum or **pediculosis** is an infestation of the eyelashes with lice. This infection is directly transmitted, usually through sexual contact, and causes a blepharoconjunctivitis with intense itching. The significant findings on exam are conjunctival follicles and

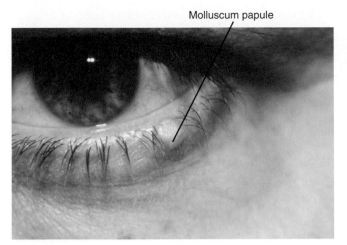

Molluscum papule

FIGURE 8–8
Molluscum contagiosum, demonstrating characteristic shiny, domed papule with central umbilication of the lower eyelid.

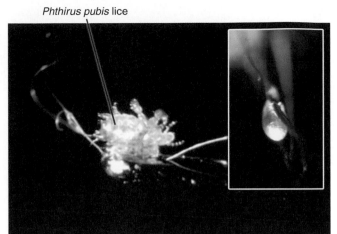

Phthirus pubis lice

FIGURE 8–10
Close-up of eyelash with *Phthirus pubis*.

injection, and small white eggs (nits) and lice attached to the lashes (Figures 8–9 and 8–10). Pediculosis is treated by manually removing nits and lice, suffocating lice with topical ointment, and delousing with creams and shampoo.

Inflammation

CHALAZION/HORDEOLUM (STYE)

Definition

Chalazion and hordeolum are similar in appearance and are often confused. Although these terms are usually used interchangeably and indiscriminately when referring to an eyelid nodule, they are distinct processes that should be differentiated.

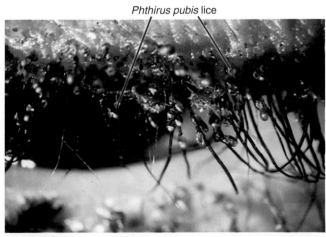

Phthirus pubis lice

FIGURE 8–9
Infestation of eyelashes with *Phthirus pubis*. Note the chronic skin changes at the base of the lashes.

Chalazion is a lipogranuloma resulting from leakage of sebum from an obstructed meibomian gland. A chalazion often emerges from an internal hordeolum and is associated with meibomitis and/or rosacea.

Hordeolum (stye) is an acute bacterial infection of an eyelid sebaceous gland, most commonly a meibomian gland (internal hordeolum) or a gland of Zeis or Moll (external hordeolum), associated with *Staphylococcus aureus*.

Symptoms

A chalazion/hordeolum presents acutely as a warm, tender, swollen, red eyelid lump. The eyelid may be droopy. As the inflammation resolves, chronic chalazia become non-tender. Patients may experience blurred vision.

Signs

One or more erythematous, often tender subcutaneous eyelid nodules, sometimes with visible pointing or drainage, is the characteristic appearance (Figures 8–11 and 8–12). Local swelling may prevent visualization or palpation of a discrete nodule. A large chalazion may produce ptosis as well as blurred vision from astigmatism (due to deformation of the cornea from a mass effect). Signs of blepharitis/meibomitis can also be present.

Differential diagnosis

It is important to rule out preseptal cellulitis in cases with severe lid swelling, erythema, and tenderness. Sebaceous cell carcinoma is commonly misdiagnosed as a recurrent chalazion. A pyogenic granuloma may also present in a similar fashion.

Evaluation

• Important aspects of the **history** are previous episodes, constitutional symptoms (i.e., fever), and the timing and character of the symptoms.

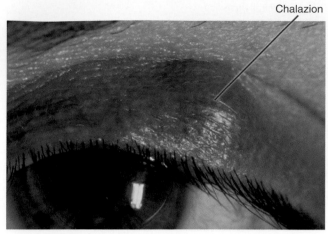

Chalazion

FIGURE 8–11
Chalazion of the upper eyelid.

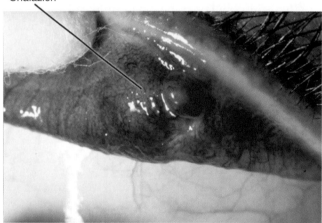

Chalazion

FIGURE 8–12
Everted eyelid of the same patient as in Figure 8–11, demonstrating the chalazion.

- The **eye exam** should pay particular attention to facial skin (rosacea), lids (blepharitis, meibomian gland evaluation, eyelid eversion), and cornea (astigmatism).
- **Biopsy** recurrent lesions to rule out malignancy.

Management

- Initial treatment is with warm compresses and gentle massage (10 minutes qid for 1 month). A topical antibiotic or combination antibiotic/steroid ointment (erythromycin, bacitracin, or Tobradex bid to tid) may be instilled in the inferior fornix during the first 2 weeks, especially if the lesion is draining.
- Consider incision and curettage or intralesional steroid injection (triamcinolone acetate 40 mg/ml; inject 0.5 ml with a 30-gauge needle) if there is no improvement to conservative therapy after 1 month.
- Treat underlying meibomitis and rosacea.
- Recurrent chalazia may respond to oral medication (doxycycline 100 mg PO bid or erythromycin 250 mg

PO qid). Tetracyclines must not be used in children and during pregnancy.

Prognosis

Most lesions fully resolve within weeks to months with conservative treatment, but recurrence is common (20%). Scarring may complicate surgical drainage, and steroid injection can cause hypopigmentation or local fat atrophy.

ACNE ROSACEA

Definition

Acne rosacea or "rosacea" is a chronic inflammatory disorder affecting the facial skin, with ocular involvement in >50%.

Etiology

Rosacea is idiopathic, but there is a genetic predilection (more common in persons of northern European ancestry). This disorder may be due to perivascular collagen degeneration with blood vessel dilatation and leakage of inflammatory substances into the skin. An inflammatory response to *Demodex folliculorum* may also be a contributing factor.

Symptoms

Patients typically report facial flushing (often resulting from a trigger such as ingestion of alcohol or spicy food), tearing, dry eye, and foreign-body sensation.

Signs

The hallmark of rosacea is the characteristic distribution of the skin changes. Erythema, flushing, pustules, papules, and telangiectasia predominantly involve the nose, malar region, chin, and brow. The ocular findings consist of blepharitis, chalazia, shortened tear break-up time, conjunctivitis, keratitis, and peripheral corneal neovascularization. Rhinophyma may eventually develop (Figure 8–13).

Evaluation

- The **history** should note awareness of facial flushing and any triggers, as well as ocular symptoms.
- The **eye exam** should concentrate on the facial skin (malar rash), lids (blepharitis, meibomitis, chalazia), conjunctiva (injection), and cornea (staining, vascularization).

Management

- Dermatologic manifestations:
  - Low-dose doxycycline (100 mg PO bid for 3 weeks, followed by 100 mg PO qd for 3–4 months) is very effective in treating the skin changes. Tetracycline can be substituted but requires more frequent

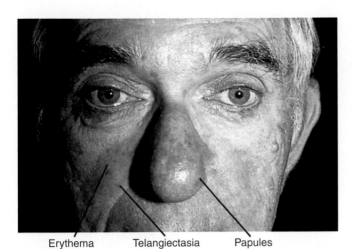

Erythema   Telangiectasia   Papules

FIGURE 8-13
Acne rosacea demonstrating rhinophyma (bulbous nose) and midline facial erythema in the malar and brow regions.

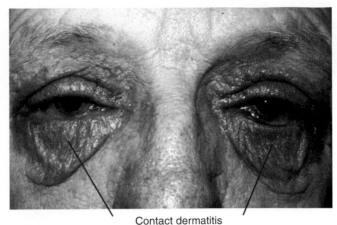

Contact dermatitis

FIGURE 8-14
Contact dermatitis, demonstrating bilateral erythematous, flaking rash.

dosing and is associated with more gastrointestinal side-effects. Neither agent is prescribed in children or during pregnancy.
- Topical metronidazole (0.75% bid for 2–4 weeks) is applied directly to the affected areas.
- Avoid agents that trigger flushing (i.e., alcohol, spicy foods, extreme temperatures, prolonged sunlight exposure, caffeine).
- Consider CO_2 laser, incisional surgery, or electro-cauterization for advanced rhinophyma.
- Ophthalmic manifestations:
  - Treat associated blepharitis and dry eye: oral doxycycline, flaxseed oil and omega-3 fatty acids, lid hygiene, Restasis, and artificial tear drops.

Prognosis

Acne rosacea is a chronic disease that waxes and wanes. There is no cure, but the manifestations can usually be controlled with treatment.

CONTACT DERMATITIS

Definition

Contact dermatitis is an acute inflammation of the skin due to chemical or mechanical irritants, or an allergic hypersensitivity reaction.

Symptoms

Patients experience acute eyelid swelling, redness, and itching. They may also have tearing and a foreign-body sensation.

Signs

An eyelid rash is visible with varying degrees of erythema, scaling, crusting, and edema. There may also be vesicles and weeping lesions, or even lichenified plaques, which suggest chronic exposure to the irritant (Figure 8–14).

Differential diagnosis

Similar skin changes may be produced by herpes simplex, herpes zoster, preseptal cellulitis, and burns.

Evaluation

- The **history** requires a thorough review of exposure to irritants such as soaps, fragrances, cosmetics, hairspray, nail polish, jewelry, medications, poison ivy, and chemical, ultraviolet, or thermal exposure.
- A careful **skin and eye exam** should be conducted with attention to the scalp, hair, hands, fingers, lids (rash), conjunctiva (injection), and cornea (staining).

Management

The treatment of eyelid dermatitis utilizes a stepwise strategy depending on the severity:
- Identify and eliminate the inciting agent(s).
- Apply cool compresses to the affected area.
- Topical antibiotic ointment (erythromycin or bacitracin bid) is used on crusted or weeping lesions.
- Consider using a mild steroid cream (<1% hydrocortisone bid to tid for 7–10 days) on the eyelids but avoid the lid margins and ocular exposure (therefore, it is safer to use an ophthalmic preparation such as FML ointment). Alternatively, an ophthalmic steroid solution may be massaged on to the affected eyelids. Periocular steroids should not be used for longer than 2 weeks without monitoring the intraocular pressure.
- Consider Protopic or Eladil, which are also very effective for eyelid dermatitis.
- An oral antihistamine (diphenhydramine 25–50 mg PO tid to qid) is prescribed for extensive lesions or itching.

- Consider short-term oral steroids (prednisone 40–80 mg PO qd tapered over 10–14 days) in severe cases.

Prognosis

Contact dermatitis typically resolves 1–2 weeks after removing the inciting agent. Steroids should be tapered gradually to avoid a rebound.

Malpositions

Proper eyelid position is important for maintaining a healthy ocular surface. Structural lid abnormalities may cause not only cosmetic deformities but also increased risk of ocular infection and trauma. These conditions require early recognition to prevent potential complications. **Dermatochalasis** may affect any of the lids but tends to be more symptomatic when the upper eyelids are involved. **Ptosis** occurs in the upper eyelids while **ectropion** and **entropion** are more common in the lower lids. **Blepharospasm** and **Bell's palsy** (see Ch. 5) are two other abnormalities of eyelid function that primarily affect the upper lids.

DERMATOCHALASIS

Dermatochalasis refers to redundant eyelid skin and subcutaneous tissue. This is caused by laxity from involutional changes with aging. The orbital fat frequently prolapses through an attenuated septum as discrete bulges, giving the lids a lumpy appearance. This condition is also associated with upper-eyelid ptosis (droopy lid) or pseudoptosis (mechanical effect from the dermatochalasis) (Figure 8–15). In severe cases, there may be a superior visual field defect. Dermatochalasis is managed surgically with blepharoplasty.

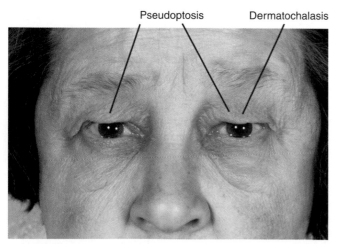

Pseudoptosis   Dermatochalasis

FIGURE 8–15
A patient with pseudoptosis from dermatochalasis.

BLEPHAROPTOSIS (PTOSIS)

Definition

Blepharoptosis, more commonly known as ptosis, is drooping of the upper eyelid.

Etiology

Ptosis is classified according to the underlying mechanism:

Involutional (aponeurotic): due to disinsertion, central dehiscence, or attenuation of the levator aponeurosis. This is the most common type of ptosis, and is associated with aging, eye surgery or trauma, pregnancy, and chronic eyelid swelling. Levator function is good.

Mechanical: due to the mass effect of tumors, dermatochalasis, or blepharochalasis, or to tethering of the eyelid by scarring (cicatricial ptosis). Levator function is good.

Myogenic: due to muscle disorders such as chronic progressive external ophthalmoplegia, myotonic dystrophy, and myasthenia gravis. This is an uncommon form of ptosis with extremely poor levator function.

Neurogenic: due to faulty innervation to the levator (cranial nerve III palsy) or Müller's muscle (Horner's syndrome), or to multiple sclerosis. Levator function is variable depending on the underlying defect.

Congenital: usually myogenic and unilateral due to fibrosis and fat infiltration of the levator muscle. Levator function is poor from birth.

Symptoms

Patients may complain that one or both eyelids droop. In more advanced cases, they may see their upper eyelashes or report a noticeable defect in their superior vision. Use of the orbicularis muscle to elevate the lids may result in brow ache. Decreased vision can occur in congenital cases due to deprivation amblyopia.

Signs

By definition, the upper eyelid droops and does not elevate fully on upgaze (Figures 8–16–8–19). The eye appears smaller on the affected side, and the lid crease may be higher (involutional) or absent (congenital). In downgaze, the ptosis is usually accentuated (acquired cases), but in congential cases, the ptotic lid is higher than the unaffected lid (lid lag). If the visual axis is obscured, the patient may have decreased vision or may adopt a head tilt with chin-up position to improve vision (bilateral congenital ptosis). Other muscular and neurologic deficits may be present in patients with myogenic and neurogenic ptosis, respectively. Congenital ptosis is sometimes associated with lagophthalmos, astigmatism, strabismus, amblyopia, epicanthus, or blepharophimosis.

Acquired ptosis

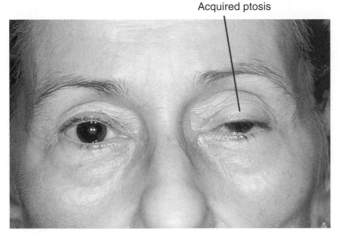

FIGURE 8–16
Significant acquired ptosis of the left eye. Most commonly caused by levator aponeurosis attenuation or dehiscence.

Congenital ptosis

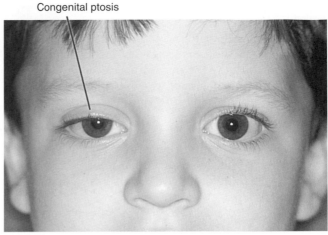

FIGURE 8–18
Congenital ptosis of the right eye in a child.

Acquired myogenic ptosis

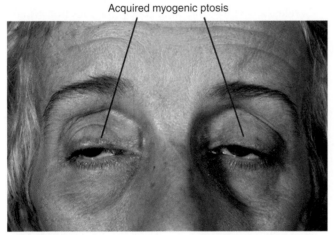

FIGURE 8–17
Bilateral acquired myogenic ptosis due to myasthenia gravis.

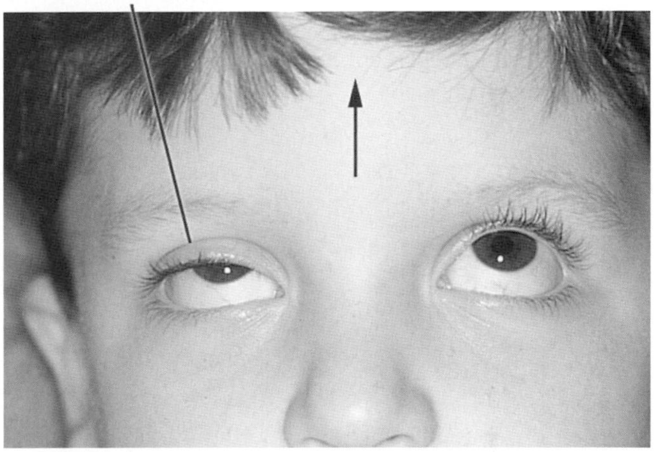

Poor levator function

FIGURE 8–19
Same patient as shown in Figure 8–18, demonstrating poor levator function with upgaze of the right eye. Note reduced levator excursion.

Differential diagnosis

When ptosis is suspected, it is also important to consider other processes that may cause pseudoptosis: dermatochalasis, lid swelling, enophthalmos, hypotropia, contralateral eyelid retraction or proptosis, or a small eye (e.g., phthisis bulbi, microphthalmia, nanophthalmos, anophthalmia).

Evaluation

- The **history** must include the age of onset, previous surgeries or trauma, degree of functional impairment and time of day when the ptosis is worst, associated symptoms such as generalized fatigue, breathing problems, and diplopia.
- A complete **eye exam** is performed with attention to visual acuity (amblyopia in children), lids (margin–reflex distance, palpebral fissure height, upper lid crease height, and levator function), pupillary response (Horner's syndrome, cranial nerve III palsy), and ocular motility (restricted). Ptosis surgery can sometimes be complicated by exposure keratopathy; therefore, it is also important to document the patient's ability to protect the cornea by evaluating the Bell's phenomenon, corneal sensation, and cornea (staining).
- **Visual field testing** is performed with and without the lids being held open by tape or finger (ptosis visual fields) to assess and record any visual impairment prior to surgery.
- Consider a **neurologic evaluation** and **Tensilon test** to rule out myasthenia gravis.
- Consider **pharmacologic pupil testing** to rule out Horner's syndrome.

Management

- Ptosis is corrected surgically with a variety of procedures depending upon the extent of levator function:
  - **Good levator function**: levator aponeurosis advancement, levator resection, Fasanella–Servat tarsoconjunctival resection, or superior tarsal (Müller's muscle) resection (also used for Horner's syndrome).
  - **Poor levator function**: usually frontalis suspension with silicone rods, fascia lata, or frontalis flap, but maximal levator resection can sometimes be helpful.
- Ptosis surgery should be performed by an experienced eyelid surgeon.
- Treat any underlying medical problems.

Prognosis

The prognosis is based on the etiology: excellent for acquired mechanical and involutional forms, fair to excellent for congenital ptosis, and variable for myogenic and neurogenic types. Ptosis repair may be complicated by over- or undercorrection, lid lag, lagophthalmos, and corneal exposure.

ECTROPION

Definition

Ectropion is the outward turning or eversion of the eyelid margin.

Etiology

Ectropion is classified by the underlying mechanism:

Cicatricial: due to contraction of the anterior eyelid lamella (skin and orbicularis muscle) as occurs with burns, trauma, or chronic inflammation.

Congenital: due to vertical shortening of the anterior lamella. This form is rarely isolated and may be associated with blepharophimosis syndrome.

Inflammatory: due to chronic inflammation such as atopic dermatitis, herpes zoster infection, or rosacea.

Involutional: due to horizontal lid laxity and tissue relaxation, which causes lid elongation, sagging, and conjunctival hypertrophy. This is the most common type of ectropion in adults and usually affects the lower eyelids.

Mechanical: due to eyelid edema, bulky lid tumors, orbital fat herniation, or poor-fitting glasses.

Paralytic: due to cranial nerve VII (Bell's) palsy.

Symptoms

Patients may be asymptomatic or present with tearing, redness, and chronic eyelid or ocular irritation.

Signs

By definition, the eyelid margin is everted with conjunctival keratinization, injection, and hypertrophy. There is often a superficial punctate keratitis (corneal staining) as well as dermatitis from chronic tearing and rubbing (Figure 8–20).

Evaluation

- The **history** should document any facial burns, trauma, surgery, or palsy.
- The **eye exam** focuses on orbicularis function, lids (position, laxity, herniated fat, scarring), conjunctiva (injection, hypertrophy), and cornea (staining).

Management

- Definitive treatment is surgical repair, which should be performed by an oculoplastic surgeon. The principles of surgery are to shorten the lid horizontally and lengthen the anterior lamella vertically. Any scar tissue is released. Mild congenital ectropion does not usually require treatment.
- Temporizing measures include taping the temporal side of the eyelid, suture tarsorrhaphy, moisture chamber goggles, and topical lubrication with non-preserved artificial tears (up to q1h) and ointment (qhs).
- Treat any underlying inflammatory dermatologic condition.
- Remove any contributing mechanical force (i.e., tumor or fat excision, eyeglass adjustment, etc.)

Prognosis

Surgical treatment is usually curative, but cicatricial or inflammatory ectropion is prone to recurrence. Paralytic ectropion is usually temporary and tends to resolve spontaneously within 6 months.

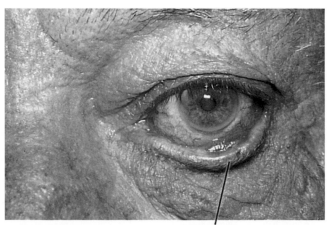

Ectropion

FIGURE 8–20
Involutional ectropion of the left lower eyelid.

ENTROPION

Definition

Entropion is the inward turning or inversion of the eyelid margin.

Etiology

Entropion is classified by the underlying mechanism:

Cicatricial: due to shortening of the posterior eyelid lamella (tarsus and conjunctiva), which occurs with Stevens–Johnson syndrome, ocular cicatricial pemphigoid, trachoma, herpes zoster, surgery, trauma, and chemical burns. This form is more common in the upper eyelid.

Congenital: due to structural tarsal plate defects, shortened posterior lamella, or eyelid retractor dysgenesis. It usually affects the upper eyelid.

Involutional: due to horizontal (canthal tendon) and vertical (eyelid retractor dehiscence) lid laxity, over-riding preseptal orbicularis muscle, and involutional enophthalmos. This is the most common type of entropion in older patients and usually affects the lower eyelids.

Spastic: due to ocular inflammation or irritation, this form often occurs after ocular surgery in patients with early underlying involutional changes or after prolonged patching. Squeezing the eyelids closed causes inward rolling of the lid margin.

Symptoms

The characteristic symptoms are tearing, foreign-body sensation, and red eye.

Signs

By definition, the eyelid margin is inverted. The eyelashes contact the ocular surface, causing conjunctival injection and corneal staining (Figure 8–21). Symblepharon (adhesion between the palpebral and bulbar conjunctiva) may also be seen in the cicatricial form.

Differential diagnosis

The differential diagnosis includes trichiasis, distichiasis, and blepharospasm.

Evaluation

- When recording the **history** it is important to ask about previous eye surgery, trauma, burns, and infections.
- The **eye exam** should focus on the lids (position, laxity, unusually deep inferior fornix), conjunctiva (injection), and cornea (staining).

Management

- Definitive treatment is surgical repair, which should be performed by an oculoplastic surgeon. The options

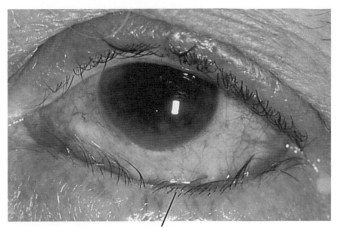

Entropion

FIGURE 8–21
Involutional entropion of the left lower eyelid.

for surgery are anterior lamellar resection or recession, horizontal lid tightening, lid retractor repair, eyelid margin rotation, and tarsal, conjunctival, or mucous membrane grafts.
- Temporizing measures to break the entropion/irritation cycle include techniques such as taping, thermal cautery, or sutures to evert the lid temporarily.
- Topical antibiotic ointment (erythromycin or bacitracin bid to qid) is recommended for corneal involvement.

Prognosis

The outcome is usually good, except for the cicatricial form.

TRICHIASIS

Definition

Trichiasis refers to misdirected eyelashes that touch the ocular surface.

Etiology

Trichiasis is caused by entropion, cicatricial eye disease, chronic eyelid inflammation, or may be idiopathic.

Symptoms

Patients have a red eye with foreign-body sensation and tearing.

Signs

By definition, eyelashes are seen directed toward and rubbing against the eye (Figures 8–22 and 8–23). There is also focal conjunctival injection and corneal staining in the areas of lash contact with the globe. Corneal scarring can develop in chronic cases.

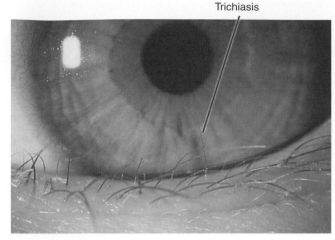

FIGURE 8-22
Trichiasis, demonstrating posterior misdirection of eyelid lashes touching the corneal epithelium. Not to be confused with distichiasis (see Figure 8–23).

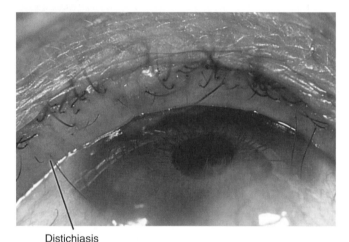

FIGURE 8-23
Distichiasis with lashes originating from meibomian gland orifice.

Differential diagnosis

Trichiasis and distichiasis (ectopic eyelashes) are distinct conditions that are sometimes mistaken for one another. They may exist simultaneously, but ectopic lashes do not necessarily cause trichiasis, and vice versa.

Evaluation

- The **history** should include questions about previous eye surgery, trauma, burns, and infections.
- The **eye exam** should focus on the lids (position, lashes), conjunctiva (injection), and cornea (staining, scarring).

Management

- Topical lubrication with non-preserved artificial tears (up to q1h) and ointment (qhs).

- Topical antibiotic ointment (erythromycin or bacitracin bid to qid for 5–7 days) for corneal involvement.
- For trichiasis with only a few misdirected lashes, mechanical epilation using fine forceps works temporarily.
- For extensive or recurrent trichiasis, consider electroepilation.
- For segmental trichiasis, consider cryotherapy or a full-thickness wedge resection, which should be performed by an oculoplastic surgeon.

Prognosis

Trichiasis eventually recurs after mechanical epilation. The other techniques are permanent; however, lid edema, eyelid notching, and skin depigmentation may complicate cryotherapy, while electroepilation has the potential for scarring adjacent follicles and eyelid tissue.

Tumors

A multitude of different types of tumors can affect the eyelids. These neoplasms, consisting of benign and malignant growths, are conveniently classified according to their cell of origin. The majority of lid tumors are pigmented, non-pigmented, vascular, or malignant growths of epithelial origin.

BENIGN TUMORS

Acquired nevus

Acquired nevus is a flat or elevated, pigmented lesion composed of modified melanocytes (Figure 8–24). Nevi arise in the epidermis (junctional), dermis (dermal) or both (compound), and tend to migrate deeper (into the dermis) with time. Growth during puberty is not

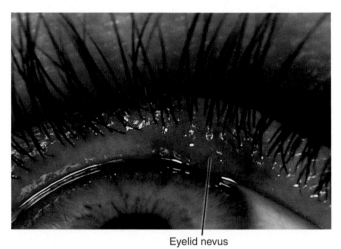

FIGURE 8-24
Nevus of the upper eyelid along the lid margin.

uncommon, but malignant transformation is rare. Excision is considered for cosmesis, chronic irritation, or evidence of malignancy.

Seborrheic keratosis

Seborrheic keratosis is a pigmented, plaque-like, growth with a "stuck-on" appearance commonly seen in the elderly (Figure 8–25). The tumor is comprised of basal epithelioid cells that proliferate within the dermis. Seborrheic keratoses frequently become irritated, but have no malignant potential. They can be excised if desired.

Squamous papilloma

Squamous papilloma, the most common benign eyelid tumor, is caused by hyperplasia of the squamous epithelium (Figure 8–26). The etiology is unclear, but some are viral (**verruca vulgaris**), associated with human papillomavirus (strains 6, 11, and 16) and having malignant potential (Figure 8–27). These occur in clusters, usually in children, while the non-viral variety are typically solitary and affect elderly individuals. Papillomas grow slowly as a sessile or pedunculated mass with a color similar to that of skin. They are frequently asymptomatic and may resolve spontaneously. Treatment is with surgical excision, cryotherapy, cautery, or laser ablation.

Xanthelasma

Xanthelasma refers to non-specific xanthomas of the eyelids that appear as flat or slightly elevated yellow plaques (Figure 8–28). Xanthelasma usually affects older patients, occurring on the medial aspect of the upper

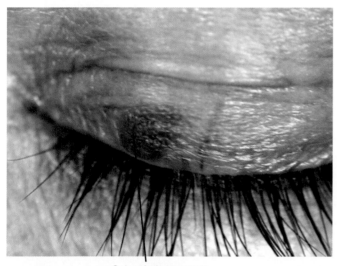

Seborrheic keratosis

FIGURE 8–25
Seborrheic keratosis at the lash line.

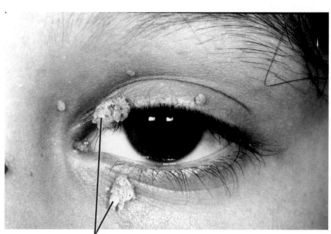

Verruca vulgaris

FIGURE 8–27
Verruca vulgaris, demonstrating multiple large and small lesions of the eyelids.

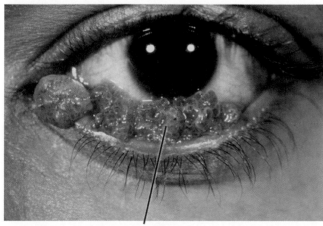

Squamous papilloma

FIGURE 8–26
Squamous papilloma demonstrating abundant multiple lesions of the lower eyelid.

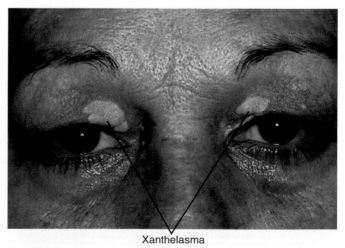

Xanthelasma

FIGURE 8–28
Xanthelasma, demonstrating characteristic yellow plaques on upper eyelids bilaterally.

eyelids bilaterally. A common misconception is that this lesion is related to hyperlipidemia. In fact, the majority of patients with xanthelasma have normal serum lipids. However, xanthomatosis is associated with certain systemic diseases, such as biliary cirrhosis, diabetes, pancreatitis, renal disease, and hypothyroidism. In severe cases, serum cholesterol and triglycerides should be evaluated. Unfortunately, the lesions usually recur after excision.

Epidermal inclusion cyst

Epidermal inclusion (**epidermoid**) cyst is a firm, round, mobile, subepithelial mass, which probably arises from occluded surface epithelium or pilosebaceous follicles carried into the subepithelium by trauma (Figure 8–29). The cyst contains cheesy keratin debris produced by the epithelial lining, and may produce a foreign-body granulomatous reaction upon rupture. Puncturing the cyst merely collapses it but eventually the lesion will reform. The cyst lining, responsible for producing the keratin, must be removed, so treatment requires complete surgical excision.

Milia

Milia are multiple, tiny, round, elevated, white nodules believed to be retention follicular cysts caused by obstructed pilosebaceous units (Figure 8–30). Milia occur spontaneously, or following trauma, radiation, herpes zoster ophthalmicus, or epidermolysis bullosa. These lesions are commonly treated by curettage with a 25–30-gauge needle, but other options include surgical excision, electrolysis, or diathermy.

Sebaceous cyst

Sebaceous (**pilar**) cyst is a smooth, elevated, subcutaneous yellow tumor with a central plug produced by an obstructed

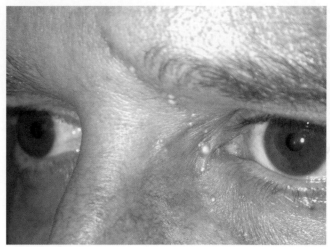

FIGURE 8–30
Milia, appearing as small white bumps in the medial canthus.

sebaceous or meibomian gland (Figure 8–31). This type of cyst is less common than the epidermoid type. It occurs in elderly patients and may be associated with chalazia. Definitive therapy is complete excision, including the epithelial lining.

Hemangioma

Hemangioma (see Ch. 6), the most common eyelid tumor in children, represents an abnormal collection of capillary blood vessels that usually appears within the first month of life as a blue subcutaneous mass or a superficial vascular lesion known as a "strawberry

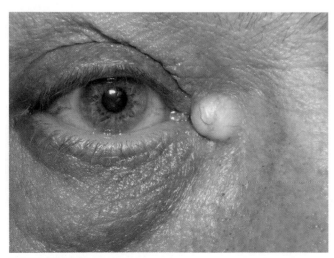

FIGURE 8–29
Epidermal inclusion cyst, appearing as a smooth round mass in the medial canthus.

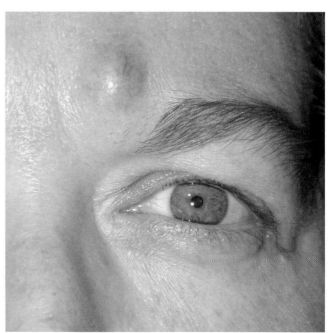

FIGURE 8–31
Sebaceous cyst, appearing as a solid nodule above the eyebrow.

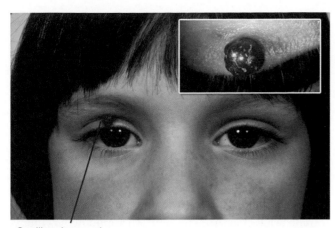

Capillary hemangioma

FIGURE 8–32
Capillary hemangioma involving right upper eyelid.

nevus" (Figure 8–32). The tumor rapidly grows during the first year of life, and then undergoes spontaneous involution. An eyelid lesion must be followed carefully, since ptosis and astigmatism can cause amblyopia and strabismus. Treatment of large hemangiomas is with intralesional steroid injection, systemic corticosteroids, or surgical excision. A pulsed dye laser can sometimes be helpful for treating the superficial component of the tumor.

Port wine stain

Port wine stain (**nevus flammeus**) is a congenital venular malformation that is often confused with a hemangioma. The port wine stain is distinguished by its lighter, purplish color, presence at birth, and dermatomal distribution along any or multiple branches of cranial nerve V (Figure 8–33). Furthermore, it does not blanch on palpation and does not involute, but instead grows with

the patient. With V_1 and V_2 involvement there is an increased risk of glaucoma (due to increased venous pressure) and Sturge–Weber syndrome (facial port wine stain, choroidal "hemangioma," intracranial vascular anomalies). Affected children must be examined early for choroidal involvement and glaucoma. A brain magnetic resonance imaging (MRI) scan is indicated for V_2 involvement. Treatment with a pulsed dye laser is recommended as early as 1 month of life.

MALIGNANT TUMORS

Risk factors for malignancy include increased age, sun exposure, fair skin, and a previous history or family history of skin cancer.

Basal cell carcinoma

Basal cell carcinoma (BCC) is the most common eyelid malignancy, constituting 90% of all malignant eyelid tumors. The tumor develops on sun-exposed areas in older adults, and is most frequently seen on the lower lid and medial canthus, followed by the upper lid and lateral canthus. BCC has two growth patterns:

1. **Nodular**: this is the more common, less invasive form, which appears as a firm, raised, pearly nodule usually with central ulceration, telangiectasia, lash loss (madarosis), and inflammation (Figures 8–34 and 8–35).
2. **Morpheaform**: this less common but more aggressive type presents as a firm, flat sclerosing lesion with indistinct borders and can penetrate by pagetoid spread (discontinuous areas of tumor spread) into the dermis.

BCC is locally invasive, but rarely metastatic. Treatment requires complete surgical excision with margin controls,

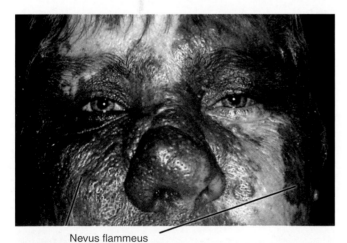

Nevus flammeus

FIGURE 8–33
Extensive nevus flammeus in a patient with encephalotrigeminal angiomatosis (Sturge–Weber syndrome).

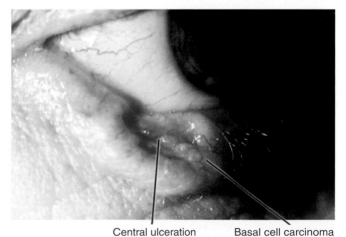

Central ulceration   Basal cell carcinoma

FIGURE 8–34
Basal cell carcinoma of the lower eyelid, demonstrating central ulceration with pearly, nodular border containing telangiectatic vessels.

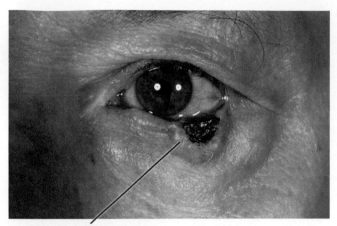

Basal cell carcinoma

FIGURE 8–35
Basal cell carcinoma of the lower eyelid, demonstrating central ulceration with scab and pearly, nodular borders.

so Moh's micrographic surgery is helpful. Orbital CT scan is performed for canthal tumors in order to evaluate posterior (orbital) involvement. Radiation and cryotherapy are not recommended for these lesions because posterior portions of the tumor may go untreated. Exenteration is necessary for orbital extension. The prognosis is excellent, but up to 10% recur locally.

Squamous cell carcinoma

Squamous cell carcinoma (SCC) is a less common cancer, comprising <5% of malignant eyelid tumors. This tumor, usually found on the lower eyelid as a flat or slightly elevated, scaly, ulcerated, erythematous plaque, is associated with solar or radiation injury, or other irritative insults (Figures 8–36). It often originates from an actinic keratosis, but may also arise from Bowen's disease or radiation dermatosis. SCC is locally invasive

and potentially metastatic. Spread to regional lymph nodes occurs in up to 25% of cases. The prognosis depends on tumor size, differentiation, etiology, and depth of invasion. Management is incisional or excisional biopsy with wide surgical margins and adjunctive radiation, cryotherapy, and/or chemotherapy. Exenteration is performed for orbital involvement.

Actinic keratosis

Actinic keratosis is the most common precancerous skin lesion; up to 25% develop SCC. It is associated with sun exposure and occurs in older adults, particularly those having fair complexions. Actinic keratosis appears as a round, scaly, flat growth with surrounding erythema (Figure 8–37). Histologically, it is squamous carcinoma-in-situ. Eyelid lesions are biopsied to rule out SCC, and then cryotherapy or surgical excision can be performed.

Keratoacanthoma

Keratoacanthoma, previously considered a form of pseudoepitheliomatous hyperplasia, is now classified as a squamous carcinoma. This lesion can be recognized by its distinctive presentation: rapid onset and growth (1–2 months) of a dome-shaped lesion with a central, ulcerated, keratin-filled crater and elevated rolled edges (Figure 8–38). Clinically, it resembles BCC, and is usually found in sun-exposed areas of older individuals. Eyelid involvement may cause madarosis and permanent damage to the lid margin. Keratoacanthoma often resolves spontaneously, but surgical excision is the treatment of choice.

Sebaceous cell carcinoma

Sebaceous cell carcinoma (**sebaceous adenocarcinoma**) is an extremely malignant tumor of the sebaceous glands in the eyelids or caruncle, and is the second most

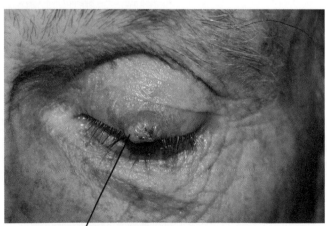

Squamous cell carcinoma

FIGURE 8–36
Squamous cell carcinoma of the left upper eyelid, demonstrating erythematous lesion with central scaly plaque.

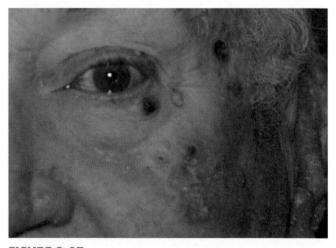

FIGURE 8–37
Actinic keratosis of the malar region demonstrating flat, erythematous, scaly appearance. The pigmented lesions are seborrheic keratoses.

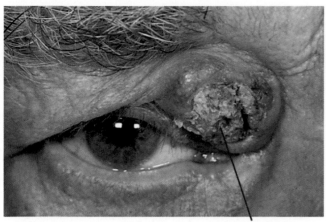

FIGURE 8–38
Keratoacanthoma of the right upper eyelid, demonstrating central keratin-filled crater with hyperkeratotic margins

common eyelid malignancy after BCC. This cancer most often presents in the 6th to 7th decade of life, more commonly in women, and usually in the upper eyelid (since it contains more meibomian glands than the lower lid). Sebaceous cell carcinoma may masquerade as chronic blepharitis (20–50% of patients) or a recurrent chalazion. The cardinal features are madarosis, poliosis (white eyelashes), and thick, red lid margin inflammation. The tumor is typically a hard, orange-yellow nodule, and pagetoid spread is common, as are regional lymphadenopathy and hematogenous metastasis (Figure 8–39). Treatment is with wide excision, frozen section, and conjunctival map biopsy. Exenteration is performed for orbital extension or pagetoid spread, and radiotherapy is used for palliation. The 5-year mortality rate is 30%, and poor prognostic factors include symptoms for longer than 6 months, size >2 cm, involvement of both upper and lower lids, poor differentiation, and local vascular or lymphatic infiltration.

Malignant melanoma

Malignant melanoma, the most lethal primary skin tumor, is fortunately quite rare, accounting for <1% of all eyelid malignancies. The lesion appears as a variably pigmented macule with irregular, notched borders, and can rapidly grow with color changes and nodule formation (Figure 8–40). There are three types of malignant melanoma:

1. **Nodular melanoma** (10%) is the most common type of melanoma affecting the eyelid. It typically occurs in the 5th decade of life, more frequently in men, and is always palpable. It is aggressive, with early vertical invasion and a 5-year survival rate of 44%.
2. **Superficial spreading melanoma** (80%) is not directly related to actinic damage and also originates on non-sun-exposed skin. This form usually occurs in individuals <60 years of age. The growth phase is initially horizontal before invading deeper. The 5-year survival rate is 69%.
3. **Lentigo maligna melanoma** (10%) arises from the precancerous lesion lentigo maligna found in sun-exposed areas of elderly patients. This is the least aggressive form, with a 5-year survival rate of 90%.

Melanoma can arise de novo or from nevi (20% of nodular and 50% of superficial spreading). Signs of malignant transformation include a change in color, shape, or size, crusting, and bleeding. Tumor growth is orderly and the staging is as follows:

- Stage 1: localized disease.
- Stage 2: regional lymph nodes (preauricular from the upper lid and submandibular from the lower lid).
- Stage 3: distant metastases.

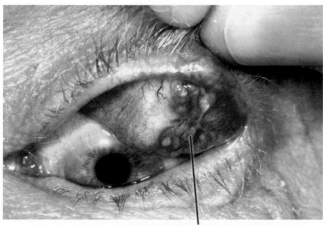

FIGURE 8–39
Sebaceous cell carcinoma with chronic lid changes of the left upper eyelid.

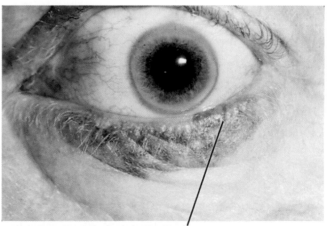

FIGURE 8–40
Malignant melanoma of the lower eyelid.

The cancer is excised with wide margins, lymph node dissection is carried out if microscopic evidence of lymphatic or vascular involvement exists, and orbital exenteration and neck dissection may be necessary in some cases. Depth of invasion is the most important prognostic factor; <0.75 mm indicates a favorable outcome.

Kaposi's sarcoma

Kaposi's sarcoma is a soft-tissue malignancy that occurs more commonly in immunocompromised patients and those of Mediterranean descent. The lesions, which are non-tender, violaceous nodules and plaques, may cause eyelid distortion with entropion, edema, and misdirected lashes (Figure 8–41). Treatment is complete surgical excision, but Kaposi's sarcoma is also responsive to other modalities such as cryotherapy, radiotherapy, chemotherapy, and immunotherapy.

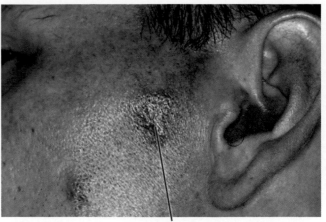

Kaposi's sarcoma

FIGURE 8–41
Kaposi's sarcoma, demonstrating characteristic purple skin lesion.

ADNEXA

Introduction

The ocular adnexa refer to the periocular structures, specifically the lacrimal drainage system and the lacrimal gland. The adnexa may be affected by congenital disorders, infection, inflammation, and tumors. It is important to recognize these conditions and determine whether or not they are isolated abnormalities or associated with eye or orbit involvement.

Canaliculitis

Definition

Canaliculitis refers to infection and inflammation of the canaliculus, the duct between the punctum and the lacrimal sac.

Etiology

Canaliculitis is classically caused by *Actinomyces israelii* (streptothrix), a filamentous Gram-positive rod; however, it may also be produced by *Candida albicans*, *Aspergillus*, *Nocardia asteroides*, and herpes simplex or zoster virus.

Symptoms

Patients are usually middle-aged women presenting with medial eyelid tenderness, tearing, redness, and discharge.

Signs

The prominent feature of this condition is erythema and swelling of the punctum and adjacent tissue ("pouting punctum"; Figure 8–42). There is also a follicular conjunctivitis near the medial canthus, expressible discharge from the punctum, concretions in the canaliculus, and a

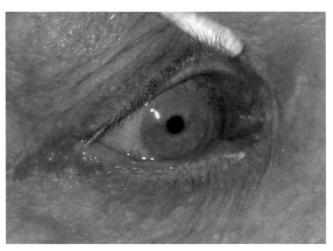

FIGURE 8–42
Canaliculitis, demonstrating swollen, erythematous, pouting upper punctum with discharge.

grating sensation on lacrimal duct probing. Patients may also have recurrent conjunctivitis.

Differential diagnosis

Canaliculitis may be mimicked by conjunctivitis, dacryocystitis, nasal lacrimal duct obstruction, and carunculitis.

Evaluation

- Important elements of the **history** are recurrent conjunctivitis and tearing.
- The **eye exam** should focus on the lids (punctum, lacrimal system) and conjunctiva (injection, follicles). Observe for discharge from the punctum while compressing the area medial to the punctum.
- **Lab tests** include culture and Gram stain (for organisms and sulfur granules).
- **Probing ± irrigation** to rule out an obstruction of the canalicular system.

- Consider **dacryocystography** to confirm a dilated canaliculus, concretions, or normal outflow function in the lower drainage system.

Management

- Warm compresses to the canalicular region (bid to qid).
- Marsupialization of the involved canaliculus.
- Systemic therapy with the appropriate antimicrobial agents:
  - *Actinomyces israelii*: canalicular irrigation with antibiotic solution (penicillin G 100 000 U/ml) and systemic antibiotic (penicillin V 500 mg PO qid for 7 days).
  - *Candida albicans*: systemic antifungal (fluconazole 600 mg PO qd for 7–10 days).
  - *Aspergillus*: topical antifungal (amphotericin B 0.15% tid) and systemic antifungal (itraconazole 200 mg PO bid for 7–10 days).
  - *Nocardia asteroides*: topical antibiotic (sulfacetamide tid) and systemic antibiotic (trimethoprim/sulfamethoxazole (Bactrim) one double-strength tablet PO qd for 7–10 days).
  - **Herpes simplex/zoster virus**: topical antiviral (trifluridine 0.1% (Viroptic) 5 times a day for 2 weeks).

Prognosis

The prognosis depends on the infecting organism but is usually good.

Dacryocystitis

Definition

Dacryocystitis is an infection of the lacrimal sac, which may be acute or chronic, and is often accompanied by an overlying cellulitis.

Etiology

The organisms commonly responsible for dacryocystitis are *Streptococcus pneumoniae*, *Staphylococcus* species, and *Pseudomonas* species. *Haemophilus influenzae* in children is less common now that they are vaccinated against it. Other pathogens include *Klebsiella*, *Actinomyces*, and *Candida*. Dacryocystitis is associated with conditions that cause lacrimal sac tear stasis and predispose to infection, such as strictures, long and narrow nasolacrimal ducts, lacrimal sac diverticulum, trauma, dacryoliths, congenital or acquired nasolacrimal duct obstruction (NLDO), and inflammatory sinus and nasal problems.

Symptoms

Lacrimal sac infections present with pain, swelling, and redness over the nasal portion of the lower eyelid, tearing, crusting, and sometimes fever.

Signs

Dacryocystitis causes edema and erythema below the medial canthal tendon (Figures 8–43 and 8–44). There is tenderness on palpation of the lacrimal sac and discharge can be expressed from the punctum. Fistula formation or a lacrimal sac cyst is also possible.

Differential diagnosis

Other conditions to be considered are ethmoid sinusitis, preseptal or orbital cellulitis, lacrimal sac tumor, facial abscess, dacryocystocele, and encephalocele.

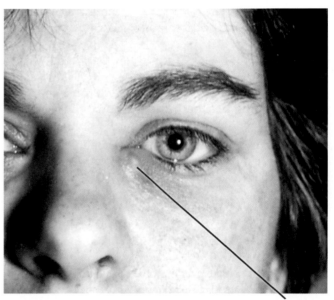

Dacryocystitis

FIGURE 8–43
Dacryocystitis demonstrating erythema and swelling of the lacrimal sac of the left eye.

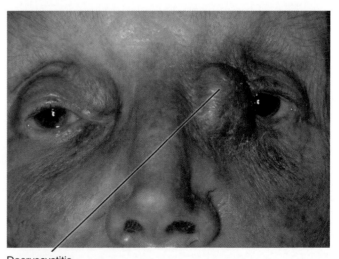

Dacryocystitis

FIGURE 8–44
Dacryocystitis with massive medial canthal swelling.

Evaluation

- It is essential to ask about a **history** of tearing (the absence of tearing calls the diagnosis into question) and previous sinus and/or upper respiratory infection.
- The **eye exam** is performed with attention to the lids (medial canthal swelling, expression of discharge from the punctum, lacrimal sac tenderness), ocular motility (normal), exophthalmometry (no proptosis), and conjunctiva (no injection).
- **Lab tests** include culture and Gram stain of any punctal discharge.
- **Nasolacrimal duct probing** is *not* performed during an acute infection.
- **Orbital CT scan** for restricted extraocular motility, proptosis, sinus disease, or atypical cases that do not respond to treatment.

Management

Treatment of dacryocystitis is with warm compresses (tid) and appropriate antibiotic therapy.

- **Acute infection:**
  - Systemic antibiotics (amoxicillin/clavulanate (Augmentin) 500 mg PO tid for 10 days or amoxicillin/sulbactam (Unasyn) 15–30 mg IV q6h). In penicillin-allergic patients, use trimethoprim/sulfamethoxazole ((Bactrim) one double-strength tablet PO bid for 10 days).
  - Topical antibiotic (erythromycin ointment bid) for conjunctivitis.
  - Percutaneous aspiration of the lacrimal sac contents with an 18-gauge needle for culture and Gram stain.
  - Consider incision and drainage for a pointing abscess.
  - Consider dacryocystorhinostomy (anastomosis between lacrimal sac and nasal cavity through a bony ostium) with silicone intubation once the acute infection has resolved. This procedure should be performed by an oculoplastic surgeon.
- **Chronic infection:**
  - Obtain cultures to determine antibiotic therapy (see above).
  - Dacryocystorhinostomy is required to relieve the obstruction, although lacrimal probing with intubation is occasionally effective.

Prognosis

Dacryocystitis typically responds to therapy, but surgery is almost always necessary. Without treatment, possible sequelae include mucocele formation, recurrent lacrimal sac abscess, orbital cellulitis, and infectious keratitis.

Nasolacrimal Duct Obstruction

Definition

NLDO is a blockage of the nasolacrimal duct.

Etiology

This may be acquired or congenital (see Ch. 6).

Acquired cases, which affect women more often than men (2:1), are due to chronic sinus disease, involutional stenosis, dacryocystitis, or naso-orbital trauma, and may be associated with granulomatous diseases such as Wegener's granulomatosis and sarcoidosis.

Symptoms

NLDO presents with tearing, discharge, and crusting.

Signs

Patients have watery eyes, eyelash crusting and debris, mucus reflux from the punctum with compression over the lacrimal sac, and medial lower-eyelid erythema (Figure 8–45).

Differential diagnosis

Other causes of acquired tearing are conjunctivitis, trichiasis, entropion, ectropion, corneal abnormalities, dry-eye syndrome, punctal stenosis, and canalicular stenosis.

Evaluation

- The **history** should note any history of sinus problems, trauma, or granulomatous disease, as well as the timing and onset of symptoms.
- The **eye exam** concentrates on the lids (margins, lashes, punctum), conjunctiva (no injection), and cornea (normal).
- **Digital pressure** over the lacrimal sac producing mucoid reflux from the punctum indicates an obstruction.
- The **dye disappearance test** with fluorescein is helpful. A drop of fluorescein dye is instilled in each

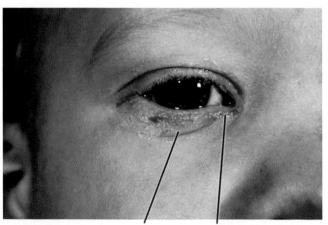

Erythema   Crusting

FIGURE 8–45
Nasolacrimal duct obstruction with tearing, crusting of eyelids, and lower-lid erythema.

eye and the time for the dye to vanish is monitored. Prolonged or asymmetric dye clearance is found in NLDO.

- **Jones I test**: fluorescein is instilled in the conjunctival cul-de-sac, and a cotton-tipped applicator is used to attempt fluorescein retrieval via the external naris. A positive test indicates a functional blockage.
- **Jones II test**: nasolacrimal irrigation with saline following positive Jones I test, and fluorescein retrieval is attempted once again. A positive test indicates an anatomic blockage.
- **Nasolacrimal irrigation**: a 23-gauge cannula mounted on a 3–5 cc syringe is inserted into the canaliculus, and irrigation is attempted. Retrograde flow through the opposite canaliculus and punctum indicates a nasolacrimal blockage. Reflux through the same punctum indicates a canalicular obstruction. Successful irrigation into the nose and throat eliminates an anatomic blockage but does not rule out a functional blockage.

Management

- Treat dacryocystitis, if present.
- Treat partial NLDO with a topical antibiotic/steroid combination (Maxitrol qid).
- Consider silicone intubation of the NLD or dacryoplasty for persistent partial obstruction.
- Complete NLDO with patent canaliculi and a functional lacrimal pump requires a dacryocystorhinostomy by an oculoplastic surgeon.

Prognosis

The outcome is usually good but depends on the cause of obstruction. There is an increased risk of dacryocystitis.

Dacryoadenitis

Definition

Dacryoadenitis is inflammation of the lacrimal gland.

Etiology

Dacryoadenitis is usually of idiopathic, non-infectious origin, viral, bacterial, or rarely parasitic etiology. There are two forms:

1. **Acute**: this type usually occurs in children and young adults and is most commonly due to infection (*Staphylococcus* species, mumps, Epstein–Barr virus, herpes zoster, or *Neisseria gonorrhoeae*). Most cases are associated with systemic infection.
2. **Chronic**: this is the more common form and is usually due to inflammatory disorders such as idiopathic orbital inflammation, sarcoidosis, thyroid-related ophthalmopathy, Sjögren's syndrome, and benign lymphoepithelial lesions. It can also occur with syphilis and tuberculosis.

Symptoms

Patients note lateral upper-eyelid swelling.

- **Acute**: also causes redness, pain, tearing, and discharge.
- **Chronic**: occasionally causes redness and discomfort.

Signs

- **Acute**: edema, tenderness, and erythema of the upper eyelid, enlarged and erythematous lacrimal gland (palpebral lobe), preauricular lymphadenopathy, and fever. The globe may be displaced inferonasally, and proptosis may be present if the orbital lobe is involved (Figure 8–46).
- **Chronic**: upper-eyelid tenderness, globe displacement, ocular motility restriction, and lacrimal gland enlargement.

Differential diagnosis

Other disorders presenting with upper-eyelid swelling and tenderness include malignant lacrimal gland neoplasm,

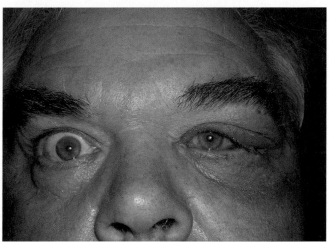

A

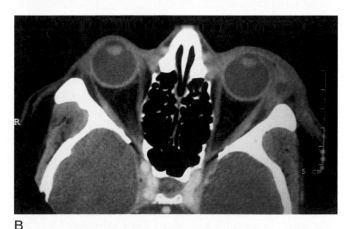

B

FIGURE 8–46
Dacryoadenitis, demonstrating erythema and edema of the left upper eyelid laterally and conjunctival injection (**A**), and lacrimal gland enlargement on CT scan (**B**).

preseptal or orbital cellulitis, chalazion, dermoid tumor, and lacrimal gland cyst (dacryops).

Evaluation

- It is important to ask about the timing of onset and presence of any constitutional symptoms when taking the **history**.
- The **eye exam** must include palpation of the parotid glands, lymph nodes, and upper eyelids, as well as assessment of the palpebral lacrimal lobe (lift upper lid) for enlargement, globe retropulsion (may have resistance), exophthalmometry (may have proptosis), and ocular motility (may be restricted).
- **Lab tests** depend on the form:
  - **Acute**: culture and Gram stain of discharge, complete blood count (CBC) with differential, and consider blood cultures for suspected systemic involvement.
  - **Chronic**: chest radiographs, CBC with differential, angiotensin-converting enzyme, Venereal Disease Research Laboratory test, fluorescent treponemal antibody absorption test, purified protein derivative, and anergy panel.
- **Orbital CT scan** for proptosis, restricted motility, or suspected mass.
- Consider **lacrimal gland biopsy** if the diagnosis is uncertain or malignancy is suspected.

Management

- Appropriate treatment for the underlying infection or inflammatory disorder:
  - **Mumps/Epstein–Barr virus**: warm compresses (bid to tid).
  - **Herpes simplex/zoster virus**: systemic antiviral (acyclovir (Zovirax) 800 mg PO 5 times a day for 10 days or famciclovir (Famvir) 500 mg PO tid for 7 days. For immunocompromised patients use acyclovir 10–12 mg/kg per day IV divided into three doses for 7–10 days).
  - *Staphylococcus* and *Streptococcus* **species**: systemic antibiotic (amoxicillin/clavulanate (Augmentin) 500 mg PO q8h. For severe cases use ampicillin/sulbactam (Unasyn) 1.5–3 g IV q6h).
  - *Neisseria gonorrhoeae*: systemic antibiotic (ceftriaxone 1 g IV), warm compresses, and incision and drainage if suppurative.
  - *Mycobacterium* **species**: surgical excision and systemic treatment with isoniazid (300 mg PO qd) and rifampin (600 mg PO qd) for 6–9 months. Consider adding pyrazinamide (25–35 mg/kg PO qd) for the first 2 months.
  - *Treponema pallidum*: systemic antibiotic (penicillin G 24 million U/day IV for 10 days).

Prognosis

Most infections respond well to treatment.

Lacrimal Gland Tumors

Lacrimal gland masses are inflammatory (50%) or neoplastic (50%). Of the tumors, approximately half are of epithelial origin, while the other half are primarily lymphoproliferative. The epithelial tumors are divided equally between benign and malignant varieties:

Benign mixed cell tumor (pleomorphic adenoma) is the most common epithelial tumor of the lacrimal gland, usually presenting insidiously in middle-aged adults. The tumor contains mucinous, osteoid, and cartilaginous components. There is often bony remodeling evident on radiographic images. Complete resection is imperative in order to avoid malignant transformation.

Malignant mixed cell tumor (pleomorphic adenocarcinoma) occurs in the elderly, with pain and rapid progression. The tumor contains the same features as the benign form but with malignant components. It is associated with long-standing or incompletely excised pleomorphic adenomas.

Adenoid cystic carcinoma (cylindroma) is the most common malignant tumor of the lacrimal gland. It is a rapidly infiltrative tumor associated with pain due to perineural invasion, bony erosion, and proptosis. CT scan shows adjacent bony destruction.

Symptoms

Patients may notice upper-lid fullness, diplopia, and pain.

Signs

Lacrimal gland tumors present with a palpable mass under the superotemporal orbital rim causing inferomedial globe displacement, eyelid edema and erythema, and limited ocular motility (Figure 8–47).

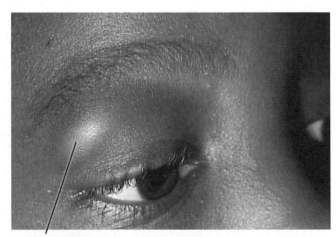

Lacrimal gland tumor
FIGURE 8–47
Lacrimal gland tumor of the right orbit.

Differential diagnosis

Other entities that may have a similar external appearance include dermoid cyst, sarcoidosis, idiopathic orbital inflammation, lymphoid tumor, and lacrimal gland cyst (dacryops).

Evaluation

- The **history** must note the duration of onset, rate of progression, and presence of pain, visual complaints, and constitutional symptoms.
- The **eye exam** is performed with attention to the lids (edema, erythema), lacrimal gland (tenderness, mass), and ocular motility (restricted).
- **Orbital CT scan** to look for a well-circumscribed mass with lacrimal gland fossa enlargement (pleomorphic adenoma) or an irregular mass with or without adjacent bony erosion (adenoid cystic carcinoma).
- **Fine-needle aspiration biopsy** may be useful in some cases; however, incisional biopsy should be avoided.
- Consider **oncology consultation**.

Management

- **Benign mixed tumor (pleomorphic adenoma):** en bloc excision is mandatory because rupture of the pseudocapsule may result in recurrence and malignant transformation.
- **Pleomorphic adenocarcinoma and adenoid cystic carcinoma (cylindroma):** ranges from en bloc resection with wide margins including the orbital rim to orbital exenteration with adjunctive chemotherapy and radiation.

Prognosis

- **Benign mixed tumor (pleomorphic adenoma):** excellent if the tumor is completely excised.
- **Pleomorphic adenocarcinoma:** similar to adenoid cystic carcinoma.
- **Adenoid cystic carcinoma (cylindroma):** the 5-year survival rate approaches 50% but is less than 25% at 15 years. Intracranial extension is the major cause of death.

CHAPTER NINE

Conjunctiva

Introduction

The conjunctiva covers the white of the eye and inner surface of the eyelids. This transparent mucous membrane is usually inconspicuous until it becomes inflamed, causing the eye to appear red and swollen. Although the conjunctiva has a limited way in which to respond to irritation, the pattern of inflammation and the associated symptoms are helpful in determining the diagnosis.

Trauma

As the outermost layer of the globe, the conjunctiva is usually the first tissue affected by ocular trauma. The most common conjunctival injuries are foreign bodies, lacerations, and subconjunctival hemorrhages. The presence of any one of these findings is reason to suspect more extensive eye involvement, and therefore, a detailed history and exam must be performed.

CONJUNCTIVAL FOREIGN BODY

A conjunctival foreign body refers to exogenous material, commonly dirt, glass, metal, or cilia (eyelash), on, under, or embedded within the conjunctiva. This often produces a foreign-body sensation and red eye. If the foreign body is not readily visible on the bulbar conjunctiva, then the eyelids must be everted to check the palpebral (tarsal) surface (Figure 9–1). Instilling a drop of fluorescein may enhance visualization of very small or clear substances. The foreign body is removed under topical anesthesia and a topical broad-spectrum anti-biotic (polymyxin B sulfate–trimethoprim (Polytrim) or bacitracin ointment qid) is prescribed for several days.

CONJUNCTIVAL LACERATION

A conjunctival laceration is a partial or full-thickness cut in the conjunctiva. Subconjunctival hemorrhage is present around the laceration and a foreign body may be present as well (Figure 9–2). A careful history and exam are very important to rule out an open globe. A conjunctival laceration is treated with a topical broad-spectrum antibiotic (polymyxin B sulfate–trimethoprim (Polytrim) or bacitracin ointment qid) until the wound is healed, and rarely requires surgical repair.

SUBCONJUNCTIVAL HEMORRHAGE

A subconjunctival hemorrhage is a diffuse or focal collection of blood under the conjunctiva. The hemorrhage appears bright or dark red, flat or elevated, depending on the quantity of blood (Figure 9–3). It often frightens the patient due to the ominous appearance of the area, but is otherwise asymptomatic. In addition to trauma, subconjunctival hemorrhage is associated with sneezing, coughing, straining, emesis, aspirin or anticoagulant use, hypertension, or may be idiopathic or due to an abnormal or fragile conjunctival vessel. Reassurance is all that is necessary if no other ocular findings exist. For non-traumatic recurrent hemorrhages, consider measuring the patient's blood pressure. A medical or hematology consultation is advisable for recurrent, idiopathic, subconjunctival hemorrhages, or other evidence of systemic bleeding (ecchymoses, epistaxis, gastrointestinal bleeding, and hematuria).

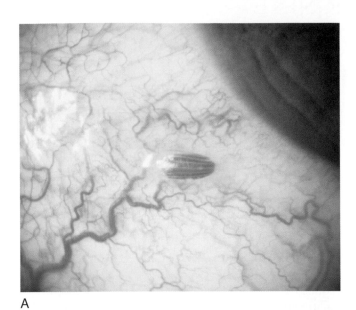

A

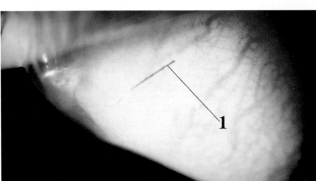

B

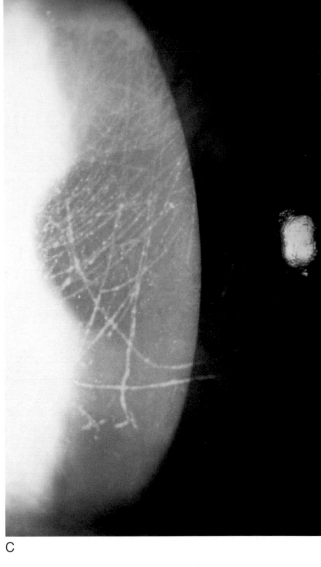

C

FIGURE 9–1
(**A**) Conjunctival foreign body, demonstrating a fragment of corn husk embedded in the conjunctiva. (**B**) Conjunctival foreign body, demonstrating a grasshopper leg embedded in the conjunctiva. (**C**) Same patient as in (**B**), demonstrating multiple vertical corneal abrasions from a grasshopper leg in the superior tarsal conjunctiva. Such a pattern of linear abrasions suggests a foreign body under the upper eyelid, and therefore the examiner should always evert the eyelid to inspect for this.

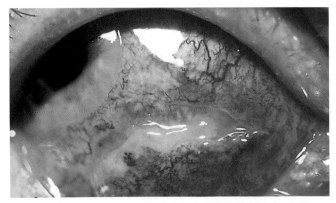

FIGURE 9–2
Conjuctival laceration with gaping edges.

Inflammation

The conjunctiva is a protective mucous membrane that responds to irritation in a limited number of ways. The signs of conjunctival inflammation include:

Injection: conjunctival redness or hyperemia, which can be minimal to severe (Figure 9–4).

Chemosis: conjunctival edema, ranging from mild with a boggy appearance to extensive with tense conjunctival ballooning (sometimes mistaken for a blister by the patient) (Figure 9–5).

Papillae: small to large fibrovascular mounds containing a central vascular tuft. Papillae, the result of

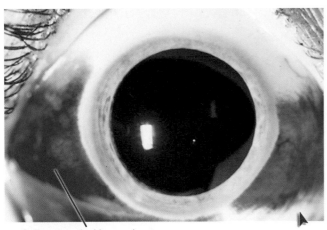

Subconjunctival hemorrhage

FIGURE 9–3

Subconjunctival hemorrhage, demonstrating bright red blood under the conjunctiva. As the hemorrhage resorbs, the edges may spread, become feathery, and turn yellowish (arrowhead).

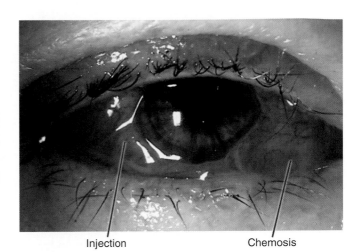

Injection   Chemosis

FIGURE 9–5

Chemosis with extensive ballooning of conjunctiva and prolapse over lower lid nasally. Temporally, the edges of the elevated conjunctiva are delineated by the light reflexes from the tear film.

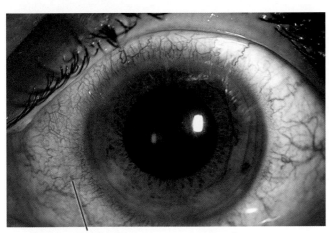

Conjunctival injection

FIGURE 9–4

Injection. The dilated conjunctival vessels produce a diffuse redness (hyperemia).

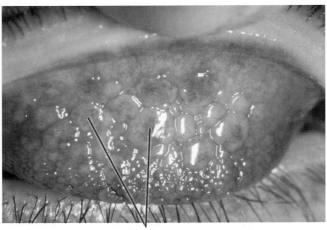

Papillae

FIGURE 9–6

Large papillae in a patient with vernal keratoconjunctivitis. The central vascular cores are clearly visible as dots within the papillae.

edema and leakage of fluid from vessels, are a non-specific finding seen on the palpebral (tarsal) conjunctiva. Large papillae >1 mm in diameter are called "cobblestones" or giant papillae (Figure 9–6).

Follicles: small, translucent, avascular mounds of plasma cells and lymphocytes that are usually most prominent in the inferior fornix, but may affect the bulbar conjunctiva (Figure 9–7). Follicles represent well-circumscribed foci of lymphoid hypertrophy due to reactive hyperplasia. They are seen in viral, chlamydial, and toxic conjunctivitis, as well as Parinaud's oculoglandular syndrome.

Membranes: a true membrane is a fibrinous exudate firmly adherent to the palpebral (tarsal) conjunctiva that bleeds and scars when removed. It occurs in bacterial conjunctivitis (*Streptococcus* species,

N. gonorrhoeae, *Corynebacterium diphtheriae*), Stevens–Johnson syndrome, and burns. A **pseudomembrane**, on the other hand, is a loosely attached, avascular, fibrinous exudate seen in epidemic keratoconjunctivitis (EKC) and mild allergic or bacterial conjunctivitis (Figure 9–8).

Preauricular lymphadenopathy: a palpable preauricular node may also be associated with certain types of conjunctivitis such as EKC, herpes simplex virus (HSV), *N. gonorrhoeae*, *Chlamydia*, Parinaud's oculoglandular syndrome, and Newcastle's disease.

Some or all of these signs may be present depending upon the underlying cause and the severity of the inflammation. It is the history, associated symptoms, and pattern of these findings that enable the examiner to determine the etiology and institute the appropriate treatment.

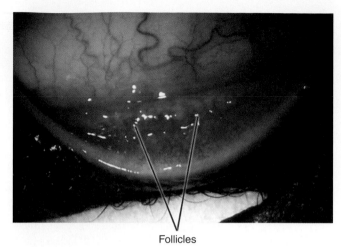

Follicles

FIGURE 9–7
Follicular conjunctivitis, demonstrating inferior palpebral (tarsal) follicles with the typical gelatinous bump appearance.

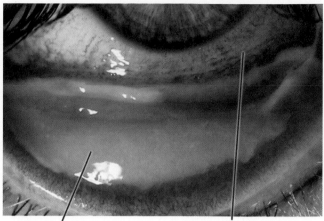

Pseudomembrane   Conjunctival injection

FIGURE 9–8
Pseudomembrane evident as a thick yellow coating in a patient with epidemic keratoconjunctivitis.

Conjunctivitis

Definition

Conjunctivitis means inflammation of the conjunctiva.

Etiology

Although most people equate conjunctivitis with "pink eye," there are many different forms of this very common eye disorder. Conjunctivitis is classified as acute (less than 4 weeks' duration) or chronic (greater than 4 weeks' duration); and infectious or non-infectious.

ACUTE CONJUNCTIVITIS

Infectious

- **Bacterial**: usually caused by *Staphylococcus aureus*, *Streptococcus pneumoniae*, *Haemophilus* species, or *Moraxella catarrhalis*, with a spectrum of presentations ranging from mild (minimal lid edema and scant purulent discharge) to moderate (significant conjunctival injection and membranes) (Figure 9–9). *N. gonorrhoeae* is noteworthy for producing a hyperacute conjunctivitis with severe purulent discharge, chemosis, papillary reaction, preauricular lymphadenopathy, and lid swelling. This organism can invade intact corneal epithelium and cause infectious keratitis.
- **Viral**: most commonly caused by adenovirus, "pink eye" presents with lid edema, serous discharge, and pseudomembranes. There may be a palpable preauricular node, subconjunctival hemorrhages, and corneal subepithelial infiltrates, which appear about 2 weeks later, can last months, and cause decreased vision, glare, and photophobia. The infection is transmitted by contact and is contagious for 12–14 days.

Mucopurulent discharge

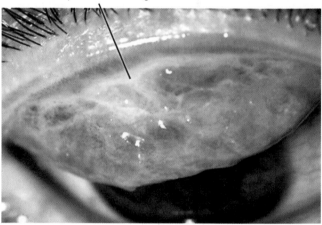

FIGURE 9–9
Bacterial conjunctivitis with mucopurulent discharge adherent to the upper palpebral (tarsal) conjunctiva.

The two most common forms are EKC due to types 8 and 19, and pharyngoconjunctival fever due to types 3 and 7 (young children with fever, pharyngitis, and follicular conjunctivitis) (Figure 9–10). Primary HSV ocular disease presents in children with lid vesicles and conjunctivitis (Figure 9–11). There may also be fever, preauricular lymphadenopathy, and an upper respiratory infection.

- **Pediculosis**: this is pubic lice eyelash infestation that causes a follicular conjunctivitis.

Allergic

- **Seasonal**: caused by airborne allergens such as pollen, mold, and dander, and associated with hayfever. The majority of patients with systemic allergies have ocular involvement.
- **Vernal keratoconjunctivitis**: see Ch. 6.

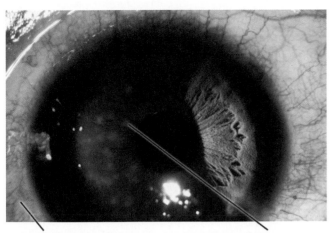

Conjunctival injection   Subepithelial infiltrates

FIGURE 9–10
Adenoviral conjunctivitis due to epidemic keratoconjunctivitis with characteristic subepithelial infiltrates.

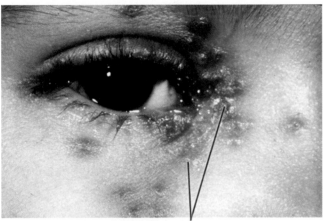

Seropurulent vesicles due to HSV

FIGURE 9–11
Herpes simplex viral (HSV) conjunctivitis with characteristic lid vesicles.

- **Atopic keratoconjunctivitis**: associated with atopy (hereditary allergic hypersensitivity, which is a clinical diagnosis consisting of rhinitis, asthma, and dermatitis). Atopic keratoconjunctivitis has similar features to vernal keratoconjunctivitis, but is distinguished from the latter because it occurs in adults and is not seasonal. It is also associated with smaller papillae, milky conjunctival edema, thickened and erythematous lids, corneal neovascularization, cataracts (10%), and keratoconus.

Toxic

Direct contact of topical medications or chemical substances with the conjunctiva causes a follicular reaction (acute or chronic). Particularly toxic eye drops include neomycin, aminoglycosides, antivirals, atropine, miotics, epinephrine, and preservatives, including contact lens solutions.

CHRONIC CONJUNCTIVITIS

Infectious

- **Bacterial**: *Staphylococcus* and *Moraxella* species may cause a chronic infection.
- **Chlamydial**: different serotypes produce different infections.
  - **Trachoma** is caused by serotypes A–C. Trachoma is the leading cause of blindness worldwide. This progressive bilateral infection of the upper tarsal and superior bulbar conjunctiva is characterized by follicles, Herbert's pits (scarred limbal follicles), superior corneal pannus, superficial punctate keratitis, upper tarsal scarring (Arlt's line), entropion, and trichiasis (Figure 9–12; Box 9–1).
  - **Inclusion conjunctivitis** is caused by serotypes D–K. This chronic, follicular conjunctivitis is notable

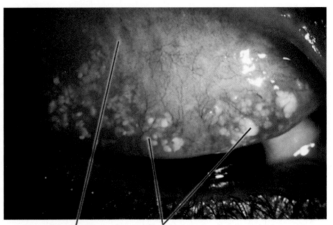

Arlt's line   Concretions

FIGURE 9–12
Trachoma demonstrating linear pattern of upper tarsal scarring. Also note the abundant concretions that appear as yellow granular aggregates.

BOX	**9–1**

World Health Organization Classification of Trachoma

TF trachomatous inflammation (follicular): >5 follicles larger than 0.5 mm on the upper tarsus
TI trachomatous inflammation (intense): inflammatory thickening obscuring >50% of the large, deep tarsal vessels
TS trachomatous cicatrization (scarring): visible white lines or sheets of fibrosis (Arlt's line)
TT trachomatous trichiasis: at least one misdirected eyelash
CO corneal opacity: obscuring at least part of the pupillary margin and causing visual acuity worse than 20/60

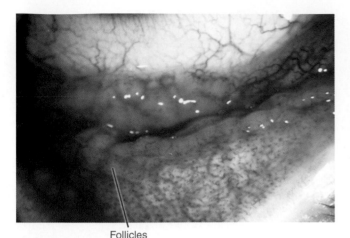

Follicles

FIGURE 9–13
Chlamydial conjunctivitis with follicles in the inferior fornix.

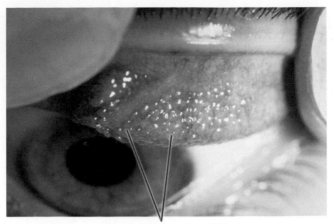

Giant papillary conjunctivitis

FIGURE 9–14
Giant papillary conjunctivitis, demonstrating large papillae on the upper palpebral (tarsal) conjunctiva.

for bulbar involvement, corneal subepithelial infiltrates, and no membrane formation (Figure 9–13). Inclusion conjunctivitis is associated with urethritis in 5% of cases.

- **Lymphogranuloma venereum** is caused by serotype L. Lymphogranuloma venereum is associated with Parinaud's oculoglandular syndrome (see below), conjunctival granulomas, and interstitial keratitis.

- **Molluscum contagiosum**: caused by a viral lid infection with multiple, umbilicated, shiny nodules. Release of toxic viral products is associated with a follicular conjunctivitis.

Allergic

- **Giant papillary conjunctivitis**: caused by an allergic reaction to material coating a foreign body on the ocular surface (i.e., contact lens (>95% of giant papillary conjunctivitis cases), exposed suture, ocular prosthesis). Patients with atopy are at higher risk. The hallmarks of giant papillary conjunctivitis are itching, ropy discharge, blurry vision, and contact lens discomfort followed by intolerance. Giant papillae are found on the upper palpebral (tarsal) conjunctiva (Figure 9–14).

Toxic

See above.

OTHER CONJUNCTIVITIS

- **Ophthalmia neonatorum**: see Ch. 6.
- **Superior limbic keratoconjunctivitis**: recurrent superior conjunctival inflammation of unknown etiology associated with contact lens wear and thyroid disease (50%). Superior limbic keratoconjunctivitis occurs most commonly in middle-aged females (70%)

Rose Bengal staining

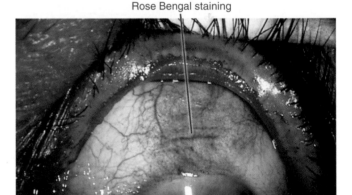

FIGURE 9–15
Superior limbic keratoconjunctivitis, demonstrating the typical staining of the central superior bulbar conjunctiva with rose Bengal dye.

and is usually bilateral and asymmetric. Characteristic findings are boggy edema, redundancy, injection, and fine punctate staining (with rose Bengal dye) of the superior bulbar conjunctiva (Figure 9–15). There is also a velvety papillary reaction of the upper palpebral (tarsal) conjunctiva, filamentary keratitis, micropannus, and no discharge. The symptoms tend to be worse than the signs.

- **Parinaud's oculoglandular syndrome**: unilateral conjunctivitis caused by cat-scratch fever, tularemia, rickettsiae, sporotrichosis, tuberculosis, syphilis, lymphogranuloma venereum, Epstein–Barr virus, mumps, fungi, malignancy, or sarcoidosis. Patients develop follicles, granulomas, lymphadenopathy (preauricular and/or submandibular), and may have fever, malaise, and a rash (Figure 9–16).

- **Other systemic diseases**: conjunctivitis can also occur in mucocutaneous disorders (Stevens–Johnson

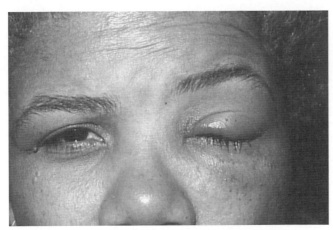

FIGURE 9–16
Parinaud's oculoglandular syndrome. There is marked eyelid swelling and erythema in this patient with an affected left eye.

syndrome, ocular cicatricial pemphigoid, bullous pemphigoid, pemphigus, epidermolysis bullosa, dermatitis herpetiform), arthropathies (Reiter's syndrome, psoriatic arthritis), and Wegener's granulomatosis.

Symptoms

Patients with conjunctivitis report variable amounts of redness, swelling, itching, burning, foreign-body sensation, tearing, discharge, and crusting of the eye lashes. If the cornea is involved, then additional symptoms may include photophobia and decreased vision.

Signs

Depending on the etiology, there is usually a characteristic pattern of findings. These include any combination of lid edema, conjunctival injection, chemosis, papillae, follicles, membranes, and discharge. The visual acuity is normal or decreased. Other signs that may be seen are preauricular lymphadenopathy, conjunctival concretions, subconjunctival hemorrhages, and corneal staining, subepithelial infiltrates, and ulcers. Corneal involvement may cause a mild anterior chamber reaction with cell and flare, and cataracts may occur in atopic keratoconjunctivitis.

Differential diagnosis

Other disorders that may mimic or cause a secondary conjunctivitis are dacryocystitis, canaliculitis, and nasolacrimal duct obstruction.

Evaluation

- When gathering the **history**, it is essential to characterize completely all of the ocular symptoms with respect to timing, quality, and severity. Patients must be questioned about constitutional symptoms, allergens, topical medications, contact lens use, skin lesions, systemic disorders, and exposure to infection.

- A careful **eye exam** is performed with attention to preauricular lymphadenopathy, lids (lesions, edema, erythema, lash crusting), conjunctiva (bulbar and palpebral (tarsal) for injection, chemosis, papillae, follicles, membranes, discharge, hemorrhages, concretions), cornea (staining, filaments, scarring, infiltrates, ulcers), anterior chamber (cell and flare), and lens (cataract).

- **Lab tests** include cultures and smears of the conjunctiva and cornea for suspected bacterial cases.

Management

- Treatment depends on the etiology and is usually supportive, with medications, cold compresses, topical lubrication, and debridement of membranes for symptomatic relief. Contact lens wearers should refrain from lens wear until the condition has completely resolved.

- **Infectious**: topical antimicrobial and may require systemic antibiotics based on the causative organism: *Neisseria gonorrhoeae*, *Chlamydia*, and Parinaud's oculoglandular syndrome (e.g., cat-scratch disease, tularemia, syphilis, tuberculosis). Patients should be warned about the contagious nature of the disease and practice contact precautions.
  - **Bacterial**:
    - Topical broad-spectrum antibiotic (moxifloxacin (Vigamox) tid, gatifloxacin (Zymar) qid, or levofloxacin (Quixin) qid).
    - Remove discharge with irrigation and membranes with sterile cotton-tipped applicator.
  - **Viral**:
    - Topical lubrication with artificial tears, and topical vasoconstrictor, non-steroidal anti-inflammatory drug (NSAID), antihistamine, mast cell stabilizer, or mast cell stabilizer/antihistamine combination (bid to qid).
    - Add topical antibiotic (polymyxin B sulfate–trimethoprim (Polytrim) qid, erythromycin or bacitracin ointment qd to tid) for corneal epithelial defects.
    - Add topical steroid (fluorometholone alcohol 0.1% (FML) qid) for subepithelial infiltrates in EKC that reduce vision below 20/40.
    - Add topical antiviral (trifluridine (Viroptic) 5 times a day) for HSV.
- **Allergic**: topical vasoconstrictor, NSAID, antihistamine, mast cell stabilizer, or mast cell stabilizer/antihistamine combination (bid to qid). Consider a topical steroid, particularly for severe allergic keratoconjunctivitis (start with a mild form like fluorometholone alcohol 0.1% (FML) qid or loteprednol etabonate 0.2% (Alrex) qid, and change to a stronger preparation like prednisolone 1% qid to q1h for severe cases. Typically, a solution (phosphate (Inflamase Mild, AK-Pred)) works better than a suspension (acetate

(Pred Mild, EconoPred))). Also, consider treatment with a systemic antihistamine (Benadryl 25–50 mg PO q6h prn). Other specific recommendations include:

- **Giant papillary conjunctivitis:**
  - Clean, change, or discontinue contact lenses, and switch to a preservative-free contact lens cleaning solution.
- **Superior limbic keratoconjunctivitis:**
  - Effective treatment usually requires scarring of the superior bulbar conjunctiva with silver nitrate solution (0.5–1.0%), conjunctival cautery, recession, or resection.
  - Consider pressure patching or a large-diameter bandage contact lens.
  - Topical steroids are not effective.
- **Atopic keratoconjunctivitis:**
  - Consider topical cyclosporine (1–2%) qid.
  - Consider supratarsal steroid injection (0.25–0.50 ml dexamethasone or triamcinolone acetate (Kenalog)).
- **Toxic:** remove the inciting agent, and institute similar supportive measures as for allergic conjunctivitis.

Prognosis

The prognosis is usually good, since most forms of conjunctivitis are benign and self-limited, but corneal infiltrates, scarring, and cataracts can cause decreased vision.

Dry-Eye Syndrome

Definition

In dry-eye syndrome there is dryness of the ocular surface.

Etiology

Dry eye is a condition with many causes. The term is used to refer to the end-state of various disorders that produce inadequate lubrication of the conjunctiva and cornea. These abnormalities usually involve one or more components of the tear film (aqueous, mucin, and lipid) or the eyelids. A classification system is helpful, but often the etiology of dry eye is multifactorial:

Aqueous deficiency: lacrimal gland dysfunction due to aplasia, surgical removal, radiation, infiltration (sarcoidosis, thyroid disease, lymphoma, amyloidosis, tuberculosis), inflammation (mumps, Sjögren's syndrome), tumor, denervation (Riley–Day (familial dysautonomia), Shy–Drager (adult dysautonomia), and Möbius syndrome), and drugs that decrease lacrimal secretion (see below).

- **Keratoconjunctivitis sicca** is an aqueous tear deficiency caused by poor lacrimal gland function and associated with **Sjögren's syndrome** (dry eye,

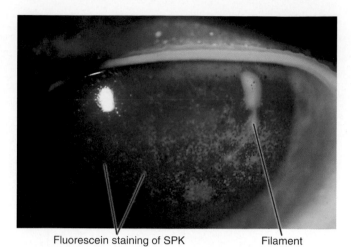

Fluorescein staining of SPK   Filament

FIGURE 9–17

Keratoconjunctivitis sicca, demonstrating superficial punctate keratitis (SPK) and filaments stained with fluorescein dye.

dry mouth, and arthritis). It may occur in isolation (primary form; >95% female) or with connective tissue disease (secondary form; rheumatoid arthritis and collagen vascular diseases) (Figure 9–17).

Mucin deficiency: goblet cell dysfunction due to conjunctival scarring and keratinization (vitamin A deficiency, Stevens–Johnson syndrome, ocular cicatricial pemphigoid, radiation, chemical burns, trachoma, graft-versus-host disease).

- **Vitamin A deficiency:** vitamin A is necessary for mucin production by the conjunctival goblet cells. Lack of mucin causes increased tear evaporation, conjunctival xerosis, and ultimately epithelial keratinization. Vitamin A deficiency is a major cause of worldwide blindness, affecting 20–40 million children, especially in developing countries. In developed countries, vitamin A deficiency is due to lipid malabsorption (short-bowel syndrome, chronic liver dysfunction, cystic fibrosis) and poor diet (chronic alcoholism). The hallmark of this disorder is night blindness (nyctalopia). Other characteristic findings are conjunctival xerosis (leathery appearance) and Bitot's spots (white, foamy patch of keratinized bulbar conjunctiva), corneal melting, ulceration, and scarring, and progressive retinal degeneration (fine white mottling) (Figure 9–18).

Lipid deficiency: meibomian gland dysfunction due to blepharitis, meibomitis, and acne rosacea.

Lid abnormality: increased evaporative tear loss due to lagophthalmos, Bell's palsy, ectropion, entropion, proptosis, and thyroid-related ophthalmopathy.

Other factors: aging (reduced basal tear secretion), environment (wind, low humidity, high altitude, indoor heating, and air conditioning), medications (antihistamines, decongestants, phenothiazines, antidepressants, anticholinergics, β-blockers, diuretics,

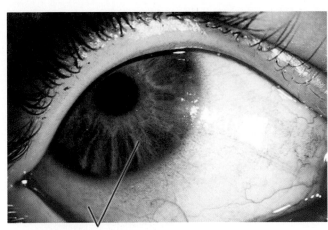

Rose Bengal staining

FIGURE 9–18
Dry eye due to vitamin A deficiency, demonstrating diffuse staining of cornea, inferior limbus, and interpalpebral conjunctiva with rose Bengal dye.

retinoids, estrogens, and eyedrop preservatives (benzalkonium chloride, thimerisol, polyquad)), extended computer work or reading (reduced blink rate), contact lens wear, and corneal surgery (denervation causing decreased tear production).

Symptoms

Patients with dry eye describe the sensation as dryness, burning, or foreign-body sensation. They frequently report tearing, redness, discharge, blurred vision, and sometimes photophobia. Their symptoms are exacerbated by wind, smoke, contact lens wear, and prolonged reading or computer work, and tend to be worse at the end of the day.

Signs

The signs of conjunctival and corneal dryness can be extremely variable. In general, there is conjunctival injection, decreased tear break-up time (<10 seconds), decreased tear meniscus (lacrimal lake), increased tear film debris, irregular or dull corneal light reflex, conjunctival and/or corneal staining with fluorescein and other dyes (rose Bengal and lissamine green), and corneal filaments. Loosened, redundant bulbar conjunctiva may be noticeable resting on or hanging over the eyelid margin (conjunctivochalasis). The presence of Bitot's spot is pathognomonic for vitamin A deficiency. Lid abnormalities and blepharitis may also be evident.

Differential diagnosis

Blepharitis and allergic conjunctivitis are sometimes misdiagnosed as dry eye. Although both these conditions can exacerbate dry eye and blepharitis can even cause dry eye, they can also present independently and in a similar fashion as dry eye. Therefore, it is important to differentiate between them.

Evaluation

- The **history** must precisely document the onset and character of the symptoms. Patients should be questioned specifically about any measures or activities that aggravate or alleviate the dryness. Standardized dry-eye questionnaires may also be useful (i.e., Ocular Surface Disease Index (OSDI)).
- The **eye exam** concentrates on the lids (malpositions, blepharitis), tear film (quantity (tear meniscus height, Schirmer's test) and quality (tear film debris, tear break-up time)), conjunctiva (injection, staining), and cornea (staining, ulceration, scarring).
- **Schirmer's test** is a method of measuring the quantity of tears and is performed with or without topical anesthesia. The test consists of drying the inferior fornix with a cotton-tipped applicator to remove excess tears, placing a strip of standardized filter paper (Whatman #41, 5 mm width) over each lower eyelid at the junction of the lateral and middle thirds, and measuring the amount of wetting after 5 minutes. Normal results are considered ≥10 mm with anesthesia (measures basal tearing only), and ≥15 mm without anesthesia (measures basal + reflex tearing). Most tests are performed with anesthesia, but unfortunately, the results are quite variable since reflex tearing can occur anyway.
- **Lab tests** to consider are tear lactoferrin and lysozyme (decreased) and tear osmolarity (>310 mosmol/l).
- Consider **impression cytology** (reduced number of goblet cells), **electroretinogram** (reduced), **electro-oculogram** (abnormal), and **dark adaptation** (prolonged) for vitamin A deficiency.
- Consider **medical consultation** for systemic diseases.

Management

- The strategies for dry-eye treatment are to lubricate the ocular surface by replacing tears, inducing tear production, and/or preserving the patient's own tears.
- The mainstay of therapy is topical lubrication. Patients may try any artificial tear preparation, but if they are using these drops more than qid, then a preservative-free formulation (up to q1h) should be used to avoid toxicity from preservatives. Lubricating ointment (qhs) is also helpful. A sustained-release product (Lacriserts) is another alternative.
- Topical cyclosporine 0.05% (Restasis) bid is effective in many inflammatory dry-eye conditions. Similarly, topical steroids may be useful but require monitoring of the intraocular pressure and should be used with caution.
- Consider topical autologous serum eyedrops for severe cases.
- Punctal occlusion (with plugs or cautery) is a simple office procedure that blocks tear drainage through the lacrimal system.

- Other options include the use of bandage contact lenses or moisture chamber goggles.
- Consider acetylcysteine 10% (Mucomyst qd to qid) for excess mucus or filamentary keratitis.
- Consider lid taping, tarsorrhaphy, or surgical repair for lid abnormalities.
- Treat any underlying conditions (i.e., vitamin A replacement (15 000 IU PO qd)).

Prognosis

Although most forms of dry eye are chronic conditions without a cure, the majority of cases are benign and can be managed effectively with current treatments. However, severe cases may be difficult to control and may cause corneal ulceration, scarring, and possible perforation.

Stevens–Johnson Syndrome (Erythema Multiforme Major)

Definition

Stevens–Johnson syndrome is a cutaneous, bullous disease with mucosal involvement resulting in acute, bilateral, membranous conjunctivitis.

Etiology

This systemic disorder is usually caused by a drug reaction (i.e., sulfonamides, penicillin, aspirin, barbiturates, isoniazid, or phenytoin) or infection (HSV, adenovirus, *Mycoplasma* and *Streptococcus* species).

Symptoms

Patients present with constitutional symptoms of fever, upper respiratory infection, headache, arthralgias, and malaise. They complain of skin eruptions and eye involvement causing decreased vision, pain, redness, and swelling.

Signs

Inspection of the skin reveals a rash consisting of characteristic target lesions. Patients have elevated temperature, and the mucous membranes show ulceration and strictures. The conjunctivitis is characterized by decreased visual acuity, conjunctival injection, discharge, membranes, symblepharon (adhesion between the palpebral and bulbar conjunctiva), trichiasis, and corneal ulceration, scarring, vascularization, and keratinization (Figures 9–19 and 9–20).

Differential diagnosis

Other diseases that can produce similar eye findings include ocular cicatricial pemphigoid, chemical burn, radiation, squamous cell carcinoma, scleroderma, infectious or allergic conjunctivitis, trachoma, sarcoidosis, and ocular rosacea.

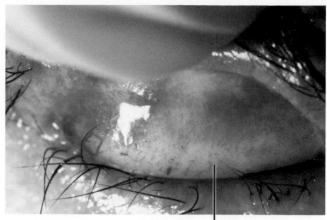

Tarsal scarring

FIGURE 9–19
Stevens–Johnson syndrome, demonstrating tarsal scarring.

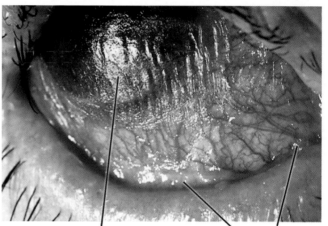

Corneal keratinization   Symblepharon

FIGURE 9–20
Stevens–Johnson syndrome, demonstrating keratinization of the ocular surface with a dry, wrinkled appearance. Note the resulting irregular, diffuse corneal reflex.

Evaluation

- A main goal of the **history** is to identify the causative agent if possible.
- The **eye exam** should focus on the lids (trichiasis), conjunctiva (injection, symblepharon, ulceration), and cornea (staining, ulceration, scarring). If the patient presents during the acute phase of the disease, it is also important to inspect the skin and oral mucosa for characteristic lesions.
- **Medical consultation**.

Management

- Treatment of Stevens–Johnson syndrome is supportive, consisting of:
  - Topical lubrication using non-preserved artificial tears (up to q1h) and ointment (qhs).

- Topical antibiotic (polymyxin B sulfate–trimethoprim (Polytrim) qid or erythromycin ointment tid) for corneal epithelial defects.
- Topical steroid (prednisolone acetate 1% up to q2h) depending on the degree of inflammation. Systemic steroids (prednisone 60–100 mg PO qd) may be necessary in very severe cases.
- Consider punctal occlusion and possibly tarsorrhaphy to control dry eye.
- Some cases may require lysis of symblepharon, and surgery for trichiasis or corneal scarring.

Prognosis

The prognosis is fair because, even though Stevens–Johnson syndrome is usually self-limited (<6 weeks) and recurrences are rare, the mucous membrane damage is permanent and can be difficult to treat. Furthermore, these patients are susceptible to secondary infection, with a mortality rate up to 30%.

Ocular Cicatricial Pemphigoid

Definition

Ocular cicatricial pemphigoid is a systemic vesiculobullous disease of mucous membranes resulting in chronic, bilateral, cicatrizing conjunctivitis.

Etiology

The etiology is usually idiopathic but probably has an autoimmune mechanism. It may also be drug-induced, occurring with epinephrine, timolol, pilocarpine, ecothiophate iodide, or idoxuridine.

Epidemiology

Ocular cicatricial pemphigoid has an incidence of 1 in 20 000 and is more common in elderly women.

Symptoms

Patients notice decreased vision, redness, dryness, foreign-body sensation, and tearing. Involvement of other mucosal surfaces may produce difficulty swallowing or breathing.

Signs

On exam, the visual acuity is normal or decreased. There is conjunctival injection, scarring, and keratinization, symblepharon, ankyloblepharon (adhesion between the upper and lower eyelids), foreshortened fornices, trichiasis, entropion, corneal ulceration, scarring, vascularization, and keratinization (Figures 9–21 and 9–22). Other mucous membranes are frequently involved (oral (up to 90%), nasal, pharyngeal, esophageal, tracheal, and genital), causing strictures and visible oral lesions. Skin involvement also occurs in up to 30% of cases, with recurrent

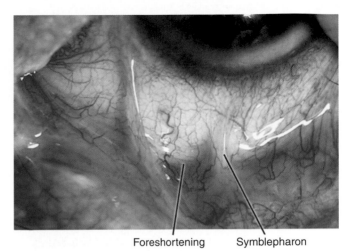

Foreshortening   Symblepharon

FIGURE 9–21
Ocular cicatricial pemphigoid, demonstrating symblepharon and foreshortening of the inferior fornix.

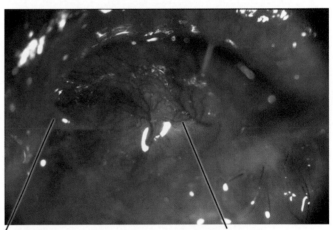

Symblepharon   Neovascularization

FIGURE 9–22
Ocular cicatricial pemphigoid, demonstrating advanced stage with corneal vascularization and symblepharon.

lesions of the inguinal region and extremities, and scarring of the scalp and face.

Differential diagnosis

Other diseases that can produce similar ocular manifestations are Stevens–Johnson syndrome, chemical burn, radiation, squamous cell carcinoma, scleroderma, infectious or allergic conjunctivitis, trachoma, sarcoidosis, and ocular rosacea.

Evaluation

- The **history** should document the course of disease and extraocular symptoms.
- The **eye exam** concentrates on the lids (trichiasis, entropion, ankyloblepharon), conjunctiva (injection, symblepharon, ulceration), and cornea (staining, ulceration, scarring). It is also important to inspect the oral mucosa and skin for lesions.

- **Conjunctival biopsy** shows immunoglobulin and complement deposition in the basement membrane.

Management

- Treatment of ocular cicatricial pemphigoid is supportive, consisting of:
  - Topical lubrication using non-preserved artificial tears (up to q1h) and ointment (qhs).
  - Topical antibiotic (polymyxin B sulfate–trimethoprim (Polytrim) qid or erythromycin ointment tid) for corneal epithelial defects.
  - Treatment with systemic steroids and/or immuno-suppressive agents (dapsone, cyclophosphamide) is commonly required and should be performed by a cornea or uveitis specialist.
  - Consider punctal occlusion and possibly tarsorrhaphy to control dry eye.
  - Consider surgery for entropion and trichiasis, lysis of symblepharon, and mucous membrane grafting.
  - Corneal tranplantation has a poor success rate and is usually avoided. End-stage disease can be treated with a keratoprosthesis but has limited success.

Prognosis

In contrast to Steven–Johnson syndrome, ocular cicatricial pemphigoid is a chronic progressive disease with remissions and exacerbations, typically initiated by surgical intervention. Therefore the prognosis is poor. Corneal perforation and endophthalmitis are possible complications.

Degenerations

Secondary degenerative changes of the conjunctiva are extremely common, particularly in individuals living in dry, warm, sunny climates. This is because two common conjunctival degenerations, **pingueculae** and **pterygia**, are associated with ultraviolet light exposure. **Concretions**, another frequent finding, are associated with aging and chronic conjunctivitis. Conjunctival degenerations are usually asymptomatic, but may produce redness, foreign-body sensation, a visible bump or growth, and, rarely, decreased vision or contact lens intolerance. Treatment is usually not necessary, but topical lubrication with artificial tears and limited use of a vasoconstrictor (naphazoline (Naphcon) qid) is useful for inflamed lesions. It is important to be able to differentiate these benign conditions from more serious conditions like phlyctenule, conjunctival intraepithelial neoplasia (CIN), squamous cell carcinoma, episcleritis, and scleritis.

CONCRETIONS

Concretions are yellow-white inclusion cysts filled with keratin and epithelial debris that are located in the palpebral (tarsal) conjunctiva and fornix (see Figure 9–12). They are associated with aging and chronic conjunctivitis. Concretions may contain calcium and can erode through the overlying conjunctiva to cause a foreign-body sensation. If symptomatic, they are easily unroofed and the contents removed with a small-gauge needle under topical anesthesia.

PINGUECULA

Pinguecula is a small, yellow-white, subepithelial nodule located at the limbus (nasal more often than temporal) and does not involve the cornea (Figure 9–23). Pingueculae are caused by actinic (ultraviolet light) damage and are composed of abnormal collagen. They may calcify with time. Pingueculitis occurs when a pinguecula becomes inflamed due to dryness and irritation. Treatment is lubrication and possibly a short course of topical steroids.

PTERYGIUM

Pterygium is an interpalpebral, triangular, fibrovascular growth that invades the cornea, destroying Bowman's membrane (Figure 9–24). Pterygia are also associated with actinic exposure and are often preceded by a pinguecula. They may induce astigmatism and cause decreased vision if they extend across the visual axis. Chronic inflammation, cosmesis, contact lens intolerance, and decreased vision are indications for surgical excision. However, there is a recurrence rate of up to 50% after simple excision. This can be reduced by the use of conjunctival autograft, amniotic membrane, beta irradiation, thiotepa, or mitomycin C.

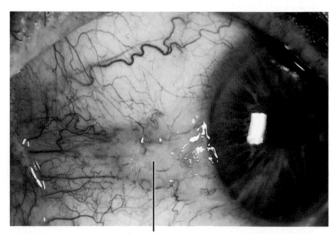

Pinguecula

FIGURE 9–23
Pinguecula seen as a yellow-white elevated mass near the medial limbus.

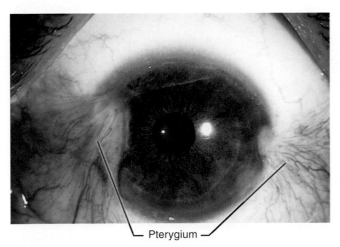

FIGURE 9–24
Large nasal and smaller temporal pterygia. Note the typical triangular, wedge-shaped configuration, and also the white corneal scarring at the leading edges.

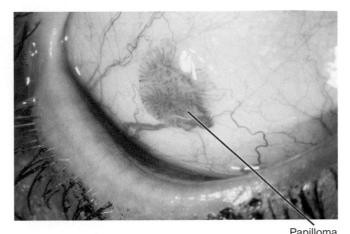

FIGURE 9–26
Papilloma, demonstrating the typical elevated appearance with central vascular fronds.

Tumors

Numerous types of neoplasms can affect the conjunctiva. They may be benign or malignant, and pigmented, non-pigmented, or vascular. Tumors can arise from the epithelium or the stroma. Many conjunctival tumors are similar to those that involve the eyelids, and some are unique to the ocular surface.

DUCTAL OR INCLUSION CYST

Ductal or inclusion cyst is a fluid-filled cavity within the conjunctiva that is defined by its lining (Figure 9–25). It is usually due to trauma, surgery, or inflammation when dislodged epithelium implanted within the stroma undergoes cavitation. Cysts are benign and may be excised, but if so, they require complete excision to prevent recurrence.

SQUAMOUS PAPILLOMA

Squamous papilloma is a benign proliferation of conjunctival epithelium that appears as a fleshy lesion with vascular tufts (Figures 9–26 and 9–27). It can be solitary or multiple, pedunculated or sessile. The pedunculated variety is associated with human papillomavirus and usually occurs in children near the caruncle. The sessile type is broad-based and usually occurs in adults near the limbus. Papillomas can regress spontaneously. There is a rare risk of malignant transformation, and therefore, treatment is excisional biopsy with cryotherapy. Multiple recurrences may occur after incomplete excision.

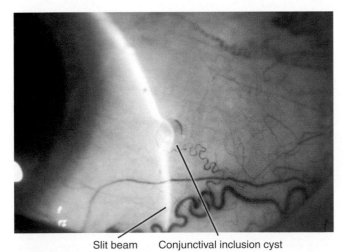

Slit beam   Conjunctival inclusion cyst

FIGURE 9–25
Conjunctival inclusion cyst appears as a clear elevation over which the slit beam bends.

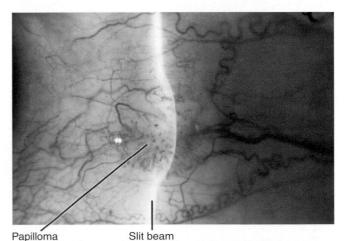

Papilloma   Slit beam

FIGURE 9–27
Squamous papilloma with elevated, gelatinous appearance.

CONJUNCTIVAL INTRAEPITHELIAL NEOPLASIA

CIN is a premalignant lesion associated with human papillomavirus (strains 16 and 18) and actinic exposure. CIN represents squamous dysplasia confined to the epithelium and is a precursor of squamous cell carcinoma. The lesion, which occurs more commonly in older fair-skinned men, has a white or translucent, gelatinous appearance (Figure 9–28). It usually begins at the limbus and spreads on to the cornea. CIN is treated by wide local excision with cryotherapy. Application of mitomycin C may also be considered. It is important to remove any involved corneal epithelium.

SQUAMOUS CELL CARCINOMA

Squamous cell carcinoma is present when malignant cells have broken through the epithelial basement membrane. The appearance is similar to CIN, as a gelatinous, papillary lesion with loops of vessels located in the interpalpebral region (Figures 9–29 and 9–30). Squamous cell carcinoma may extend on to and superficially invade the cornea. Deep invasion and metastasis seldom occur. Acquired immunodeficiency syndrome (AIDS) should be suspected when patients are <50 years old. The management of squamous cell carcinoma is wide excision, including superficial sclera and cryotherapy to reduce the recurrence rate (from 40% to less than 10%). Enucleation is performed for intraocular involvement, and exenteration is necessary for intraorbital spread. A rare, very aggressive variant, mucoepidermoid carcinoma, should be suspected in cases of recurrent squamous cell carcinoma.

NEVUS

Nevus is a discrete, elevated, variably pigmented lesion that arises from congenital nests of benign nevus cells. It is freely movable over the globe, and may contain cysts, be amelanotic (20–30%), and enlarge or become more pigmented during puberty or pregnancy (Figure 9–31). Nevi are categorized by their location as junctional (epithelial), subepithelial (substantia propria), or compound (both). They rarely become malignant.

OCULAR MELANOCYTOSIS

Ocular melanocytosis refers to unilateral, increased uveal, scleral, and episcleral pigmentation that appears as blue-gray patches and is more common in Caucasians (Figure 9–32).

If the periorbital skin is also involved, which is more common in Asians and African Americans, then the disorder is known as **oculodermal melanocytosis** (Figure 9–33).

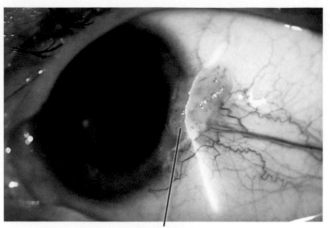

Conjunctival intraepithelial neoplasia

FIGURE 9–28
Conjunctival intraepithelial neoplasia demonstrating pink, nodular, gelatinous, vascularized appearance at the limbus.

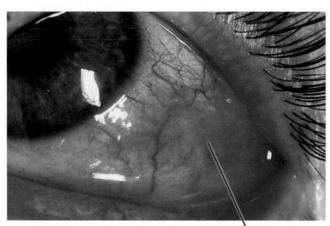

Squamous cell carcinoma

FIGURE 9–29
Squamous cell carcinoma appearing as a pink, diffuse, gelatinous growth.

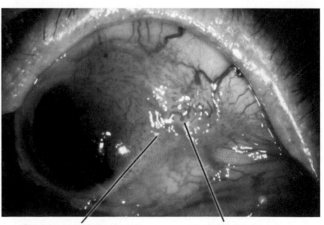

Squamous cell carcinoma   Vascular loops

FIGURE 9–30
More advanced squamous cell carcinoma with gelatinous growth and abnormal vascular loops.

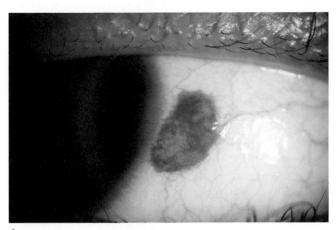

A

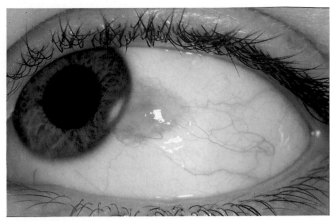

B

FIGURE 9–31
Elevated (**A**) pigmented and (**B**) non-pigmented conjunctival nevus.

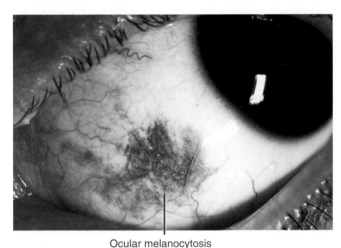

Ocular melanocytosis

FIGURE 9–32
Ocular melanocytosis, demonstrating blue-gray, patchy pigmentation.

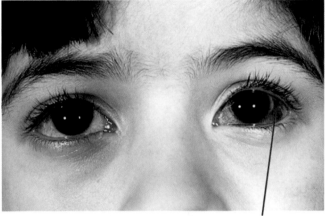

Oculodermal melanocytosis (nevus of Ota)

FIGURE 9–33
Oculodermal melanocytosis (nevus of Ota) of the left eye. Note the prominent scleral pigmentation; the periorbital skin changes are difficult to see in this photo.

PRIMARY ACQUIRED MELANOSIS

Primary acquired melanosis is a mobile, patchy, diffuse, flat brown lesion that occurs in middle-aged and elderly Caucasians (Figure 9–34). It has indistinct margins, does not contain cysts, may grow, and has malignant potential (30%). Primary acquired melanosis is analogous to lentigo maligna of the skin and should be observed with serial photographs. Nodular thickening is an indication for biopsy, and complete excision is performed if the result is malignant.

SECONDARY ACQUIRED MELANOSIS

Secondary acquired melanosis is the term applied to conjunctival hyperpigmentation due to racial variations,

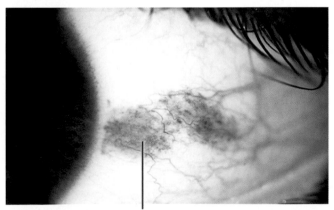

Primary acquired melanosis

FIGURE 9–34
Primary acquired melanosis, demonstrating mottled, brown, patchy pigmentation.

actinic stimulation, radiation, pregnancy, Addison's disease, or inflammation. It is usually perilimbal (Figure 9–35).

MALIGNANT MELANOMA

Malignant melanoma is a nodular, variably pigmented, elevated mass containing vessels but no cysts (Figures 9–36 and 9–37). This rare lesion may arise from primary acquired melanosis (55%), nevi (25%), or de novo. Melanoma must be completely excised (no-touch technique) with clear margins, partial lamellar sclerectomy, and cryotherapy. Recurrence is typically amelanotic. Metastases, to regional lymph nodes and the brain, occur in 25%, and the mortality rate is 20%. Exenteration does not improve survival. The prognosis depends on depth and location, and is worse for tumors >2 mm thick, and those involving the caruncle, fornices, and palpebral (tarsal) conjunctiva.

KAPOSI'S SARCOMA

Kaposi's sarcoma occurs as single or multiple, flat or elevated, deep red or purple plaques on the palpebral (tarsal) conjunctiva of immunocompromised individuals, especially those with AIDS (Figure 9–38). It is essentially malignant granulation tissue (i.e., proliferation of capillaries, endothelial cells, and fibroblast-like cells) and may involve the orbit. The tumor is treated with excision, radiation, or chemotherapy.

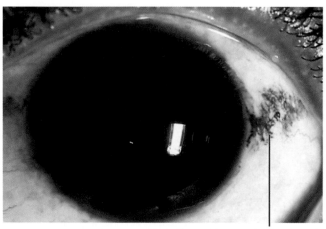

Secondary acquired melanosis

FIGURE 9–35
Secondary acquired melanosis (racial pigmentation), demonstrating typical perilimbal, brown, homogeneous pigmentation.

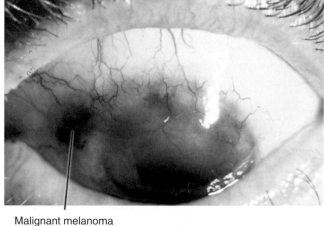

Malignant melanoma

FIGURE 9–37
Malignant melanoma, demonstrating irregular pigmented growth at limbus and on to cornea with vascularization.

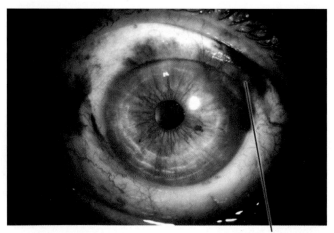

Malignant melanoma

FIGURE 9–36
Malignant melanoma, demonstrating nodular, pigmented, vascular lesion at the limbus.

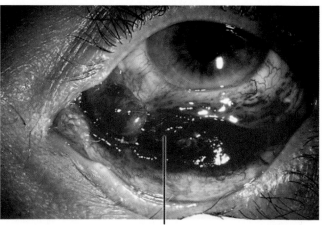

Kaposi's sarcoma

FIGURE 9–38
Kaposi's sarcoma, demonstrating beefy, red, large, nodular mass in the inferior fornix.

LYMPHOID TUMORS

Lymphoid tumors can grow in the eyelids, orbit, or conjunctiva. In the latter, they appear as single or multiple, smooth, flat, salmon-colored patches in the substantia propria, most commonly in the fornix (Figures 9–39 and 9–40). Lymphoid lesions typically occur in middle-aged adults, and represent a spectrum of disease from benign reactive lymphoid hyperplasia to malignant lymphoma (non-Hodgkin's type). These cannot be distinguished clinically, so biopsy and immunohistochemical studies are required. Patients are at risk for developing systemic lymphoma (20%), and therefore a work-up must be performed, including a computed tomography scan, bone scan, serum protein electrophoresis, and medical consultation. Treatment is with low-dose radiation, surgery, and local chemotherapy.

PYOGENIC GRANULOMA

Pyogenic granuloma is neither pyogenic nor a granuloma, but rather an exuberant proliferation of granulation tissue. The lesion presents as a smooth, red, fleshy mass at the site of chronic inflammation, often after surgery or trauma (Figure 9–41). If the lesion does not respond to topical steroids, then excision with a conjunctival graft or cryotherapy is curative.

CARUNCLE TUMORS

The same tumors that affect the conjunctiva can also appear in the caruncle. In order of frequency, they are: **papilloma**, **nevus**, **inclusion cyst**, **malignant melanoma**, **sebaceous cell carcinoma**, and **oncocytoma** (Figures 9–42 and 9–43).

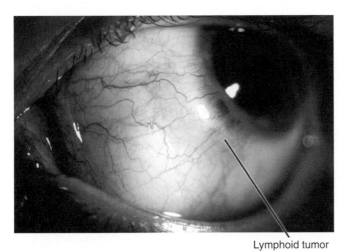

Lymphoid tumor

FIGURE 9–39
Malignant lymphoma with salmon-colored lesion.

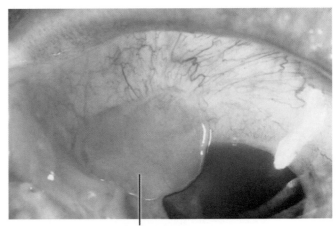

Pyogenic granuloma

FIGURE 9–41
Pyogenic granuloma, appearing as a large, fleshy, vascular, pedunculated growth.

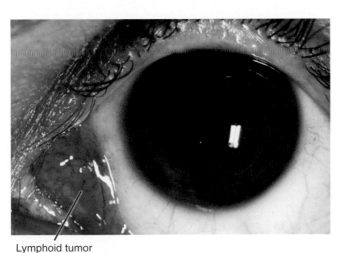

Lymphoid tumor
FIGURE 9–40
Lymphoid tumor, demonstrating typical salmon-patch appearance.

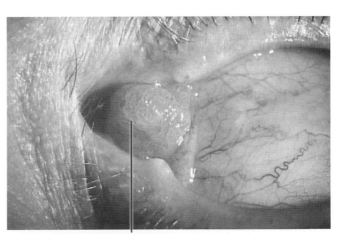

Caruncle papilloma

FIGURE 9–42
Papilloma of the caruncle, appearing as a large, vascular, pedunculated mass.

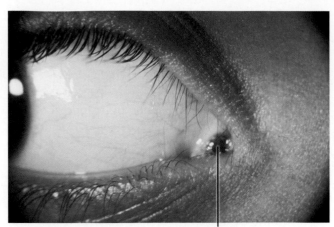

Caruncle nevus

FIGURE 9–43
Nevus of the caruncle, appearing as a brown pigmented spot on the medial side of the caruncle.

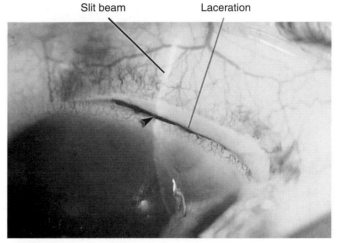

CHAPTER TEN

Sclera

Introduction

The sclera is the strong, white, avascular coat of the eye that protects the delicate inner tissues. It also serves as the attachment site for the extraocular muscles. The sclera can become damaged by trauma, inflamed by systemic disease, and discolored by various disorders.

Trauma

SCLERAL LACERATION

A scleral laceration is a partial or full-thickness cut in the sclera. It is critical to assess the extent of the laceration accurately since the treatment and prognosis are quite different for each. Partial-thickness scleral lacerations do not require surgical repair but only treatment with a topical broad-spectrum antibiotic (polymyxin B sulfate–trimethoprim (Polytrim) or bacitracin ointment qid). A full-thickness laceration produces an open globe, which is an ocular emergency with a guarded prognosis (Figure 10–1).

OPEN GLOBE

Definition

An open or ruptured globe is a full-thickness defect in the cornea or sclera.

Etiology

This is most commonly due to penetrating or blunt trauma, and the latter causes the eye to rupture at the weakest sites: the limbus, just posterior to the rectus

Slit beam   Laceration

FIGURE 10–1
Full-thickness corneoscleral limbal laceration with wound gape. Note discontinuity of slit beam as it crosses the wound edge (arrowhead).

muscle insertions, and previous surgical incisions. Other causes of an open globe include corneal or scleral melting from a chemical burn, autoimmune disease, or infection.

Symptoms

An open globe may be asymptomatic or present with variable degrees of decreased vision and/or pain depending on the etiology.

Signs

In general, there are obvious signs of trauma with concomitant lid and orbital injuries in a patient with an open globe. On examination the wound may be visible or it may be occult, obscured by overlying hemorrhage (usually bullous, subconjunctival hemorrhage), or a posterior location. The most obvious sign of globe penetration is leakage of aqueous fluid or extrusion of intraocular tissue from the wound. The former is demonstrated by a positive Seidel test (see Ch. 11). Other important clues that the eye has been ruptured are a flat or shallow anterior chamber, very low intraocular pressure, peaked pupil (toward the wound), dark uveal tissue sticking through the wound, and intraocular foreign body or air bubble (Figures 10–2 and 10–3). Depending on the severity of the injury, there may be additional signs of trauma such as subconjunctival or intraocular hemorrhage (hyphema, vitreous, retinal), angle damage (recession, iridodialysis, cyclodialysis), iris damage (transillumination defect, sphincter tear), iridodonesis or phacodonesis (looseness of the iris or lens, respectively, apparent as slight jiggling at the slit lamp), dislocated lens, cataract, retinal tear or detachment, and choroidal rupture.

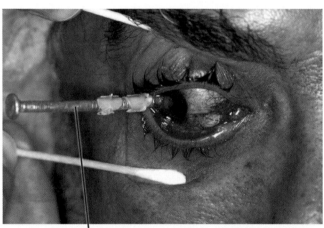

Intraocular nail

FIGURE 10–2
Penetrating injury with foreign body (nail) protruding from globe.

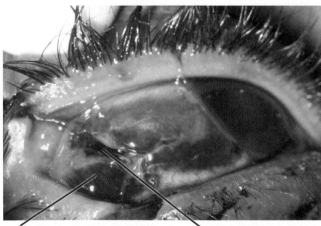

Bullous subconjunctival hemorrhage   Uveal prolapse

FIGURE 10–3
Open globe. There is a temporal full-thickness scleral laceration with uveal prolapse. Also note the extensive subconjunctival hemorrhage and upper- and lower-eyelid lacerations.

Evaluation

- The **history** must include the exact mechanism of injury, detailed past ocular history, especially any previous ocular surgery, tetanus booster history, and time the patient last had anything to eat or drink since he/she will need to go to the operating room.
- When an open globe is suspected, the **eye exam** is performed with minimal manipulation of the globe and periocular tissues to prevent causing further damage. If possible, the visual acuity, pupillary response, and any associated findings (see above) should be documented. Once the diagnosis is confirmed, the examination can be abbreviated or discontinued since further exploration is done in the operating room at the time of surgical repair.
- Consider **B-scan ultrasonography** if the fundus cannot be adequately visualized; however, this may be difficult if the globe is too soft.
- Consider **orbital computed tomography scan** or **radiographs** to rule out an intraocular foreign body. A **magnetic resonance imaging scan** is *contraindicated* if the foreign body is metallic.

Management

- An open globe is a true *ophthalmic emergency* that requires immediate diagnosis and treatment.
- Cover the eye with a metal shield for protection.
- Admit the patient to the hospital for surgical exploration and repair. The primary goal is to avoid infection by closing the wound and removing any intraocular foreign bodies.
- Systemic antibiotics (vancomycin and ceftazidime (1 g IV q12h)) are started immediately, and subconjunctival antibiotics and steroids are injected at the end of surgery. Topical antibiotics (fortified vancomycin (25–50 mg/ml q1h) and ceftazidime (50 mg/ml q1h) alternating every 30 minutes), steroid (prednisolone acetate 1% q1–2h initially), and cycloplegic (scopolamine 0.25% or atropine 1% tid) are administered postoperatively.
- Small corneal lacerations (<2 mm) that are self-sealing or intermittently Seidel-positive may be followed carefully with daily observation and treatment with a bandage contact lens, topical broad-spectrum antibiotic (moxifloxacin (Vigamox) or gatifloxacin (Zymar) q2h to q6h), cycloplegic (cyclopentolate 1% bid), and an aqueous suppressant (timolol maleate (Timoptic) 0.5% or bromonidine (Alphagan-P) 0.15% bid). If the wound has not healed at 1 week, then it should be sutured.
- Additional surgical procedures are typically required for visual rehabilitation (i.e., corneal transplant, cataract extraction, iris reconstruction, glaucoma surgery, drainage of choroidal hemorrhage, retinal detachment repair).

Prognosis

An open globe carries a very guarded prognosis despite emergent treatment, primarily because there is a 3–7% risk of infectious endophthalmitis. Factors that increase the risk of infection are a retained foreign body, delayed surgery (>24 hours), soil contamination, or lens disruption. The outcome is best for cases of limited trauma confined to the anterior segment of the eye. In severe cases, enucleation may need to be performed.

INTRAOCULAR FOREIGN BODY

An intraocular foreign body may occur with penetrating trauma from a projectile. This situation results in an increased risk of developing an intraocular infection (endophthalmitis) despite empiric therapy with systemic and topical antibiotics.

Radiographic studies are used to localize the foreign material, and if the object may be made of metal, magnetic resonance imaging must be avoided. The foreign body is removed during surgical repair of the open globe. However, like for intraorbital foreign bodies, when removal is not possible, small inert intraocular fragments may be observed since they are well tolerated. Foreign matter composed of glass, plastic, sand, stone, ceramic, gold, platinum, silver, or aluminum are inert, while those consisting of copper (>85%), iron, or organic material (i.e., wood) are reactive (Figure 10–4).

Copper

The intensity of the inflammatory response from a copper foreign body depends upon the copper content (severe endophthalmitis if >85%, chalcosis if <85%, and relatively inert if <70%). Mild intraocular inflammation due to an intraocular foreign body containing between 70 and 85% copper is called **chalcosis**. Chalcosis results in copper deposits in the anterior lens capsule (sunflower cataract), Descemet's membrane (Kayser–Fleischer ring), iris (green discoloration and sluggish pupillary response), and retina (degeneration with abnormal electroretinogram (decreased amplitude)).

Iron

Siderosis (iron toxicity) causes iris heterochromia (darker in the involved eye), mid-dilated minimally reactive pupil, lens discoloration (brown-orange dots and generalized yellowing), vitritis, and retinal degeneration.

Inflammation

Scleral inflammation can affect the episclera or the sclera. It is critical to localize the exact level of involvement because these are distinct diagnoses with different etiologies and treatments.

EPISCLERITIS

Definition

Episcleritis is inflammation of the episclera.

Epidemiology

The condition is self-limited and typically affects young adults. It is bilateral in 33% of cases.

Etiology

Episcleritis is usually idiopathic, but is also associated with tuberculosis, syphilis, herpes zoster, rheumatoid arthritis, gout, and collagen vascular disease. It is classified as sectoral (70%) or diffuse (30%), simple (80%) or nodular (20%).

Symptoms

Patients usually notice redness of the eye and sometimes mild discomfort.

Signs

Episcleritis usually presents with sectoral subconjunctival and conjunctival injection (redness), but it can be diffuse (Figure 10–5). There may be chemosis, an episcleral nodule, and anterior-chamber cell and flare.

Differential diagnosis

Episcleritis must be differentiated from more serious conditions, such as scleritis, iritis, phlyctenule, and myositis.

Evaluation

- The **history** must note any pain and history of systemic conditions, which are more consistent with scleritis.

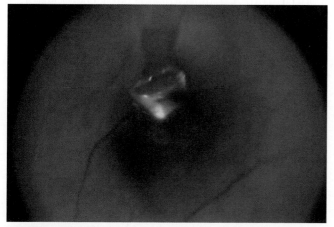

FIGURE 10–4
Intraocular foreign body with surrounding vitreous hemorrhage.

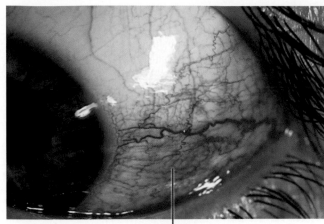

Episcleritis

FIGURE 10–5
Episcleritis, demonstrating characteristic sectoral injection.

- The **eye exam** must pay particular attention to the conjunctiva (injection, may have chemosis), sclera (episcleral injection, may have episcleral nodule), and anterior chamber (may have cell and flare). Specifically, the quality of injection (bright red and superficial), its response to topical 2.5% phenylephrine (blanches when this topical vasoconstrictor is applied), and the absence of pain on palpation help to distinguish episcleritis from scleritis.
- Consider **lab tests** (systemic work-up) for recurrent or bilateral cases (see section on scleritis, below).

Management

- Treatment is usually not required.
- Consider limited use of a vasoconstrictor (naphazoline (Naphcon) qid).
- A mild topical steroid (fluorometholone acetate (Flarex) qid) or oral non-steroidal anti-inflammatory drug (NSAID: indomethacin 50 mg PO qd to bid) can be prescribed for severe cases.

Prognosis

The prognosis is good, but recurrence is common (67%).

SCLERITIS

Definition

Scleritis is inflammation of the sclera.

Epidemiology

The condition most commonly affects women between the ages of 30 and 60 years old and is usually bilateral.

Etiology

Scleritis may be idiopathic or associated with a systemic disease (50%). Most commonly, this is a collagen vascular disease (rheumatoid arthritis, lupus erythematosus, polyarteritis nodosa), vascular disease (Wegener's granulomatosis, giant cell arteritis, Takayasu's disease), relapsing polychondritis, ankylosing spondylitis, Reiter's syndrome, Crohn's disease, ulcerative colitis, sarcoidosis, infection (syphilis, tuberculosis, leprosy, herpes simplex or zoster), gout, or rosacea.

Scleritis is classified as:

Anterior (98%)

- **Diffuse** (40%): most benign, but widespread involvement (Figure 10–6).
- **Nodular** (44%): focal involvement with an immobile nodule (Figure 10–7).
- **Necrotizing** (14%): associated with a life-threatening autoimmune disease.
  - **With inflammation**: focal or diffuse, progressive scleral thinning with vascular occlusion. The

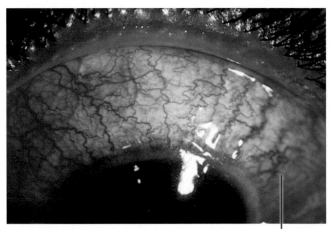

Scleritis

FIGURE 10–6
Diffuse anterior scleritis, demonstrating characteristic deep red, violaceous hue.

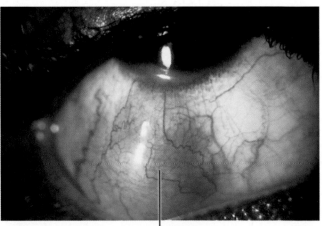

Nodular scleritis

FIGURE 10–7
Nodular anterior scleritis. Note the elevated nodule within the deep, red, sectoral injection.

underlying blue uveal tissue may become visible, imparting a violaceous hue to the involved scleral area (Figure 10–8).

- **Without inflammation** (scleromalacia perforans): this occurs in women with severe rheumatoid arthritis. It is characterized by scleral thinning and ischemia with minimal symptoms and no injection (Figure 10–9).

Posterior (2%)

Usually unilateral, idiopathic, and very painful. Anterior scleritis is also present in 80% of patients with posterior involvement (see Ch. 17).

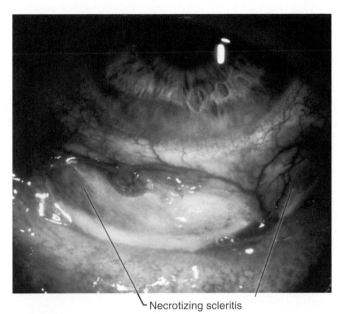

Necrotizing scleritis

FIGURE 10–8
Necrotizing scleritis, demonstrating thinning of sclera superiorly with increased visibility of the underlying blue uvea.

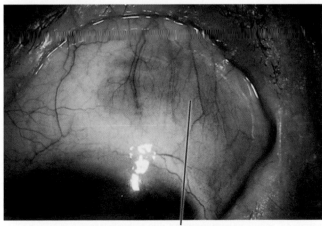

Scleromalacia perforans

FIGURE 10–9
Scleromalacia perforans, demonstrating characteristic blue appearance due to visible uvea underneath thin sclera.

Symptoms

Patients present with pain, photophobia, swelling, redness, and variably decreased vision.

Signs

The most salient feature of scleritis is deep sub-conjunctival injection, sometimes with a violaceous hue. The inflammation is also characterized by tenderness to palpation, chemosis, and scleral edema. There may be anterior-chamber cell and flare (30%), corneal infiltrates or thinning, scleral thinning (30%), and normal or decreased visual acuity. A scleral nodule is readily visible in the nodular type. Additional findings in the posterior form include chorioretinal folds, focal serous retinal detachment, amelanotic fundus lesions, macular edema, optic nerve edema, vitritis, restricted ocular motility, ptosis, proptosis, and elevated intraocular pressure.

Differential diagnosis

Anterior scleritis must be distinguished from episcleritis, iritis, phlyctenule, myositis, and scleral ectasia.

Posterior scleritis must be distinguished from choroidal tumor, orbital tumor, idiopathic orbital inflammation, posterior uveitis, and thyroid-related ophthalmopathy.

Evaluation

- The **history** must document any systemic diseases.
- The **eye exam** should concentrate on the conjunctiva (injection), sclera (may have violaceous hue, nodules, or thinning), cornea (may have infiltrates or thinning), tonometry (may have increased intraocular pressure), anterior chamber (may have cell and flare), and ophthalmoscopy (in posterior scleritis may have chorioretinal folds, focal serous retinal detachment, amelanotic fundus lesions, macular edema, optic nerve edema, and vitritis). It is essential to evaluate the pattern and depth of injection carefully, its response to topical 2.5% phenylephrine (does not blanch in response to this topical vasoconstrictor), and the presence of pain on palpation.
- **B-scan ultrasonography** reveals a thickened sclera and a "T-sign" in posterior scleritis (see Figure 17–97).
- **Lab tests** should be performed in patients without an associated systemic disease diagnosis and include a complete blood count, erythrocyte sedimentation rate, rheumatoid factor, antinuclear antibody, antineutrophil cytoplasmic antibody, uric acid, blood urea nitrogen, Venereal Disease Research Laboratory test, fluorescent treponemal antibody absorption test, purified protein derivative and controls, and chest radiographs.
- **Medical consultation** to diagnose any systemic diseases.

Management

- Scleritis requires systemic treatment.
- Depending on the severity of the inflammation, consider using one or a combination of the following systemic medications (*Note*: topical steroids and NSAIDs are *ineffective*, and subTenon's steroid injection is *contraindicated*):
    - NSAID (indomethacin 50 mg PO bid to tid).
    - Steroid (prednisone 60–100 mg PO qd).
    - Consider immunosuppressive agents (see section on anterior uveitis in Ch. 12) for severe cases. These drugs should be administered by a uveitis specialist.
- Surgery (i.e., patch graft) is required for globe perforation.
- Treat any underlying systemic disease.

Prognosis

The prognosis depends on the etiology. Scleritis commonly recurs and may be complicated by keratitis, cataract, uveitis, and glaucoma. The outcome is poor for the necrotizing form with inflammation, which causes decreased vision in 40% of patients, ocular complications in 60% (including perforation), and has a 5-year mortality rate of 25%. Scleromalacia perforans, on the other hand, rarely perforates.

Scleral Discoloration

The sclera is usually white but can become discolored as a result of various disorders. The altered scleral appearance is usually quite obvious as a unilateral or bilateral, focal or diffuse change in color. It may signify a benign process or a serious disease. It is important to rule out a foreign body or melanoma.

Ectasia is an area of scleral thinning, usually located near the limbus. The area appears blue because the underlying uveal tissue is visible and may bulge through the scleral defect. Scleral ectasia can occur in Ehlers–Danlos, Hurler's, Turner's, and Marfan's syndromes, osteogenesis impefecta, scleromalacia perforans, and congenital staphyloma (Figure 10–10).

Scleral icterus refers to the yellow discoloration of sclera caused by hyperbilirubinemia (Figure 10–11).

A **senile scleral plaque** is a focal blue-gray hyalinization of the sclera anterior to the horizontal rectus muscle insertions that occurs in elderly individuals (Figure 10–12).

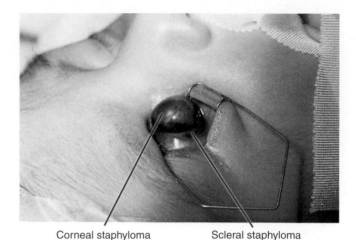

Corneal staphyloma   Scleral staphyloma

FIGURE 10–10
Scleral and corneal staphylomas with bulging blue appearance.

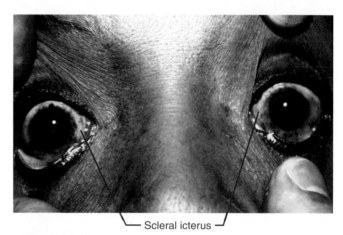

Scleral icterus

FIGURE 10–11
Scleral icterus in a patient with jaundice.

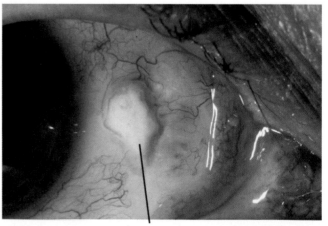

Scleral plaque

FIGURE 10–12
Senile scleral plaque, demonstrating discoloration of sclera near horizontal rectus muscle insertion due to hyalinization.

CHAPTER ELEVEN

Cornea

Introduction

The cornea is the central clear covering of the eye that merges with the conjuntiva and sclera at the limbus. In addition to focusing the entering light, this resilient tissue also serves a barrier function. Any defect in the epithelium will cause pain and foreign-body sensation, and may produce mild anterior-chamber cell and flare. Insults to deeper layers of the cornea result in edema and scarring.

Trauma

The cornea may be damaged by a variety of mechanisms. Corneal trauma is caused by chemical, thermal, blunt, or penetrating injuries. Birth trauma can occur from forceps delivery, which produces vertical or oblique breaks in Descemet's membrane with acute corneal edema and then astigmatism and amblyopia later in life. The immediate management of these situations is vital in order to minimize tissue damage. Later, additional treatment may be needed to maximize vision.

CORNEAL BURN

A corneal burn is destruction of the epithelium and stroma due to chemical (acid or base) or thermal (i.e., welding, intense sunlight, tanning lamp) injury. The conjunctiva and sclera may also be involved. Patients suffer from immediate pain, foreign-body sensation, photophobia, tearing, and redness. The visual acuity may be normal or decreased, and there are conjunctival injection, ciliary injection, and epithelial defects of the cornea and conjunctiva that stain with fluorescein dye (Figure 11–1). Corneal clouding from edema and scleral blanching from ischemia are ominous signs that indicate

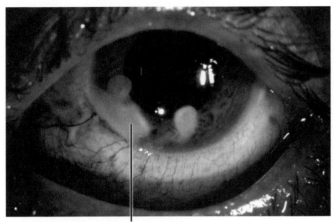

Corneal alkali burn

FIGURE 11–1

Alkali burn demonstrating corneal burns and conjunctival injection on the day of the accident.

severe damage (Figure 11–2). The severity of the burn is categorized as:

- **Grade 1**: corneal epithelial damage and no ischemia; full recovery.
- **Grade 2**: stromal haze that does not obscure iris details, and ischemia involving less than one-third of the limbus; good prognosis with some scarring.
- **Grade 3**: total corneal epithelial loss, stromal haze obscuring the iris, and ischemia involving one-third to one-half of the limbus; guarded prognosis.
- **Grade 4**: opaque cornea and ischemia involving more than one-half of the limbus; poor prognosis with risk of perforation.

In addition to the degree of tissue damage, the prognosis also depends on the etiology. It is worst for strong alkali burns, which cause the most damage and may even result in globe perforation. Other complications include

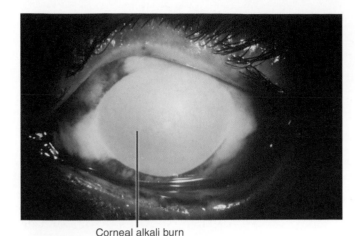

Corneal alkali burn

FIGURE 11–2
Complete corneal tissue destruction 7 days after alkali burn.

cataract, glaucoma, uveitis, symblepharon, entropion, neurotrophic keratitis, anterior-segment ischemia, and corneal ulceration, scarring, vascularization, and keratinization (Figure 11–3). Fortunately, most burns are mild (grade 1) and basically produce an abrasion of the ocular surface that heals completely without sequelae.

A corneal burn is a true *ophthalmic emergency* that requires immediate treatment:

- The eye must be copiously irrigated stat with at least 1 liter of sterile water, saline, or Ringer's solution.
- If possible, measure the pH before and after irrigation, and continue irrigation until the pH is neutral.
- Remove any chemical particulate matter from the ocular surface, evert the eyelids, and sweep the fornices with a sterile cotton-tipped applicator.
- Topical treatment includes lubrication of the eye with non-preserved artificial tears (up to q1h) and oint-

ment (qhs), a broad-spectrum antibiotic (moxifloxacin (Vigamox) or gatifloxacin (Zymar) qid), and a cycloplegic (cyclopentolate 1%, scopolamine 0.25%, or atropine 1% bid to qid depending on the severity).
- Consider topical steroids, citrate or sodium ascorbate, and a collagenase inhibitor for more serious burns.
- Treatment may be required for increased intraocular pressure (see Ch. 13).
- Severe burns may require surgery to reconstruct the ocular surface and for visual rehabilitation.

CORNEAL ABRASION

A corneal abrasion is a traumatic epithelial defect, usually resulting from a fingernail, plant branch, hairbrush, or contact lens. Patients experience variable discomfort from a mild foreign-body sensation to extreme pain, as well as photophobia, tearing, and redness. Depending on the location of the scratch, the vision may be normal or decreased. On examination, the epithelial defect is readily visible as an area that stains with fluorescein dye (Figure 11–4). The conjunctiva is injected and there may even be mild anterior-chamber cell and flare since any irritation of the cornea can produce an anterior-chamber reaction. If the patient complains of pain with blinking and there are fine, linear, vertical abrasions of the superior cornea, then the upper eyelid must be everted to look for a foreign body on the upper palpebral (tarsal) conjunctival surface (see Figure 9–1).

- Corneal epithelial defects are treated with a broad-spectrum topical antibiotic drop (polymyxin B sulfate–trimethoprim (Polytrim) or tobramycin (Tobrex) qid) or ointment (polymyxin B sulfate–bacitracin zinc (Polysporin) qid) because of the risk of infection, especially in contact lens wearers.

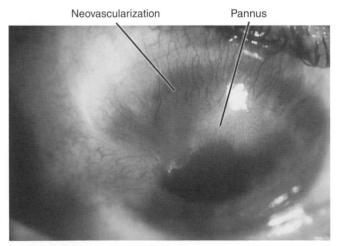

Neovascularization   Pannus

FIGURE 11–3
Large pannus demonstrating scarring and vascularization of the superior cornea in a patient with a chemical burn.

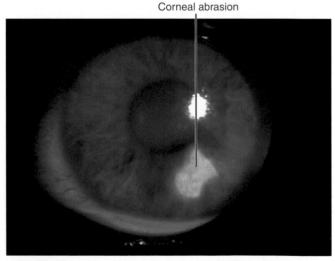

Corneal abrasion

FIGURE 11–4
Corneal abrasion demonstrating fluorescein staining of small inferior epithelial defect.

- Relief from pain may be provided by a topical non-steroidal anti-inflammatory (Acular, Voltaren, Nevanac, or Xibrom tid for 48–72 hours). A topical cycloplegic (cyclopentolate 1% bid) can also help with pain and photophobia.
- Consider using a pressure patch or bandage contact lens for comfort in patients with large abrasions; however, contact lens wear, the presence of a corneal infiltrate, or injury caused by plant material are contra-indications to patching because these scenarios are at high risk for the development of infectious keratitis if patched.
- Patients should never be given a topical anesthetic since these agents are toxic to the cornea and can cause non-healing epithelial defects and corneal melts.

CORNEAL LACERATION

A corneal laceration is a partial or full-thickness cut in the cornea (see section on open globe in Ch. 10) caused by trauma. Similar to a corneal abrasion, patients typically experience pain, foreign-body sensation, photophobia, tearing, and redness. They may have normal or decreased visual acuity, conjunctival injection, ciliary injection, intra-ocular foreign body, corneal edema, anterior-chamber cell and flare, and low intraocular pressure. The prognosis is good for partial-thickness lacerations that do not cross the visual axis. Larger, full-thickness lacerations, and those that cross the visual axis carry a more guarded prognosis (Figure 11–5).

- Perform a **Seidel test** to rule out an open globe: apply concentrated fluorescein dye directly to the laceration and observe the area at the slit lamp for a stream of dilute fluorescein (lighter color) emanating from the wound (positive test). The stream appears as a fluorescent yellow area on a dark blue background with the cobalt blue light, or a light yellow-green area on a dark orange background with the white light (Figure 11–6).
- Consider **orbital computed tomography scan** or **radiographs** to rule out an intraocular foreign body. A magnetic resonance imaging scan is *contraindicated* if the foreign body is metallic.
- Administer a topical broad-spectrum antibiotic (moxifloxacin (Vigamox) or gatifloxacin (Zymar) qid) and a cycloplegic (cyclopentolate 1% or scopolamine 0.25% tid) for a partial-thickness laceration.
- Daily follow-up is required until the laceration heals.
- Consider applying a pressure patch or bandage contact lens.
- Surgery is usually required for full-thickness lacerations (see section on open globe in Ch. 10) or for partial-thickness lacerations with wound gape.

CORNEAL FOREIGN BODY

A corneal foreign body is exogenous material, usually metal, glass, or organic, on the surface of or embedded in the cornea (Figure 11–7). Patients present with pain, foreign-body sensation, photophobia, tearing, and redness. Besides a visible foreign body, findings on exam include normal or decreased visual acuity, conjunctival injection, and ciliary injection. There may also be a rust ring surrounding a metal foreign body, epithelial defect that stains with fluorescein dye, corneal edema, and anterior-chamber cell and flare (Figure 11–8). The prognosis is good unless scarring from a central foreign body affects the visual axis. Deep, non-perforating, unexposed, inert material may be asymptomatic and well tolerated.

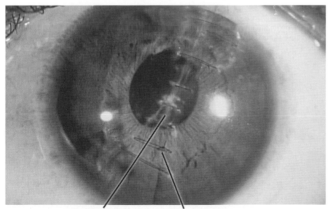

Corneal laceration   Nylon sutures

FIGURE 11–5
Large corneal laceration through the visual axis. Note the linear scar from the wound and the multiple interrupted nylon sutures of various lengths used to repair the laceration.

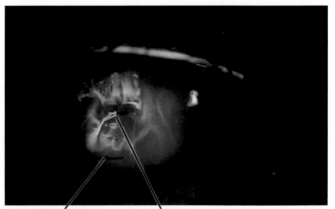

Nylon sutures   Positive Seidel test

FIGURE 11–6
Corneal laceration demonstrating positive Seidel test (bright stream of fluorescein around the central suture).

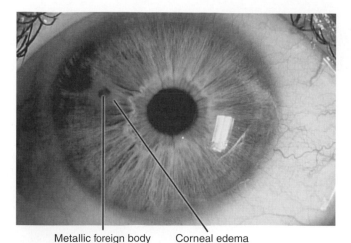

Metallic foreign body   Corneal edema

FIGURE 11–7
Metallic foreign body appears as brown spot on cornea.

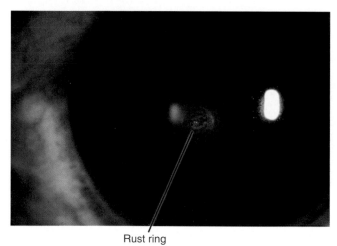

Rust ring

FIGURE 11–8
Rust ring from iron foreign body in central cornea.

- Perform a **Seidel test** for a deep foreign body to rule out an open globe.
- Remove the foreign material with a small-gauge needle or specialized instrument at the slit lamp. A rust ring is easily removed with an automated burr or Alger brush.
- Treatment of the resulting corneal epithelial defect is with a topical antibiotic and possibly a cycloplegic. Also consider a pressure patch or bandage contact lens (see section on corneal abrasion, above).

RECURRENT EROSION

A recurrent erosion is a spontaneous corneal epithelial defect due to abnormal adhesion of the epithelium to the underlying Bowman's membrane. Recurrent erosion syndrome is associated with corneal dystrophies, especially anterior basement membrane dystrophy (50% of cases) and previous traumatic corneal abrasions. Spontaneous

sloughing typically occurs upon awakening, when the mechanical trauma of the upper eyelid rubbing across the cornea dislodges an area of weak epithelium. This causes recurrent bouts of pain, foreign-body sensation, photophobia, tearing, and redness, especially in the morning. The duration and degree of symptoms depend upon the size of the erosion. On examination, the epithelial defect may be partially healed and visible with fluorescein dye as an irregular area of staining.

- Treatment is with a topical antibiotic, as for a corneal abrasion, until the erosion has completely re-epithelialized.
- Hypertonic saline ointment (Adsorbonac or Muro 128 5%) is applied to the involved eye at bedtime for 3 months to prevent recurrence, and topical lubrication is recommended during the day with non-preserved artificial tears or Muro 128 drops.
- Consider treatment with systemic doxycycline (50 mg PO bid for 2 months) and a topical steroid (tid for 2–3 weeks).
- Other options include the use of a bandage contact lens; debridement, anterior stromal puncture/reinforcement, or Nd:YAG laser reinforcement of the abnormal epithelium; or excimer laser phototherapeutic keratectomy.

Contact Lens Disorders

Contact lenses are worn primarily to correct refractive errors (myopia, hyperopia, astigmatism, and presbyopia). However, a contact lens can also be used as a therapeutic bandage lens to treat corneal surface disorders or a cosmetic appliance to appear to change iris color or create a pseudo-pupil.

TYPES OF CONTACT LENSES

Rigid lenses

Polymethylmethacrylate (PMMA) lenses are hard lenses that are impermeable to oxygen. The cornea can therefore only receive oxygen by blinking, which allows the tear film to enter the space beneath the lens. This style of lens was worn on a daily basis and provided good visual acuity, but is no longer used because of problems with corneal hypoxia and edema (Figure 11–9).

Rigid gas-permeable (RGP) lenses are rigid lenses composed of cellulose acetate butyrate, silicone acrylate, or silicone combined with PMMA. These contacts are highly permeable to oxygen and are therefore more comfortable and healthier for the eye than the older hard-style lenses. RGPs are daily-wear contacts that are the lens of choice for patients with astigmatism and irregular corneas (i.e.,

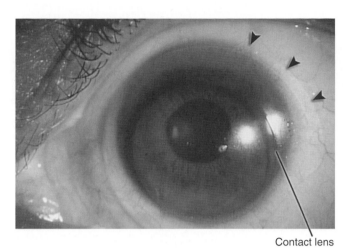

FIGURE 11–9
Hard contact lens. The edge of the lens (arrowheads) as well as the central optical portion (line) are visible.

Contact lens

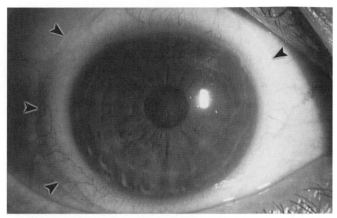

FIGURE 11–11
Soft contact lens. Note the edge of the lens overlying the sclera (arrowheads).

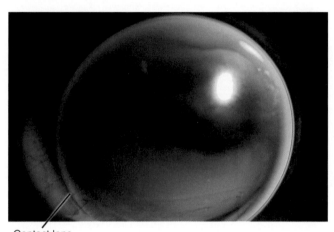

Contact lens

FIGURE 11–10
Rigid gas-permeable contact lens demonstrating fluorescein staining pattern.

keratoconus) since they provide the sharpest vision. Their smooth, regular surface essentially acts as the patient's new corneal surface (Figure 11–10).

Soft lenses

Daily-wear lenses are hydrogel lenses (hydroxymethylmethacrylate). The advantage of this material is that it is more comfortable and flexible than rigid lenses. The maximum wear time depends on the oxygen permeability and water content of each lens. However, soft contacts drape over and conform to the corneal surface, and therefore they are not ideal for correcting large degrees of astigmatism or irregular corneas (Figure 11–11).

Extended-wear lenses are disposable lenses that are removed and discarded after wearing from 1 to 4 weeks. These lenses have a significant risk of infectious keratitis with overnight wear.

CONTACT LENS PROBLEMS

Although the overwhelming majority of contact lens wearers never experience a problem, contact lens use is not without risks. Numerous complications are associated with lens wear, especially when the lenses are worn for too long (i.e., sleeping with contact lenses in) or do not fit correctly. Most contact lens-related problems are symptomatic, and patients often experience foreign-body sensation, decreased vision, redness, tearing, itching, burning, pain, lens awareness, and/or reduced contact lens wear time. It is important to take a detailed history regarding their lens wear and care habits. The contact lens appearance and fit must be assessed, and the conjunctiva and cornea are carefully inspected without the lenses. Anyone who wears contacts must be counseled to remove their lenses immediately and seek medical care if they ever experience such symptoms, since failure to do so could potentially be vision-threatening.

Corneal abrasion

Contact lens-related epithelial defects result from various causes, such as foreign bodies under the lens, damaged lens, poor lens fit, corneal hypoxia, and poor lens insertion/removal technique.

- Treatment is with a topical antibiotic, as for a traumatic corneal abrasion, except contact lens-related abrasions should never be patched because of the significant risk of developing a corneal infection.

Corneal hypoxia

A certain degree of hypoxia occurs with any type of lens wear. Usually this is minimal and does not require treatment; however, lack of oxygen can produce a number of complications.

Hard lenses may cause **acute hypoxia** with conjunctival injection and epithelial defects.

- Suspend lens wear and treat with a topical antibiotic.
- When the cornea heals, the patient should be refitted with a lens of greater oxygen transmissibility (higher-Dk/L value).

Any type of contact lens may produce **chronic hypoxia** with perilimbal punctate staining, corneal epithelial microcysts, stromal edema, and corneal neovascularization.

- Suspend contact lens use or reduce contact lens wear time.
- Consider replacing the lens with one of higher oxygen transmissibility.

Contact lens solution hypersensitivity/toxicity

Reactions to contact lens solutions commonly cause conjunctival injection and diffuse corneal punctate staining. The preservative in the solution (e.g., thimerosal) is usually responsible for this toxicity.

- It is important to identify and discontinue the offending agent.
- Lens wear should be suspended until the ocular surface heals and may be resumed after thoroughly cleaning, rinsing, and disinfecting the lens.
- Patients must be educated about proper contact lens care.
- It may be necessary to change the system of care, replace soft contact lenses, or polish rigid lenses.

Corneal neovascularization

Growth of limbal blood vessels into the cornea is due to hypoxia in patients who wear contact lenses. A 1–2 mm superior corneal vascular scar (**pannus**) is frequently seen on slit-lamp exam. The new vessels are usually superficial and sectoral, but may become deep and involve the entire corneal circumference. Neovascularization >2 mm is significant and may lead to intrastromal hemorrhage, lipid deposits, and scarring if the fragile vessels leak blood or fluid (Figure 11–12).

- Options to promote regression of the vascularization are to refit with a lens of higher oxygen transmissibility, reduce or stop lens wear, and treat with a topical steroid.

Corneal warpage

Contact lenses can alter the shape of the cornea. The amount of induced corneal irregularity is related to the lens material (hard > RGP > soft), fit, and length of time of wear. It is not associated with corneal edema. Although this condition is frequently asymptomatic, patients with contact lens-related corneal warpage may notice blurred vision with their glasses, contact lens intolerance, loss of best spectacle corrected visual acuity, or a change in refraction, particularly in the axis of astigmatism. The diagnosis is confirmed by an abnormal corneal topography (computerized videokeratography),

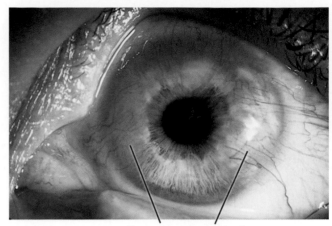

Corneal neovascularization

FIGURE 11–12
Contact lens-induced corneal neovascularization and scarring.

which usually shows an area of steepening that may mimic keratoconus.

- Discontinue contact lens wear until the patient's refraction and corneal topography are stable.

Damaged contact lens

A defective or broken contact lens will produce pain with lens insertion and prompt relief upon lens removal. The contact lens must be inspected for chips (in RGPs) and fissures or tears (in soft lenses).

- Replace the damaged lens.

Deposits on contact lens

Debris, often visible as abundant film or bumps, may accumulate on the surfaces of contact lenses (Figures 11–13 and 11–14). Patients are often aware of blurred

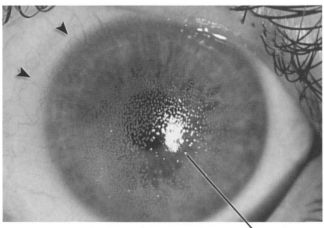

Deposits on contact lens

FIGURE 11–13
Calcium phosphate deposits on soft contact lens. Arrowheads show edge of contact lens.

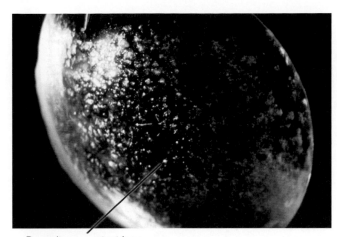

Deposits on contact lens

FIGURE 11–14
Lipid deposits on contact lens.

vision with or without discomfort. The deposits may cause conjunctival injection, corneal erosion, excess contact lens movement, and giant papillary conjunctivitis.

- Contact lens cleaning procedures should be reviewed with the patient, including regular enzyme use and frequent replacement schedule.
- Consider polishing rigid lenses or ordering new ones.

Giant papillary conjunctivitis

Giant papillary conjunctivitis is a unique form of allergic conjunctivitis due to sensitivity to contact lens material, deposits on the lens, or mechanical irritation. Exposed sutures and ocular prostheses also cause giant papillary conjunctivitis. The characteristic findings are large papillae on the superior palpebral (tarsal) conjunctiva and ropy mucous discharge in a patient with itchy eyes and contact lens intolerance (see Ch. 9).

- Temporarily decrease or suspend contact lens wear and administer a topical mast cell stabilizer (lodoxamide tromethamine 0.1% (Alomide) or cromolyn sodium 4% (Crolom) qid) or mild steroid (fluorometholone qid).
- Consider changing the cleaning regimen or the lens material.

Infiltrates

White spots in the cornea of various size and depth are a common contact lens-related problem. They are due to hypoxia, antigenic reaction to preservatives in contact lens solutions, or infection. Sterile infiltrates are typically multifocal, peripheral, small (≤1 mm), hazy, white lesions with intact overlying epithelium. An infectious etiology is the most feared, and therefore any corneal infiltrate is presumed to be infectious and is treated as such.

- Stop lens wear and start topical antibiotics.

Infectious keratitis

A corneal infection or ulcer produces an infiltrate with an overlying epithelial defect that stains with fluorescein. There is pain, redness, and anterior chamber cell and flare. Contact lens wear, especially extended wear, is a significant risk factor for microbial keratitis. In particular, infection with *Pseudomonas* or *Acanthamoeba* is more common in this patient population (see section on corneal ulcer, below).

- Immediately discontinue lens wear and begin topical broad-spectrum antibiotics (a fluoroquinolone (Vigamox or Zymar) or fortified antibiotic q1h).
- Consider culturing the cornea, contact lens, and lens case.

Poor fit

Contact lenses that fit too loosely or too tightly can become problematic.

A **loose lens** causes upper-eyelid irritation, limbal injection, excess contact lens movement with blinking, poor contact lens centration, lens edge bubbles, and lens edge elevation.

- Tighten the lens by increasing the sagittal vault, steepening the base curve, or enlarging the diameter.

A **tight lens** causes injection or indentation around the limbus, minimal contact lens movement with blinking, and corneal edema.

- Loosen the lens by decreasing the sagittal vault, flattening the base curve, or reducing the diameter.

Superior limbic keratoconjunctivitis

Superior limbic keratoconjunctivitis is a special form of conjunctivitis caused by a contact lens hypersensitivity reaction, poor contact lens fit, or toxic reaction to thimerosal. The characteristic signs on exam are micropapillae of the upper palpebral (tarsal) conjunctiva, superior limbal injection, fluorescein staining of the superior bulbar conjunctiva, and a superior micropannus (see Ch. 9).

- Suspend lens wear, use non-preserved contact lens solutions, and clean and/or replace the lenses.
- Consider additional treatment with a topical steroid (prednisolone acetate 1% or fluorometholone qid) or silver nitrate solution (0.5–1%) if the condition persists.

Superficial punctate keratitis

Superficial punctate keratitis refers to punctate staining of the corneal surface with fluorescein dye (Figure 11–15). Contact lens-related superficial punctate keratitis results from poor lens fit, dryness, and contact lens solution toxicity. Other causes include blepharitis, dry eye, trauma, foreign body, trichiasis, burn, medicamentosa, exposure, and conjunctivitis.

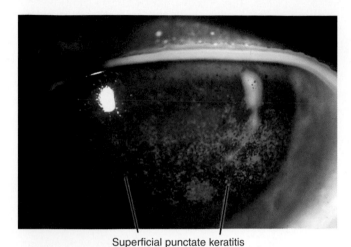

Superficial punctate keratitis

FIGURE 11–15
Superficial punctate keratitis, demonstrating diffuse epithelial staining of the central cornea with fluorescein.

- Treatment consists of topical lubrication with artificial tears and ointment.
- Consider adding a topical antibiotic for moderate to severe cases.

Exposure Keratopathy

Exposure keratopathy refers to drying of the cornea with subsequent epithelial breakdown. This condition has numerous causes, including neurotrophic (cranial nerve V palsy, aneurysm, cerebrovascular accident, multiple sclerosis, tumor, herpes simplex, herpes zoster), neuroparalytic (cranial nerve VII palsy), and lid malposition (lagophthalmos, proptosis). Protection of the corneal surface with lubrication, a bandage contact lens, or tarsorrhaphy is required to prevent complications such

as filamentary keratitis, microbial keratitis, and corneal ulceration and vascularization (Figure 11–16).

Corneal Edema

Definition

Corneal edema is focal or diffuse swelling of the corneal stroma and/or epithelium.

Etiology

Stromal edema is due to endothelial dysfunction, whereas epithelial edema is caused by increased intraocular pressure or corneal hypoxia.

Symptoms

Depending on the time course, amount of edema, and location relative to the visual axis, patients may be asymptomatic or have photophobia, foreign-body sensation, tearing, pain, halos around lights, and decreased vision.

Signs

Stromal edema appears as a thickened cornea with hazy stromal whitening and Descemet's folds (Figure 11–17). Epithelial edema is visible as superficial microcysts and bullae (epithelial "blisters"), which produce a poor corneal light reflex. Other findings may include normal or decreased visual acuity, non-healing epithelial defects, superficial punctate keratitis, tiny endothelial bumps (guttata), anterior-chamber cell and flare, decreased or increased intraocular pressure, and iris or vitreous touching the cornea.

Differential diagnosis

Any significant insult to the cornea can produce corneal edema: inflammation, infection, trauma, dystrophy,

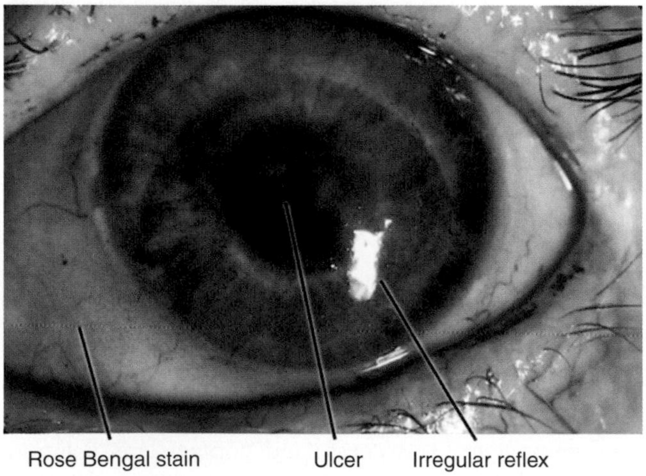

Rose Bengal stain   Ulcer   Irregular reflex

FIGURE 11–16
Exposure keratopathy with interpalpebral rose Bengal staining, a neurotrophic ulcer in the central cornea, and an irregular light reflex on the cornea.

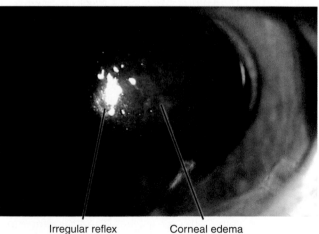

Irregular reflex   Corneal edema

FIGURE 11–17
Pseudophakic bullous keratopathy demonstrating corneal edema with central corneal folds, hazy stroma, and distorted light reflex.

hydrops, acute angle-closure glaucoma, congenital glaucoma, previous ocular surgery (i.e., bullous keratopathy due to aphakia or pseudophakia), contact lens overwear, hypotony, and anterior-segment ischemia.

Evaluation

- The **history** must include any previous ocular disease, injury, or surgery.
- The **eye exam** focuses on the cornea (extent and location of edema, thickness, contact with iris or vitreous), tonometry (altered intraocular pressure), anterior chamber (depth, cell and flare), and gonioscopy (rule out angle closure).
- Consider **pachymetry** to measure central corneal thickness (>0.610 mm indicates edema).
- Consider **specular microscopy** to measure the endothelial cells (abnormal morphology and reduced number of cells are risks for edema).

Management

- Hypertonic saline ointment (Adsorbonac or Muro 128 5% tid) can often improve or resolve epithelial edema.
- A broad-spectrum topical antibiotic (polymyxin B sulfate–trimethoprim (Polytrim) or tobramycin (Tobrex) qid) is used to treat epithelial defects. Persistent defects or painful bullae may require a bandage contact lens or tarsorrhaphy.
- A topical steroid (prednisolone acetate 1% up to qid) may be useful for stromal edema.
- Treat the underlying abnormality.
- A penetrating keratoplasty (corneal graft/transplant) may be required.

Prognosis

The prognosis depends on the underlying problem and the status of the corneal endothelium, which is the natural pump that keeps the cornea clear and compact (see Ch. 1). If the endothelium is healthy, then the edema usually resolves completely. However, corneas with reduced endothelial cell counts may not be able to recover from significant stresses and may fail.

Corneal Ulcer

Definition

A corneal ulcer refers to corneal tissue (epithelial and stromal) destruction.

Etiology

A corneal ulcer is usually due to an infection, although other conditions can sometimes produce corneal ulceration. Any defect in the corneal epithelium increases the risk of infection, especially in the setting of trauma or contact lens wear. Other risks include dry eyes, exposure

keratopathy, bullous keratopathy, neurotrophic cornea, and lid abnormalities.

INFECTIOUS (MICROBIAL KERATITIS)

Bacterial is the most common cause of infectious keratitis. The usual organisms are *Pseudomonas aeruginosa, Staphylococcus aureus, S. epidermidis, Streptococcus pneumoniae, Haemophilus influenzae,* and *Moraxella catarrhalis. Neisseria* species, *Corynebacterium diphtheriae, H. aegyptius,* and *Listeria* are especially dangerous because they can penetrate intact corneal epithelium (Figures 11–18–11–20).

Fungal keratitis is usually due to *Aspergillus, Candida,* or *Fusarium* species and is associated with trauma (especially involving tree branch or vegetable

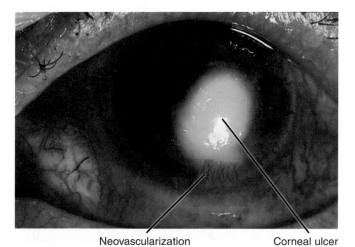

Neovascularization   Corneal ulcer

FIGURE 11–18
Bacterial keratitis demonstrating large, central, *Streptococcus pneumoniae* corneal ulcer. Note the dense, white corneal infiltrate and the extreme conjunctival injection.

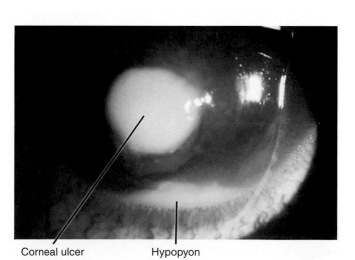

Corneal ulcer   Hypopyon

FIGURE 11–19
Bacterial keratitis demonstrating *Pseudomonas aeruginosa* corneal ulcer with surrounding corneal edema and hypopyon.

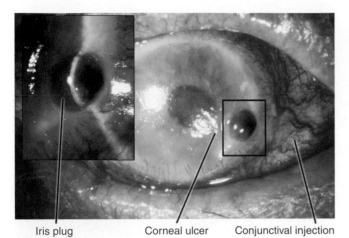

Iris plug   Corneal ulcer   Conjunctival injection

FIGURE 11–20
Perforated corneal ulcer. The cornea is opaque, scarred, and vascularized, and there is a paracentral perforation with iris plugging the wound. Inset shows slit beam over iris plugging perforated wound.

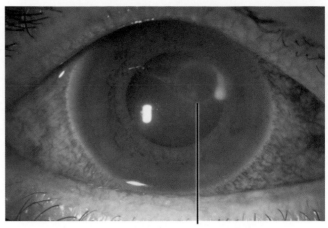

Acanthamoeba ring infiltrate

FIGURE 11–22
Acanthamoeba keratitis, demonstrating the characteristic ring infiltrate.

matter), soft contact lens wear, topical steroid use, non-healing epithelial defects, and immuno-compromised hosts. These ulcers characteristically have feathery edges, satellite infiltrates, and endothelial plaques (Figure 11–21). Fungi can penetrate Descemet's membrane.

Parasitic infection with *Acanthamoeba* is associated with poor contact lens cleaning habits (i.e., using non-sterile water) and swimming or hot tubbing while wearing contact lenses. This organism causes a serious keratitis that is often initially misdiagnosed as herpes simplex virus (HSV: see below). Patients commonly experience pain out of proportion to the signs. Initially there is a punctate keratopathy or pseudodendrite. The classic perineural and ring infiltrates appear later (Figure 11–22). Corneal edema,

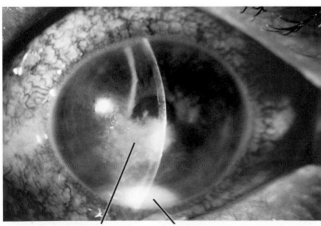

Fungal keratitis   Hypopyon

FIGURE 11–21
Fungal keratitis demonstrating a central corneal infiltrate with feathery borders, severe conjunctival injection, and a small hypopyon.

subepithelial infiltrates, iritis, hypopyon (30–40%), scleritis, and perforation may also occur.

Viral keratitis is caused by both herpes simplex and herpes zoster.

- **HSV**: recurrent HSV is the most common cause of central infectious keratitis and is caused by reactivation of latent virus in the Gasserian ganglion. Triggers include sun exposure, fever, stress, menses, trauma, illness, and immunosuppression. HSV can produce different types of corneal infection:
  - **Epithelial keratitis** is the most common manifestation of HSV, but does not always appear as a classic dendrite with ulceration and terminal bulbs (Figures 11–23 and 11–24). It can also present as a superficial punctate keratitis or geographic ulcer. Epithelial involvement is associated with scarring and decreased corneal sensation.
  - **Disciform keratitis** is a self-limited (up to 6 months), cell-mediated, immune response that causes a focal disc-like area of stromal edema, keratic precipitates (KP), and scarring (Figure 11–25).
  - **Necrotizing interstitial keratitis** is an antigen–antibody–complement-mediated reaction that results in severe stromal destruction and iritis.
  - **Endotheliitis** causes corneal edema, KP, increased intraocular pressure, and anterior chamber cell and flare.
- **Herpes zoster virus (HZV)**: HZV can also affect the eye (herpes zoster ophthalmicus: HZO), and particularly the cornea, in various ways. In fact, the most common single dermatome involved with shingles is cranial nerve V: ophthalmic (V_1) > maxillary (V_2) > mandibular (V_3). Involvement of the tip of the nose (nasociliary nerve) is known

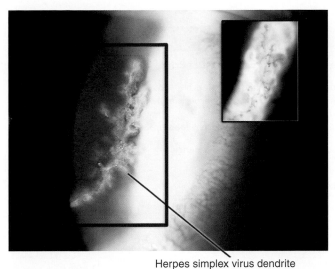

FIGURE 11–23
Herpes simplex epithelial keratitis demonstrating dendrite with terminal bulbs; inset shows staining of dendrite with rose Bengal.

Herpes simplex virus dendrite

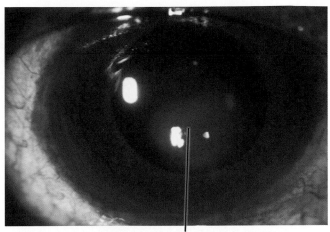

Herpes simplex virus disciform keratitis

FIGURE 11–25
Herpes simplex disciform keratitis, demonstrating central round area of hazy edema.

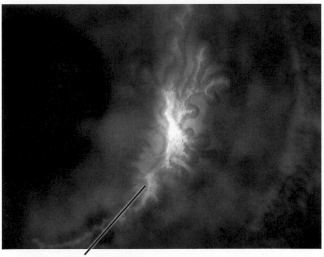

Herpes simplex virus dendrite

FIGURE 11–24
Same patient as shown in Figure 11–23, demonstrating staining of herpes simplex virus dendrite with fluorescein.

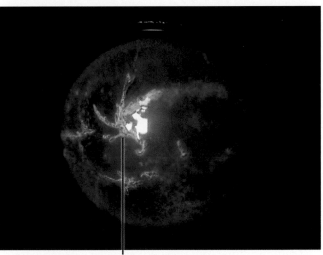

Herpes zoster virus pseudodendrite

FIGURE 11–26
Herpes zoster ophthalmicus, demonstrating staining of coarse pseudodendrites with fluorescein. The pseudodendrite has heaped-up epithelium without terminal bulbs.

as Hutchinson's sign and increases the risk of ocular involvement. Acutely, HZV can cause a pseudodendrite (a coarser, raised epithelial lesion without terminal bulbs) or superficial punctate keratitis with iritis and increased intraocular pressure (Figure 11–26 and Table 11-1). Subsequent corneal manifestations result in scarring:

- **Stromal keratitis** (50%) represents an immune response. It occurs within the first 3 weeks as nummular subepithelial infiltrates and disciform keratitis beneath the initial epithelial lesion.
- **Endotheliitis** (10%) appears as bullous keratopathy and iritis.

- **Neurotrophic keratopathy** (20%) is ulceration due to decreased corneal sensation.

NON-INFECTIOUS

Non-immune-mediated: traumatic, eyelid abnormalities (entropion, ectropion, trichiasis, exposure, lagophthalmos), neurotrophic cornea, and acne rosacea.

Localized immune-mediated: staphylococcal marginal ulcer (hypersensitivity reaction to *Staphylococcus*), vernal keratoconjunctivitis (shield ulcer), and Mooren's ulcer (Figures 11–27 and 11–28).

TABLE 11-1

Comparison of Herpetic Epithelial Keratitis

Lesion	Herpes simplex virus dendrite	Herpes zoster virus pseudodendrite
Appearance	Delicate, fine, lacy ulcer	Coarse, ropy, elevated, "painted-on" lesion Smaller, less branching than herpes simplex virus dendrite
	Terminal bulbs	Blunt ends (no terminal bulbs)
	Epithelial cells slough	Epithelial cells are swollen and heaped-up
Staining	Base with fluorescein Edges with rose Bengal	Poor with fluorescein and rose Bengal
Treatment	Do not use steroids	Good response to steroids

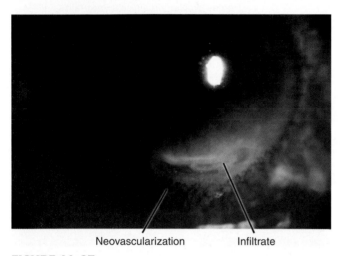

Neovascularization   Infiltrate

FIGURE 11–27
Staphylococcal marginal keratitis, demonstrating circumlimbal location of ulceration and infiltrate with intervening clear zone.

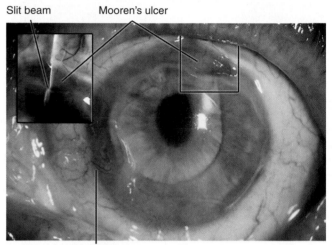

Slit beam   Mooren's ulcer

Neovascularization

FIGURE 11–28
Mooren's ulcer, demonstrating circumferential thinning and ulceration of almost the entire peripheral cornea. The leading edge of the ulcer can be seen as the thin, white, irregular line above the midsection of the iris from the 2 o'clock to 8 o'clock positions (counterclockwise) and then extending to the peripheral cornea. Neovascularization is most evident extending from the limbus at the 8 o'clock position. The inset demonstrates undermining of the ulcer's leading edge seen with a fine slit beam.

Systemic immune-mediated (marginal keratolysis/peripheral ulcerative keratitis): typically autoimmune or collagen vascular, like Sjögren's syndrome, rheumatoid arthritis, Wegener's granulomatosis, polyarteritis nodosa, systemic lupus erythematosus, scleroderma, relapsing polychondritis, inflammatory bowel disease, Behçet's disease, ocular cicatricial pemphigoid, and Stevens–Johnson syndrome. The ulceration is usually peripheral and unilateral, but it can be central and bilateral. Peripheral ulcerative keratitis progresses rapidly and may perforate, but melting resolves once the overlying epithelium heals.

Symptoms

Corneal ulcers typically cause pain, redness, discharge, tearing, photophobia, and decreased vision. Patients may notice a white spot on the cornea.

Signs

The hallmark of a corneal ulcer is corneal thinning with an overlying epithelial defect that stains with fluorescein dye. There may be normal or decreased visual acuity, conjunctival injection, ciliary injection, a white corneal infiltrate (bacterial, fungal), satellite lesions (fungal), dendrite (HSV), pseudodendrite (HZV), cutaneous herpes vesicles, perineural and ring infiltrates (*Acanthamoeba*), corneal edema, Descemet's folds, descemetocele, anterior chamber cell and flare, hypopyon, KP, mucopurulent discharge, and increased intraocular pressure.

Differential diagnosis

An ulcer must be differentiated from other corneal pathology, such as a sterile infiltrate, epidemic keratoconjunctivitis subepithelial infiltrates, Terrien's marginal degeneration, corneal abrasion, recurrent erosion, stromal scar, interstitial keratitis, Thygeson's superficial punctate keratitis, metaherpetic/trophic ulcer (noninfectious, non-healing epithelial defect with heaped-up

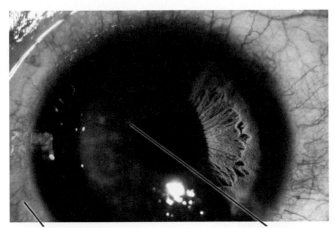

Conjunctival injection   Subepithelial infiltrates

FIGURE 11–29
Adenoviral conjunctivitis due to epidemic keratoconjuctivitis with characteristic subepithelial infiltrates.

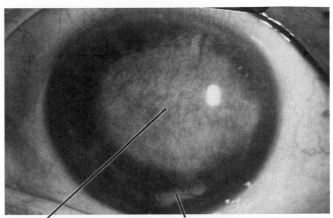

Central scarring   Ghost vessels

FIGURE 11–31
Interstitial keratitis, demonstrating ghost vessels that appear as clear, linear, branching lines within the dense, white corneal scarring.

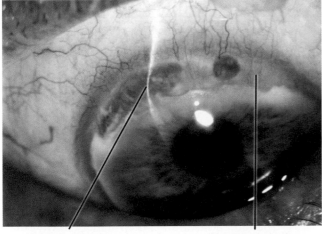

Peripheral thinning   Neovascularization

FIGURE 11–30
Terrien's marginal degeneration with superior thinning (note how slit beam dives downward), bounded by white scarring.

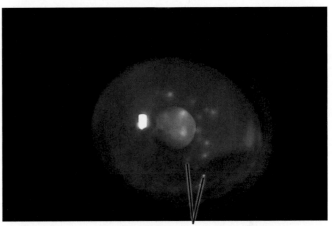

Thygeson's superficial punctate keratitis

FIGURE 11–32
Thygeson's superficial punctate keratitis, demonstrating multiple white, stellate corneal opacities with cobalt blue light.

gray edges due to HSV basement membrane disease with possible neurotrophic component), anesthetic abuse (non-healing epithelial defect, usually with ragged edges and "sick"-appearing surrounding epithelium with or without haze or an infiltrate), and tyrosinemia (pseudodendrite) (Figures 11–29–11–32).

Evaluation

- The **history** must include information about contact lens use and care regimen, ocular trauma and surgery, and systemic diseases.
- The **eye exam** concentrates on the cornea (sensation, size and depth of ulcer, character of infiltrate, fluorescein staining, edema, scarring, KP), sclera (ulcer-

ation), tonometry (may have increased intraocular pressure), and anterior chamber (may have cell and flare, hypopyon).
- **Lab tests** include cultures and smears if an infectious etiology is suspected (always culture before starting antibiotics), and a systemic work-up (complete blood count, erythrocyte sedimentation rate, rheumatoid factor, antinuclear antibodies, antineutrophil cytoplasmic antibody) for patients with non-infectious melts without an associated systemic diagnosis.
- Consider a **corneal biopsy** for progressive keratitis, culture-negative ulcer, or deep abscess.
- **Medical or rheumatology consultation** for underlying systemic disorders.

Management

- **Infectious:** the goal of therapy is to kill the organism and promote healing:
  - Suspend contact lens use.
  - *Never* patch a corneal ulcer. Consider a bandage contact lens or tarsorrhaphy to heal a persistent epithelial defect.
  - Corneal perforation requires emergent treatment. Glue may be adequate to seal a small hole; otherwise a lamellar or penetrating keratoplasty surgery is necessary.
  - Daily follow-up is required initially, and severe infections may require hospitalization.
  - Topical medication depending on the organism:
  - **Bacterial:**
    - **Small infiltrates (<2 mm):** empiric therapy with a broad-spectrum topical antibiotic (moxifloxacin (Vigamox) or gatifloxacin (Zymar) q1h initially, then taper slowly).
    - **Larger ulcers:** broad-spectrum fortified topical antibiotics (tobramycin 13.6 mg/ml and cefazolin 50 mg/ml or vancomycin 50 mg/ml (in penicillin- and cephalosporin-allergic patients) alternating q1h (i.e., instill a drop every 30 minutes) for 24–72 hours, then taper slowly). Subconjunctival antibiotic injections may be required in non-compliant patients.
    - Adjust antibiotics as necessary depending on culture and Gram stain results.
    - Topical cycloplegic (scopolamine 0.25% or atropine 1% bid to qid).
    - Topical steroid (prednisolone acetate 1% with lower frequency than topical antibiotics) may be added once improvement is noted (usually after 48–72 hours).
    - Systemic antibiotics for corneal perforation or scleral involvement.
  - **Fungal:**
    - Topical antifungal (natamycin 50 mg/ml q1h, amphotericin B 1–2.5 mg/ml q1h, or miconazole 10 mg/ml q1h for 24–72 hours, then taper slowly).
    - Systemic antifungal (ketoconazole 200–400 mg PO qd or amphotericin B 1 mg/kg IV over 6 hours) for severe infection.
    - Topical cycloplegic (scopolamine 0.25% or atropine 1% bid to qid).
    - Topical steroids are *contraindicated.*
  - **Parasitic:**
    - *Acanthamoeba:* this pernicious organism requires chronic therapy with a combination of topical antiparasitic, antifungal, and antibacterial agents. Choices include propamidine isethionate (Brolene) 0.1% or hexamidine 0.1%, and miconazole 1% or clotrimazole 1%, and polyhexamethylene biguanide (Baquacil) 0.02% or chlorhexidine 0.02% (q1h for 1 week and then taper very slowly over 2–3 months); neomycin or paromomycin (q2h); and oral ketoconazole (200 mg) or itraconazole (100 mg PO bid).
      - Topical cycloplegic (scopolamine 0.25% or atropine 1% bid to qid).
      - Topical steroids are controversial, but may be considered for severe necrotizing keratitis (prednisolone phosphate 1% qid).
      - Debridement may be curative for infection limited to the epithelium.
      - Prevent with contact lens heat disinfection (75°C).
  - **Viral:**
    - **HSV epithelial keratitis:** this active viral infection requires a topical antiviral (trifluridine (Viroptic) 9 times a day or vidarabine monohydrate (Vira-A) 5 times a day for 10–14 days).
      - Debridement of the dendrite reduces the viral load.
      - Consider an oral antiviral (acyclovir 400 mg PO tid for 10–21 days, then prophylaxis with 400 mg bid for up to 1 year to prevent recurrence (or longer after penetrating keratoplasty)). The **Herpetic Eye Disease Study (HEDS)** showed that chronic suppressive therapy with acyclovir (400 mg PO bid for 1 year) reduces the incidence of recurrent keratitis by almost 50%.
    - **HSV disciform or endotheliitis:** this immune-mediated keratitis is treated with a topical steroid (prednisolone phosphate 0.12–1.0% qd to qid depending on the severity of inflammation; adjust and then taper slowly over months depending on the response).
      - Consider a topical cycloplegic (scopolamine 0.25% bid to qid).
      - Topical antiviral (trifluridine (Viroptic) qid) for concomitant epithelial keratitis or prophylactically when using steroid doses greater than prednisolone phosphate 0.12% bid. Alternatively, oral acyclovir (400 mg PO bid) can be used.
    - **HSV metaherpetic/trophic ulcer:** this non-healing epithelial defect is managed with topical lubrication with non-preserved artificial tears (up to q1h) and ointment (qhs), a broad-spectrum topical antibiotic (polymyxin B sulfate–trimethoprim (Polytrim), tobramycin (Tobrex), moxifloxacin (Vigamox), or gatifloxacin (Zymar) qid), and a bandage contact lens.
      - Topical mild steroid (fluorometholone qd to bid) for stromal inflammation.
    - **HZV:** shingles is treated with systemic antivirals (acyclovir 800 mg PO 5 times a day for 10 days)

to reduce the risk and severity of ocular involvement (if started within 2–3 days of the cutaneous eruption).

- HZO requires a topical steroid (prednisolone acetate 1% qid to q4h, then taper slowly over months) and cycloplegic (scopolamine 0.25% bid to qid).
- Topical antibiotic ointment (erythromycin or bacitracin tid) for conjunctival or corneal involvement.
- Treatment of increased intraocular pressure may be required (see Ch. 13).
- Oral steroids (prednisone 60 mg qd for 1 week, then 30 mg qd for 1 week, then 15 mg qd for 1 week) reduce the time course, duration, and severity of acute pain, and the incidence of postherpetic neuralgia.
- Treatment options for postherpetic neuralgia include capsaicin cream (Zostrix), cimetidine, tricyclic antidepressants (amitriptyline, desipramine), carbamazepine (Tegretol), pregabalin (Lyrica), gabapentin (Neurontin), and lidoderm patch.

- **Non-infectious**: the goal of therapy is to reduce the inflammation and heal the epithelium to stop the ulceration.
  - Lubrication with non-preserved artificial tears and ointment. Consider punctal occlusion or tarsorrhaphy for non-healing epithelial defects.
  - Topical steroid (prednisolone acetate 1% or fluorometholone initially qid).
  - Topical cycloplegic (cyclopentolate 1% bid) for anterior-chamber cell and flare.
  - Topical broad-spectrum antibiotic (polymyxin B sulfate–trimethoprim (Polytrim) or tobramycin (Tobrex) qid) to prevent infection while an epithelial defect exists.
  - Consider a topical collagenase inhibitor (acetylcysteine (Mucomyst) qd to qid).
  - Oral steroids (prednisone 60–100 mg PO qd), ⁓⁓⁓⁓⁓⁓⁓⁓⁓⁓⁓⁓⁓⁓⁓⁓⁓⁓⁓⁓⁓⁓⁓, conjunctival recession or resection, or penetrating keratoplasty may be required for significant, progressive thinning.
  - Treat the underlying disease.

Prognosis

The prognosis depends on the etiology and ulcer size, location, and response to treatment.

Infectious: variable prognosis with complications ranging from an asymptomatic corneal scar to corneal perforation requiring an emergent graft. The prognosis is poor for fungal and *Acanthamoeba* keratitis, and both HSV and *Acanthamoeba* commonly recur in corneal grafts. Multiple recurrences of herpetic infections are associated with damage to other ocular structures.

- **HSV** complications include uveitis, glaucoma, episcleritis, scleritis, secondary bacterial keratitis, corneal scarring, corneal perforation, and punctal stenosis (due to topical antiviral therapy).
- **HZO** complications include corneal scarring, uveitic glaucoma (45%), segmental iris atrophy (due to vasculitis and necrosis), Argyll Robertson pupil (ciliary ganglion involvement), central retinal artery occlusion, ischemic optic neuropathy, cranial nerve palsies (cranial nerve III, IV, or VI palsy occurs in 25%, is self-limited, and may involve the pupil), Ramsay Hunt syndrome (cranial nerve V and VII involvement with facial paralysis), and postherpetic neuralgia (pain persisting after resolution of rash; occurs in 10–20% of patients with HZO and >50% who are >60 years old; 50% resolve in 1 month, and 80% within 1 year).

Non-infectious: poor for marginal keratolysis and Mooren's ulcer, which may perforate.

Degenerations

Aging or previous corneal insults may cause degenerative changes in the cornea.

ARCUS SENILIS

Arcus senilis is a benign, partial or complete, peripheral, white corneal ring that occurs bilaterally in elderly individuals, and is due to lipid deposition at the level of Bowman's and Descemet's membranes (Figure 11–33). A clear zone separates the arcus from the limbus. Carotid occlusive disease may cause a unilateral arcus (absent on

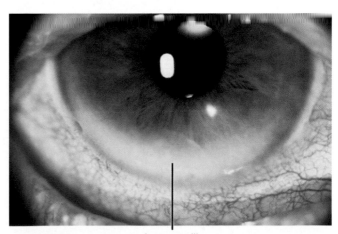

Arcus senilis

FIGURE 11–33

Arcus senilis evident as a peripheral white ring in the inferior cornea.

the side of the stenotic artery). A lipid profile should be checked if the patient is <40 years old. Arcus juvenilis is the congenital form.

LIPID KERATOPATHY

Lipid keratopathy is subepithelial and stromal lipid deposition caused by chronic inflammation and vascularization. Lipid extravasates from vessels and appears as a yellow-white infiltrate with feathery edges (Figure 11–34). Vision may be affected if the central cornea is involved.

BAND KERATOPATHY

Band keratopathy refers to interpalpebral, subepithelial, patchy, calcific changes in Bowman's membrane with a characteristic Swiss-cheese pattern (Figure 11–35).

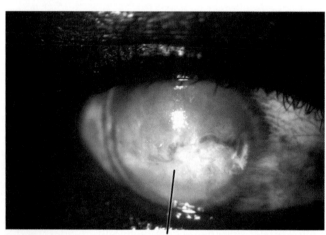

Lipid keratopathy

FIGURE 11–34
Lipid keratopathy, demonstrating dense white corneal infiltration.

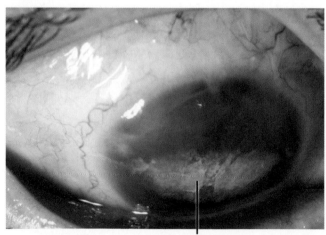

Band keratopathy

FIGURE 11–35
Band keratopathy, demonstrating characteristic Swiss-cheese pattern of central corneal opacification.

This condition is most commonly caused by chronic inflammation from corneal edema, uveitis, glaucoma, interstitial keratitis, phthisis, and dry-eye syndrome. Other etiologies include hypercalcemia, gout, and mercury vapors. If vision is reduced by involvement of the central cornea, then the calcium can easily be removed by chelation (the epithelium overlying the affected area is debrided and a solution of sodium ethylenediaminetetraacetic acid (EDTA) is applied). When the calcium band eventually recurs, the procedure can be repeated.

Keratoconus

Definition

Keratoconus is a bilateral, asymmetric, progressive thinning of the cornea that causes a central or paracentral cone-shaped deformity.

Etiology

This corneal ectasia is usually sporadic, but 10% of patients may have a positive family history. It is associated with atopy and vernal keratoconjunctivitis (due to eye rubbing), Down syndrome, Marfan's syndrome, and hard contact lens wear.

Symptoms

Patients report blurred vision and frequent changes in their glasses prescription. They may experience sudden loss of vision, pain, redness, photophobia, and tearing in hydrops.

Signs

The hallmark of keratoconus is corneal steepening and thinning. This results in decreased visual acuity, scarring (from breaks in Bowman's membrane), deep, stromal, vertical stress lines at the apex of the cone (Vogt's striae), epithelial iron deposition around the base of the cone (Fleischer's ring), and protrusion of the lower eyelid on downgaze (Munson's sign) (Figures 11–36–11–38). Patients may also present with **hydrops**: acute corneal edema and clouding due to a break in Descemet's membrane (Figure 11–39). Hydrops is often painful and accompanied by ciliary injection, anterior-chamber cell and flare, and decreased intraocular pressure.

Evaluation

- The **history** should note the frequency of changes in corrective lenses and whether or not the vision is adequate with correction.
- The **eye exam** must concentrate on the visual acuity (loss of best spectacle corrected visual acuity, ability to improve with a rigid contact lens) and cornea (shape, thinning, striae, scarring, irregular keratometer mires).

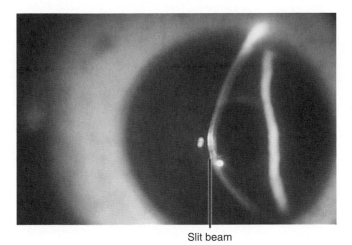

FIGURE 11–36
Keratoconus, demonstrating central "nipple" cone as seen with a fine slit beam. Note the central scarring at the apex of the cone.

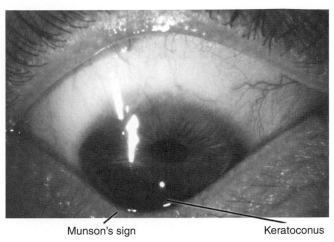

FIGURE 11–38
Munson's sign in a patient with keratoconus, demonstrating protrusion of the lower eyelid with downgaze.

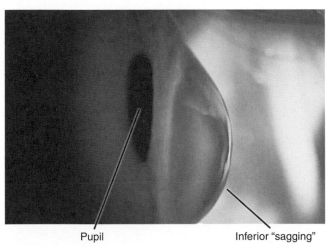

FIGURE 11–37
Keratoconus, demonstrating inferior "sagging" cone as viewed from the side. Note that the apex of the cone is below the center of the pupil.

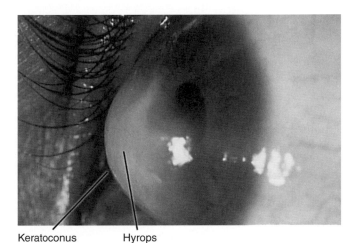

FIGURE 11–39
Hydrops in a patient with keratoconus, demonstrating hazy, white, central corneal edema.

- **Corneal topography** (computerized videokeratography) confirms the diagnosis by demonstrating a steep, abnormal corneal curvature.

Management

- Correct refractive errors with glasses (initially) or contact lenses (later).
- Consider corneal transplant (penetrating keratoplasty) when adequate vision cannot be achieved or if the patient is intolerant of contact lenses. Intracorneal ring segment (Intacs) implantation is an alternative that may stabilize or slow progression of the ectasia.
- Corneal refractive surgery (i.e., laser-assisted in situ keratomileusis (LASIK), photorefractive keratectomy, radial keratotomy) is absolutely *contraindicated* in these unstable corneas.
- Hydrops is managed acutely with supportive treatment: hypertonic saline ointment (Adsorbonac or Muro 128 5% qid), topical broad-spectrum antibiotic (polymyxin B sulfate–trimethoprim (Polytrim) or tobramycin (Tobrex) qid) if there is an epithelial defect, and topical steroid (prednisolone acetate 1% qid) and cycloplegic (cyclopentolate 1% tid) for pain.

Prognosis

Keratoconus is a spectrum of disease, from mild and asymptomatic (forme fruste) to severe and visually debilitating. However, penetrating keratoplasty is highly successful in these patients.

CHAPTER TWELVE

Anterior Chamber

Introduction

The anterior chamber (AC) is the space between the cornea and the iris. This compartment and the smaller posterior chamber, between the iris and the lens, are filled with aqueous fluid. Many ocular conditions produce changes in the aqueous and AC. These findings are helpful in determining the diagnosis as well as monitoring the patient's response to treatment.

Hypotony

Definition

Hypotony means low intraocular pressure (IOP), specifically <10 mmHg.

Etiology

Reduced IOP can be caused by any condition that increases aqueous outflow or decreases aqueous production. Hypotony is associated with trauma (blunt, penetrating, or surgical), wound leak after ocular surgery, overfiltration through a bleb (after glaucoma surgery), ciliary body shutdown, cyclodialysis, choroidal effusion, retinal detachment, medication (ocular hypotensive agents), uveitis, cyclitic membrane, and phthisis.

Symptoms

Hypotony is usually asymptomatic until the pressure is <5 mmHg. At this point, functional and structural ocular changes occur, and patients may have pain and decreased vision.

Signs

By definition, the IOP is low. The visual acuity may be normal or decreased depending on the level and duration of the hypotony, which can produce a range of findings from AC cell and flare to corneal folds, chorioretinal folds, choroidal effusion, cystoid macular edema (CME), and optic disc edema (Figure 12–1). If the eye is phthisical, then the globe shrinks and may have a squared-off appearance (see Figure 7–17).

Evaluation

- The **history** must include any ocular trauma and surgery, and medication use.

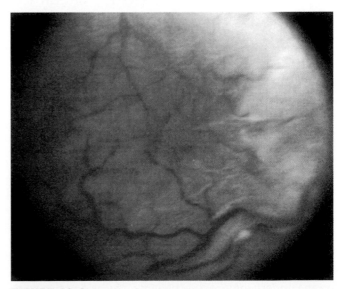

FIGURE 12–1

Hypotony maculopathy with choroidal folds after trabeculectomy surgery.

- The **eye exam** should pay particular attention to the conjunctiva (may have a filtering bleb), cornea (folds, may have surgical wounds), tonometry (decreased IOP), AC (cell and flare, depth of chamber), gonioscopy (rule out cyclodialysis), and ophthalmoscopy (may have chorioretinal folds, choroidal effusion, CME, optic disc edema, retinal detachment).
- Perform a **Seidel test** (see Ch. 11) to rule out an open globe or wound leak in traumatic or postsurgical cases.

Management

- Treatment depends on the etiology. The mainstay of therapy is a topical cycloplegic (cyclopentolate 1%, scopolamine 0.25%, or atropine 1% bid to tid) and steroid (prednisolone acetate 1% qid).
- If a wound leak is present, preventing secondary infection is important with a topical broad-spectrum antibiotic (moxifloxacin (Vigamox) or gatifloxacin (Zymar) qid).
- Surgery may be required for a wound leak, retinal detachment, ciliary body detachment, or choroidal effusion.

Prognosis

Most cases of hypotony are mild and self-limited, resolving with conservative medical management. The outcome is very poor for chronic cases with reduced vision from maculopathy and corneal folds.

Anterior-Chamber Cell and Flare

Definition

Cell and flare refers to the presence of cells and increased protein (flare) in the aqueous fluid. The cells are usually white blood cells, but sometimes they are red blood cells (microhyphema) or pigment cells (from the iris after dilation and in pigment dispersion syndrome). Abundant cells may settle inferiorly to form a visible layer (hypopyon, hyphema, or pseudohypopyon, respectively) in the AC.

Etiology

Aqueous cells and flare are caused by breakdown of the blood–aqueous barrier due to infection, inflammation from uveitis, trauma, scleritis, or keratitis, and post-operatively after eye surgery.

Symptoms

Cell and flare can be asymptomatic or cause blurry vision and photophobia (pain/sensitivity to light). Depending on the underlying process, patients may also notice pain, tearing, and redness.

Signs

By definition, there are cells and flare in the AC. These are best appreciated when viewed with a short narrow slit lamp beam directed at an oblique angle through the pupil. This technique produces an effect similar to shining a flashlight through a dark room. Cells demonstrate Brownian motion and appear as small particles floating in the AC. Flare makes the aqueous fluid appear hazy or cloudy and looks like smoke in the light beam. Severe flare is a fibrinous exudate that has a jelly-like or plasmoid appearance. Cell and flare are graded on a 1+ to 4+ scale depending on the amount per slit beam field (i.e., 1+ = 0–10 cells; 2+ = 11–20 cells; 3+ = 21–50 cells; 4+ = >50 cells) (Figure 12–2). Additional findings on exam include normal or decreased visual acuity, ciliary injection, miosis, keratic precipitates (KP: aggregates of white blood cells adherent to the corneal endothelium, most often inferiorly and centrally), keratitis, iris nodules, posterior synechiae (iris adhesions to the underlying crystalline lens near the pupillary margin), increased or decreased IOP, hypopyon (see below), hyphema (see below), pseudohypopyon (see below), vitritis, or a retinal or choroidal lesion (Figure 12–3).

Evaluation

- The **history** must ask specifically about systemic diseases, previous ocular diseases, and any recent eye trauma or surgery.
- The **eye exam** is performed with attention to the cornea (may have keratitis, KP), tonometry (altered IOP), AC (cell and flare), iris (may have nodules, synechiae), and ophthalmoscopy (may have vitritis, retinal or choroidal lesions).
- May require **lab tests** for uveitis (see section on anterior uveitis, below).

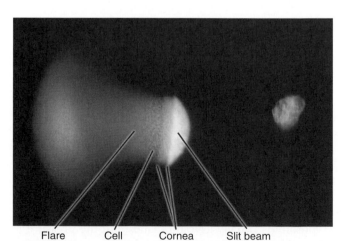

Flare Cell Cornea Slit beam

FIGURE 12–2

Grade 4+ anterior-chamber cells and flare visible with fine slit beam between the cornea and iris.

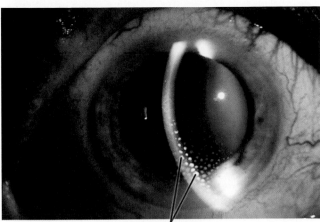

Keratic precipitates

FIGURE 12–3
White, mutton-fat, granulomatous, keratic precipitates on the central and inferior corneal endothelium in a patient with toxoplasmosis.

Management

- Treatment of cell and flare is directed at stabilizing the blood–aqueous barrier with a topical steroid (prednisolone acetate 1% up to q1h initially, then taper slowly) and cycloplegic (cyclopentolate 1%, scopolamine 0.25%, or atropine 1% bid to tid).
- Treatment of elevated IOP may be required (see Ch. 13). Miotics and prostaglandin analogues, both of which can exacerbate inflammation, should be avoided.
- Most importantly, AC cell and flare are due to some underlying disorder that must be treated.

Prognosis

Most processes that cause cell and flare are self-limited, and the AC reaction resolves with appropriate therapy. However, chronic AC inflammation may result in complications such as glaucoma, cataract, synechiae, band keratopathy, and CME. The prognosis depends on the underlying cause.

Hyphema

Definition

A hyphema is blood in the AC that forms a layer that is visible with the naked eye. In contrast, a microhyphema is blood in the AC where the hemorrhage is so small that only red blood cells floating in the AC are seen with the slit lamp, and no layer is visible.

Etiology

The majority of hyphemas result from trauma when the vascular iris and/or angle tissue tears, causing bleeding. Bleeding can also occur spontaneously from iris or angle neovascularization, intraocular tumors, or a mal-positioned or loose intraocular lens (IOL) implant that erodes into or chafes vascular tissue.

Symptoms

Patients report blurry vision and sometimes pain, photophobia, and redness.

Signs

A hyphema appears as a layer of blood or blood clot in the AC (Figure 12–4). The visual acuity may be decreased, the IOP is often elevated, and there may be other signs of trauma. The iris or angle damage (i.e., angle recession (60%), iridodialysis, cyclodialysis: see Ch. 14) in traumatic cases is usually obscured by the blood and cannot be visualized until after the blood clears. In non-traumatic cases, anterior-segment neovascularization, an iris lesion, or movement of an IOL implant may be observed.

Differential diagnosis

There are only a few diagnoses that produce a layer of cells in the AC. The color of the layer differentiates the various entities. Hyphema produces a red layer, hypopyons are white or cream-colored, and psuedohypopyons usually appear darker than hypopyons (i.e., tan).

Evaluation

- When gathering the **history**, it is important to ask about trauma, previous ocular surgery, and any ocular or systemic diseases that can produce anterior-segment neovascularization.
- The **eye exam** focuses on the cornea (may have edema, blood staining), tonometry (may have increased IOP), AC (height and color of the hyphema), iris (may have tears), gonioscopy (to evaluate angle structure damage is delayed 2–4 weeks in traumatic

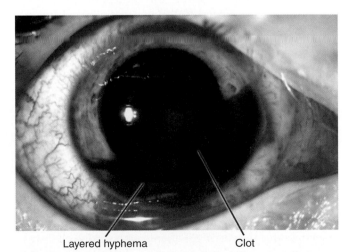

Layered hyphema   Clot

FIGURE 12–4
Hyphema, demonstrating layered blood inferiorly and suspended red blood cells and clot.

cases to prevent clot disruption and rebleeding), and ophthalmoscopy (may have other signs of ocular trauma).

- **Lab tests** include a sickle-cell prep and hemoglobin electrophoresis to rule out sickle-cell disease in high-risk patients, since this disease is a risk factor for developing increased IOP (rigid, sickled cells clog the trabecular meshwork).
- **B-scan ultrasonography** is performed to rule out an open globe or other traumatic injuries when the fundus cannot be directly visualized.

Management

- In general, the blood will be reabsorbed; thus, the goal of therapy is to prevent complications, including rebleeding and elevated IOP. Daily examination is required for the first 5 days, when the risk of elevated IOP and a rebleed are greatest.
- While the blood is visible in the AC, patients should be treated with a topical steroid (prednisolone acetate 1% up to q1h initially, then taper over 3–4 weeks as the hyphema and inflammation resolve) and cyclo-plegic (scopolamine 0.25% or atropine 1% bid to tid).
- To prevent a rebleed, advise patients to stay at bedrest for the first 5 days, avoid aspirin-containing products, sleep with the head elevated, and protect the involved eye with a metal shield at all times.
- The use of aminocaproic acid (Amicar; 50–100 mg/kg q4h) to stabilize the clot is controversial.
- Treatment of elevated IOP may be required (see Ch. 13). Miotics and prostaglandin analogues, both of which can exacerbate inflammation, should be avoided. Carbonic anhydrase inhibitors are contraindicated in patients with sickle-cell disease because these agents produce an acidic environment that promotes red blood cell sickling.
- Surgical evacuation of the blood, with an AC washout, may be required, for corneal blood staining, uncontrolled elevated IOP, persistent clot (>15 days), or **eight-ball hyphema** (complete hyphema composed of dark blood/clot, indicating poor resorption). If a problematic IOL is responsible for recurrent hyphemas, then the implant must be removed.

Prognosis

The prognosis depends on the height and duration of the hyphema as well as the IOP. The outcome is good for small, uncomplicated hyphemas. Rebleeding may occur in up to one-third of cases. The risk of glaucoma is 27% with a hyphema >50% of the AC volume, and the risk is 52% with a total hyphema. Traumatic cases with significant angle recession are at risk for future angle recession glaucoma due to scarring. Patients with sickle-cell disease and hyphema have more elevation in IOP and a higher risk of central artery occlusion and optic nerve infarction due to vascular sludging when the IOP is elevated.

Hypopyon

Definition

A hypopyon is white blood cells in the AC that form a layer that is visible with the naked eye.

Etiology

A hypopyon is caused by inflammation (uveitis) or infection (e.g., corneal ulcer, endophthalmitis).

Symptoms

Patients commonly experience pain, photophobia, redness, and blurry vision.

Signs

A hypopyon appears as a layer of white or cream-colored cells in the AC (in contrast to a hyphema, that appears red) (Figure 12–5). Other characteristic findings are normal or decreased visual acuity, conjunctival injection, and AC cell and flare. There may also be a corneal infiltrate, KP, iris nodules, vitritis, or a retinal or choroidal lesion.

Differential diagnosis

A hypopyon must be distinguished from a **pseudohypopyon** (a layer of pigment cells, ghost cells, tumor cells, or lipid- or protein-laden macrophages) and a hyphema (Figure 12–6).

Evaluation

- The **history** should document information about systemic diseases, medications, ocular disorders, and recent eye surgery.
- The **eye exam** must include the cornea (may have infiltrate, KP), tonometry (may have altered IOP), AC (height of the hypopyon, cell and flare), iris (may

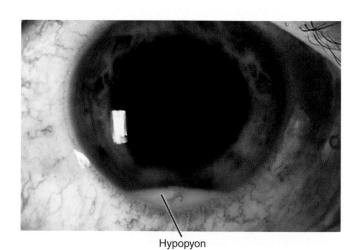

Hypopyon

FIGURE 12–5
Hypopyon, demonstrating layered white blood cells inferiorly.

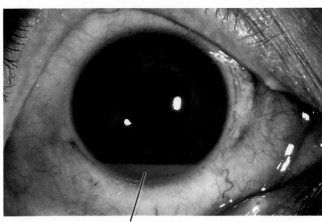

Pseudohypopyon

FIGURE 12–6
Pseudohypopyon, composed of khaki-colored ghost cells layered inferiorly.

have nodules, synechiae), and ophthalmoscopy (may have vitritis, retinal or choroidal lesions).
- **B-scan ultrasonography** is performed if the fundus cannot be visualized to rule out retinal or choroidal lesions.
- **Lab tests** may be required, including cultures and smears for infectious keratitis or endophthalmitis (see section on endophthalmitis, below), or a systemic work-up for uveitis (see section on anterior uveitis, below).

Management

- The treatment for hypopyon depends on the underlying cause. If it is inflammatory, then topical steroids are the mainstay of treatment (see section on anterior uveitis, below). If it is infectious than topical antimicrobials are administered (see sections on infectious keratitis in Ch. 11, and endophthalmitis, below). A topical cycloplegic (cyclopentolate 1%, scopolamine 0.25%, or atropine 1% bid to tid) is used to stabilize the blood–aqueous barrier.
- Monitor the response to treatment by the clearance rate of the hypopyon.

Prognosis

A hypopyon is the result of a severe inflammatory response. The white cells will eventually resorb completely, but the prognosis depends on the underlying process and its associated complications.

Anterior Uveitis

Definition

Anterior uveitis refers to inflammation of the iris (**iritis**) and/or ciliary body (**cyclitis**). The inflammation leads to

breakdown of the blood–aqueous barrier and increased vascular permeability with exudation of inflammatory cells and proteins into the aqueous fluid. Uveitis may be classified according to:

- **Etiology**: see below.
- **Pathology**: non-granulomatous (lymphocyte and plasma cell infiltrates) or granulomatous (epithelioid and giant cell infiltrates).
- **Location**: keratouveitis, sclerouveitis, anterior uveitis, intermediate uveitis, posterior uveitis, or panuveitis.
- **Course**: acute, chronic (>6 weeks' duration), or recurrent.

Etiology

Anterior uveitis is most commonly idiopathic or autoimmune. The most common etiology is also age-dependent. For example, iritis is most commonly due to juvenile rheumatoid arthritis (JRA) in children, human leukocyte antigen (HLA)-B27 associated uveitis in young adults, and idiopathic uveitis in older adults.

INFECTIOUS ANTERIOR UVEITIS

Herpes simplex and herpes zoster produce iritis characterized by KP, elevated IOP, and iris atrophy (at the pupillary border in simplex and segmental atrophy in zoster).

Lyme disease is caused by *Borrelia burgdorferi*, which is transmitted by the *Ixodes dammini* or *I. pacificus* tick. Patients develop a characteristic skin lesion (erythema chronicum migrans) at the site of the tick bite, and 1–3 months later they may have neurologic and ophthalmologic manifestations, including encephalitis, meningitis, follicular conjunctivitis, stromal keratitis, chronic granulomatous iritis, vitritis, and optic neuritis. In late stages, there can be cardiovascular and musculoskeletal changes.

Syphilis causes a chronic or recurrent granulomatous anterior uveitis. This infection must always be ruled out because it is a treatable disease with significant morbidity (see Ch. 17).

Tuberculosis produces a chronic granulomatous iritis associated with conjunctival nodules, phlyctenules, interstitial keratitis, and scleritis (see Ch. 17).

NON-INFECTIOUS ANTERIOR UVEITIS

Non-granulomatous

Idiopathic is the most common form of acute anterior uveitis, accounting for 50% of cases.

HLA-B27-associated anterior uveitis accounts for almost 50% of acute iritis. It is more common in young men and 25% of patients have a seronegative spondyloarthropathy. These **seronegative spondyloarthropathies** are a group of HLA-B27-associated disorders with the following common features: radiographic sacroiliitis (with or without spondylitis), peripheral arthritis, negative rheumatoid factor (RF) and antinuclear antibody (ANA), variable mucocutaneous lesions, and acute anterior uveitis.

- **Ankylosing spondylitis** is characterized by low-back pain and stiffness after inactivity (i.e., morning stiffness). Ninety percent of patients are HLA-B27-positive. Patients may also have cardiac (aortitis, heart block) and pulmonary (apical fibrosis) involvement. Sacroiliac radiographs often show sclerosis and narrowing of the joint spaces, and, if left untreated, patients progress to debilitating spinal fusion. Anterior uveitis develops in 30% of patients and is recurrent in 40%. Episcleritis and scleritis may also occur.

- **Reiter's syndrome** is a triad of mucopurulent conjunctivitis, non-specific urethritis, and polyarthritis (80%). Other findings include recurrent iritis, keratoderma blenorrhagicum, circinate balanitis, plantar fasciitis, Achilles tendinitis, sacroiliitis, oral ulcers, nail pitting, prostatitis, cystitis, and diarrhea. This syndrome is associated with HLA-B27 in up to 95% of cases and may be triggered by infection with *Chlamydia*, *Ureaplasma*, *Yersinia*, *Shigella*, or *Salmonella*.

- **Psoriatic arthritis** causes psoriatic skin and nail changes plus arthritis of the hands, feet, and sacroiliac joints. This disease is associated with HLA-B27, and patients can develop anterior uveitis as well as conjunctivitis and dry eyes. Iritis is rare in psoriasis without arthritis.

- **Inflammatory bowel disease** can cause a bilateral uveitis with a posterior component. This occurs in Crohn's disease (3%) and ulcerative colitis (5–10%), and is associated with dry eyes, conjunctivitis, episcleritis, scleritis, orbital cellulitis, and optic neuritis, as well as sacroiliitis, erythema nodosum, pyoderma gangrenosum, hepatitis, and sclerosing cholangitis. Sixty percent of inflammatory bowel disease patients with sacroiliitis are HLA-B27-positive.

- **Whipple's disease**, a rare systemic disorder associated with *Tropheryma whippelii* infection, is characterized by chronic diarrhea, arthritis (sacroiliitis and spondylitis), central nervous system involvement, and anterior uveitis. Patients have an increased incidence of HLA-B27.

Behçet's disease is a triad of recurrent iritis with enough cells to produce a hypopyon, aphthous stomatitis, and genital ulcers. Patients may also develop arthritis, thromboemboli, and central nervous system manifestations. The hallmark of this uveitis is bilateral retinal vasculitis (see Ch. 17). It is more common in Asians and Middle-Easterners, and is associated with HLA-B5 (subtypes Bw51 and B52) and HLA-B12.

Glaucomatocyclitic crisis (Posner–Schlossman syndrome) refers to self-limited episodes of mild recurrent unilateral iritis with markedly elevated IOP and pain. Other characteristics of this disorder include corneal edema, few or no KP, and no synechiae. It is associated with HLA-Bw54.

Medications, specifically rifabutin and cidovir, can cause an acute anterior uveitis.

Interstitial nephritis causes an acute bilateral anterior uveitis, typically in children, and may be due to an allergic reaction to medicine (non-steroidal anti-inflammatory drugs (NSAIDs) or antibiotics). Patients also have constitutional symptoms (fever, malaise, and arthralgias) and white blood cells without infection on urinalysis. Treatment with oral steroids is required to prevent renal failure.

Trauma and ocular surgery produce variable degrees of AC inflammation. It is important to rule out other etiologies such as an exacerbation of pre-existing uveitis, retained lens material (after cataract surgery), uveitis–glaucoma–hyphema syndrome, endophthalmitis, and sympathetic ophthalmia.

Other autoimmune diseases like systemic lupus erythematosus (SLE), relapsing polychondritis, and Wegener's granulomatosis can cause acute or chronic anterior uveitis.

JRA (see Ch. 6).

Fuchs' heterochromic iridocyclitis is a chronic low-grade iritis that is usually unilateral (90%) and occurs in young adults. It is characterized by small white stellate KP, fine vascularization of the angle, diffuse iris atrophy, and no synechiae (Figure 12–7). There is a predilection for blue-eyed patients, and the iris of the involved eye may be lighter in color. Complications include glaucoma (15%) and cataracts (70%). This form of iritis responds poorly to topical steroids, and therefore they should not be used.

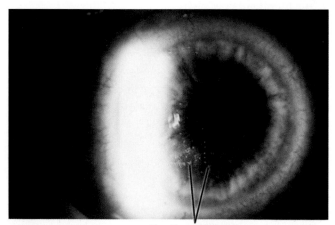

Keratic precipitates

FIGURE 12–7
Fuchs' heterochromic iridocyclitis with fine white stellate keratic precipitates.

Granulomatous

Autoimmune disorders that cause anterior uveitis are most often sarcoidosis, Vogt–Koyanagi–Harada syndrome, sympathetic ophthalmia, and lens-induced (phacoanaphylactic endophthalmitis, an immune-mediated (type 3) hypersensitivity reaction to lens particles after trauma or surgery).

Symptoms

Patients complain of pain, photophobia, and redness. They may also experience blurry vision.

Signs

Visual acuity may be normal or decreased, but the hallmark of anterior uveitis is ciliary injection, pupillary miosis, and AC cell and flare. Other typical findings include fine (non-granulomatous) or mutton-fat (granulomatous) KP, iris nodules (at the pupillary margin (Koeppe) or on the anterior iris surface (Busacca)), increased or decreased IOP, peripheral anterior synechiae (peripheral iris adhesions to the cornea that cover and obstruct the trabecular meshwork), posterior synechiae, and hypopyon (especially HLA-B27-associated and Behçet's) (Figures 12–8–12–12). There may also be keratitis, scleritis, cataract, vitritis, CME, and retinal or choroidal infiltrates.

Differential diagnosis

When making the diagnosis of anterior uveitis, it is essential to rule out the masquerade syndromes: retinal detachment, retinoblastoma, malignant melanoma, leukemia, large cell lymphoma (reticulum cell sarcoma), juvenile xanthogranuloma, intraocular foreign body, anterior-segment ischemia, ocular ischemic syndrome, multiple sclerosis, and spill-over syndromes from any posterior uveitis (most commonly toxoplasmosis).

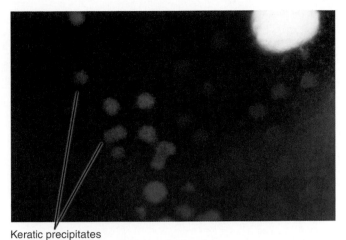

Keratic precipitates

FIGURE 12–9
Close-up of granulomatous keratic precipitates.

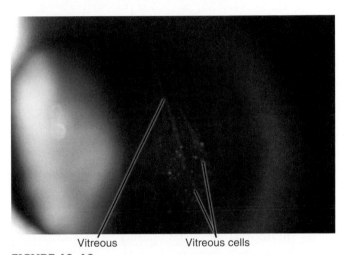

Vitreous   Vitreous cells

FIGURE 12–10
Anterior vitreous cells visible with fine slit beam behind the lens. The cells are seen here as fine white specks among the vitreous strands.

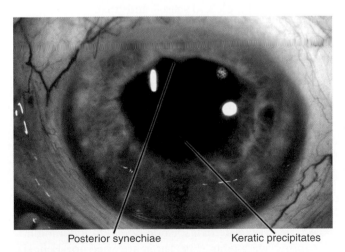

Posterior synechiae   Keratic precipitates

FIGURE 12–8
Granulomatous uveitis, demonstrating keratic precipitates and posterior synechiae.

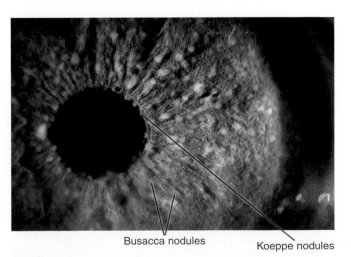

Busacca nodules   Koeppe nodules

FIGURE 12–11
Busacca and Koeppe nodules are small, lightly colored collections of inflammatory cells.

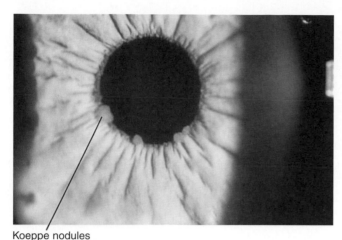

Koeppe nodules

FIGURE 12-12
Koeppe nodules.

Evaluation

- The **history** should carefully characterize the symptoms, especially the character of the pain (ache), location of the redness (diffuse or perilimbal), absence of discharge, and presence of photophobia, all of which help to differentiate uveitis from other conditions that produce a red eye. The patient must be asked about previous episodes, systemic diseases, medications, ocular trauma or surgery, and recent travel.

- The **eye exam** must evaluate the conjunctiva (injection, ciliary flush), cornea (sensation, presence and character of KP, may have scarring or edema), tonometry (altered IOP), AC (cell and flare, may have hypopyon), iris (pupillary miosis, may have posterior synechiae and nodules), gonioscopy (to look for PAS and fine-angle vessels (Fuchs')), and ophthalmoscopy (may have vitritis, CME, retinal or choroidal infiltrates).

- **Lab tests** are based upon the history and exam findings. Unilateral, non-granulomatous iritis is often idiopathic and treated without an extensive work-up, but if the uveitis is recurrent, bilateral, granulomatous, or involving the posterior segment, consider a work-up.

  - **Non-granulomatous anterior uveitis with a negative history, review of systems, and medical examination**: basic lab testing including a complete blood count, erythrocyte sedimentation rate, Venereal Disease Research Laboratory and fluorescent treponemal antibody absorption test (syphilis), and HLA-B27.

  - **Suggestive history and/or evidence of granulomatous inflammation**: consider one or more of the following, including ANA, RF (JRA), serum lysozyme, angiotensin-converting enzyme (sarcoidosis), purified protein derivative and controls (tuberculosis), herpes simplex and herpes zoster titers, Lyme titer, enzyme-linked immunosorbent assay (ELISA) for Lyme immunoglobulin M and immunoglobulin G, human immunodeficiency virus (HIV) antibody test, chest radiographs (sarcoidosis, tuberculosis), sacroiliac radiographs (ankylosing spondylitis), knee radiographs (JRA), chest computed tomography scan (sarcoidosis), urinalysis (interstitial nephritis), and urethral cultures (Reiter's syndrome).

  - **Other special diagnostic lab tests**: HLA typing, antineutrophil cytoplasmic antibody (Wegener's granulomatosis, polyarteritis nodosa), Raji cell and C1q binding assays for circulating immune complexes (SLE, systemic vasculitides), complement proteins: C3, C4, total complement (SLE, cryoglobulinemia, glomerulonephritis), and soluble interleukin-2 receptor.

- **Medical or rheumatology consultation**.

Management

- The mainstay of therapy is a topical steroid (prednisolone acetate 1% up to q2h initially, then taper very slowly over weeks to months depending on etiology and response) and cycloplegic (cyclopentolate 1%, scopolamine 0.25%, homatropine 2%, or atropine 1% bid to qid). Both of these drops stabilize the blood–aqueous barrier, and the cycloplegic also acts to relieve pain (by relaxing the ciliary muscle spasm) as well as to prevent the formation of and break existing posterior synechiae. It is imperative to monitor the patient's IOP since steroids can cause an elevation in pressure. In steroid responders, consider changing to a preparation with less tendency to raise the IOP (i.e., rimexolone 1% (Vexol) or loteprednol etabonate 0.5% (Lotemax)).

- Treatment of elevated IOP may be required, especially glaucomatocyclitic crisis (see Ch. 13). Miotics and prostaglandin analogues, both of which can exacerbate inflammation, should be avoided.

- Systemic antibiotics for Lyme disease, tuberculosis, syphilis, Whipple's disease, and toxoplasmosis are recommended.

- Topical antiviral (trifluridine (Viroptic) 9 times a day) is administered for herpes simplex virus infections with concomitant corneal epithelial involvement.

- Systemic antiviral (acyclovir 800 mg 5 times a day for 10 days) is prescribed for the initial episode of herpes zoster ophthalmicus.

- Consider oral (prednisone 60–100 mg PO qd), subTenon's (triamcinolone acetonide 40 mg/ml), intravitreal (triamcinolone acetonide 4 mg/0.1 ml) steroids, or intravitreal sustained-release implant (Retisert implant delivers intraocular fluocinolone for up to 3 years).

- Alternatives to steroids include NSAIDs and immunosuppressive agents. The latter are used for Behçet's disease, sympathetic ophthalmia, Vogt–Koyanagi–Harada syndrome, rheumatoid necrotizing scleritis and/or peripheral ulcerative keratitis, Wegener's granulomatosis, polyarteritis nodosa, relapsing polychondritis, JRA, or sarcoidosis unresponsive to conventional therapy, and should be managed by a uveitis specialist or internist familiar with these medications.

Prognosis

The prognosis for uveitis depends on the etiology, but most cases are benign and resolve without ocular complications. The outcome is poor if sequelae of chronic inflammation develop, such as cataract, glaucoma, posterior synechiae, band keratopathy, iris atrophy, CME, retinal detachment, retinal vasculitis, optic neuritis, neovascularization, hypotony, and phthisis.

Endophthalmitis

Definition

Endophthalmitis refers to intraocular infection, and may be acute, subacute, or chronic.

Etiology

Infection inside the eye usually results from surgical or traumatic penetration of the globe, but it can also occur endogenously. It is the most feared complication of ocular surgery.

Postoperative (70% of cases): has been associated with all types of eye surgery, most commonly cataract and glaucoma filtering surgeries.

- **Acute** (<6 weeks after surgery): usually caused by Gram-positive bacteria (94%), including coagulase-negative staphylococci (70%), *Staphylococcus aureus* (10%), and *Streptococcus* species (11%). Gram-negative organisms account for only 6% of acute postoperative endophthalmitis cases.
- **Delayed** (>6 weeks after surgery): usually caused by *Propionibacterium acnes*, coagulase-negative staphylococci, or fungi (*Candida* species).

Filtering bleb-associated: most frequently *Streptococcus* species (47%), coagulase-negative staphylococci (22%), and *Haemophilus influenzae* (16%).

Posttraumatic (20%): usually caused by *Staphylococcus* species (39%), *Bacillus* (i.e., *B. cereus*) species (24%), and Gram-negative organisms (7%).

Endogenous (8%): is rare and often fungal (*Candida* species) or, less commonly, bacterial (*Staphylococcus aureus* and Gram-negative bacteria).

Epidemiology

Postoperative endophthalmitis following cataract surgery occurs in <0.1% of cases and is associated with the following risk factors: blepharitis, diabetes mellitus, posterior-capsule disruption, vitreous loss, wound leak, iris prolapse, and prolonged operative time. The most common cause of postoperative endophthalmitis is after glaucoma filtering surgery, especially when the filtering bleb is placed inferiorly.

Posttraumatic endophthalmitis following penetrating trauma has an incidence of 3–7%, but may be as high as 30% after injuries in rural settings. Other risk factors include a retained intraocular foreign body, delayed surgery (>24 hours), and disruption of the crystalline lens.

Endogenous endophthalmitis affects debilitated, septicemic, and immunocompromised patients, often following abdominal surgical procedures.

Symptoms

Patients characteristically present with pain, photophobia, discharge, redness, and blurry vision; however, mild, delayed, or endogenous cases may be asymptomatic.

Signs

The classic findings on examination are dramatically decreased visual acuity (only 14% of patients in the **Endophthalmitis Vitrectomy Study (EVS)** had vision better than 5/200, which is worse than the big E on the Snellen eyechart), eyelid edema, proptosis, conjunctival injection and chemosis, wound abscess, corneal edema, KP, AC cell and flare, hypopyon, vitritis, and poor red reflex (Figures 12–13 and 12–14). There may also be a positive Seidel test due to a leaking surgical wound, or signs of an open globe (see Ch. 10).

Differential diagnosis

In the postoperative period various conditions may be confused with endophthalmitis, including sterile inflammation, toxic anterior-segment syndrome (from contaminants), retained lens material, and rebound inflammation (from tapering or discontinuing topical

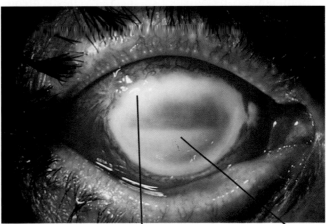

Corneal infiltrate   Hypopyon

FIGURE 12–13
Endophthalmitis with large hypopyon (almost 50% of anterior-chamber height). There is severe inflammation with 4+ conjunctival injection and a white ring corneal infiltrate at the limbus.

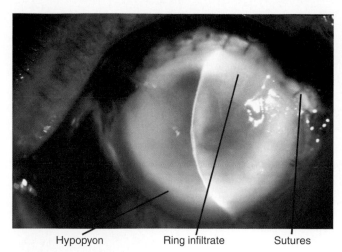

Hypopyon   Ring infiltrate   Sutures

FIGURE 12-14
Staphylococcus endophthalmitis with ring infiltrate. There is marked corneal edema and the corneal sutures across the surgical wound are visible at the superior limbus.

steroids too quickly). Uveitis, intraocular foreign body, intraocular tumor, sympathetic ophthalmia, and anterior-segment ischemia can also mimic endophthalmitis.

Evaluation

- The **history** must document systemic diseases and ocular trauma or surgery, including the type of trauma or surgery, any complications, and when it occurred.
- The **eye exam** must include the visual acuity (decreased), evaluation of the surgical incision (integrity), Seidel test (often positive), conjunctiva (injection, chemosis, discharge, evaluation of filtering bleb for signs of infection), cornea (may have edema, KP, infiltrates), tonometry (may have altered IOP), AC (depth, cell and flare, may have hypopyon), IOL (position, evidence of complicated surgery), and ophthalmoscopy (quality of the red reflex, vitreous cells, may have retinal or choroidal infiltrates).
- **B-scan ultrasonography** is performed to rule out an open globe, intraocular foreign body, retinal detachment, or posterior-segment lesion if the fundus cannot be visualized.
- **Lab tests** include stat intraocular fluid cultures and smears. Conjunctival and nasal cultures can also be collected but have a low yield.
- **Medical consultation** for endogenous endophthalmitis.

Management

- Endophthalmitis is a true *ophthalmic emergency* that must be recognized and treated immediately with the appropriate antibiotics.
- Treatment consists of a combination of intravitreal, subconjunctival, and topical antibiotics and steroids, and should be managed by a vitreoretinal specialist.

- Patients should be evaluated daily until improvement is seen. If no improvement or worsening occurs, then reinjection of antibiotics and/or pars plana vitrectomy should be performed by a vitreoretinal specialist.
- **Acute postoperative** endophthalmitis:
  - The **EVS** concluded that for endophthalmitis after cataract extraction, if the patient's vision is better than light perception, then an AC and vitreous tap is performed to acquire specimens for culture and to inject intravitreal antibiotics (vancomycin 1 mg/0.1 ml and either ceftazidime 2.25 mg/0.1 ml or amikacin 0.4 mg/0.1 ml). If the vision is light perception only or after glaucoma filtering procedures, then a pars plana vitrectomy to debulk the vitreous debris is also performed.
  - Systemic antibiotics (vancomycin 1 g IV q12h and ceftazidime 1 g IV q12h) for marked inflammation, posttrauma, severe cases, or rapid onset are controversial because they were found to be of no benefit in the EVS.
  - Intravitreal steroids (dexamethasone 0.4 mg/ 0.1 ml) at the same time as the surgery were not evaluated in the EVS and are also controversial.
  - Subconjunctival antibiotics (vancomycin 25 mg and either ceftazidime 100 mg or gentamicin 20 mg) and steroid (dexamethasone 12–24 mg), topical broad-spectrum fortified antibiotics (vancomycin 50 mg/ml q1h and ceftazidime 50 mg/ml q1h, alternating every 30 minutes), topical steroid (prednisolone acetate 1% q1–2h initially), and topical cycloplegic (atropine 1% tid or scopolamine 0.25% qid) are also administered.
- **Subacute, delayed, endogenous, filtering bleb-associated**, and **posttraumatic endophthalmitis**:
  - These types of endophthalmitis were not studied in the EVS; thus, the EVS guidelines do not apply. Nonetheless, the treatment is similar with culture and injection of intravitreal antibiotics with or without a pars plana vitrectomy.
  - Intravitreal (amphotericin B 0.005 mg/0.1 ml) and topical (amphotericin B 1–2.5 mg/ml q1h or natamycin 50 mg/ml q1h) antifungal are prescribed for presumed fungal etiology. Add a systemic antifungal (amphotericin B 0.25–1.0 mg/kg IV divided equally q6h) for disseminated disease.
  - Surgery (partial or total capsulectomy, pars plana vitrectomy, and/or IOL removal or exchange) may be required for the delayed postoperative form.

Prognosis

The prognosis depends on the etiology, duration, and organism, but is usually poor. This is particularly true for posttraumatic cases, since these organisms are especially virulent and can cause severe ocular damage.

CHAPTER THIRTEEN

Glaucoma

Introduction

Glaucoma is a form of optic neuropathy with many causes. It is classified according to etiology. The two main categories are distinguished by whether or not the anterior-chamber (AC) drainage angle is open or closed. Open-angle varieties include primary open-angle glaucoma (POAG), the most common form of glaucoma, as well as many types of secondary open-angle glaucomas. Normal-tension glaucoma is another form in which the angle is open but the intraocular pressure (IOP) is within normal limits.

The less common closed-angle glaucomas also have primary and secondary forms. It is the acute angle-closure attack that causes the classic symptoms of pain, blurred vision, headache, and nausea that are often associated with the word glaucoma. It is important that physicians be familiar with the differences between open- and closed-angle glaucoma because the treatments are quite distinct. Furthermore, high IOP (ocular hypertension) is frequently equated with glaucoma. This is a common misconception that needs to be corrected. Increased IOP is the biggest risk factor for developing glaucoma, but in order to make the diagnosis of glaucoma, optic nerve damage with visual field loss must exist. (See Ch. 6 for a discussion of childhood glaucoma.)

Primary Open-Angle Glaucoma

Definition

POAG refers to progressive, bilateral optic nerve damage with a typical pattern of nerve fiber bundle visual field loss, increased IOP (IOP >21 mmHg) that is not caused by another systemic or ocular disease (see section on secondary open-angle glaucoma, below), and open AC angles.

Etiology/mechanism

Genes for adult POAG have been identified on various chromosomes, and a mutation in the *OPTN* gene is responsible for almost 20% of cases. However, the actual pathogenesis of POAG is unknown. Elevated IOP results from mechanical resistance to aqueous outflow that may be caused by an abnormality of the trabecular meshwork or collapse of Schlemm's canal. Theories to account for the resulting optic nerve damage from ganglion cell necrosis or apoptosis include:

Mechanical: interruption of axoplasmic flow from compression of the nerve fibers against the lamina cribrosa.
Vascular: poor optic nerve perfusion or disturbed blood flow autoregulation, possibly from vasospasm.
Other pathways: damage to the nerve may also occur from excitotoxicity (glutamate), neurotrophin starvation, autoimmunity, abnormal glial–neuronal interactions, or defects in endogenous protective mechanisms (heat shock proteins).

Epidemiology

POAG is the most common type of glaucoma (60–70%). It is the second leading cause of blindness in the USA, occurring in up to 2% of the population >40 years old.

Risk factors for POAG include increased IOP (7% of the population has ocular hypertension), race (more common and more severe in African Americans, who are 3–6 times more likely to develop POAG than Caucasians), increased age (>60 years old), increased cup-to-disc ratio, thinner central corneal thickness (<545 μm), and positive family history in first-degree relatives (parent or sibling, which raises the risk sixfold). Other potential risk factors are myopia, diabetes mellitus, hypertension, and cardiovascular disease.

Symptoms

POAG is asymptomatic. Patients only notice decreased vision or constricted visual fields in late stages of the disease.

Signs

The hallmarks of POAG are elevated IOP, optic nerve cupping, characteristic visual field defects, and an open AC angle. The enlarged cup-to-disc ratio is usually noticeable as vertical elongation of the optic cup, notching of the disc, or asymmetry between the patient's two nerves (Figure 13–1). Careful evaluation of the retinal nerve fiber layer may reveal one or more defects visible as dull sectors lacking the characteristic nerve fiber layer sheen (particularly evident on examination with a green light). Occasionally a splinter hemorrhage is visible on the disc margin, followed by a notch in the same region (Figure 13–2). Peripapillary atrophy is also common. In advanced disease, the visual acuity is decreased.

Differential diagnosis

POAG must be differentiated from secondary open-angle glaucoma, normal-tension glaucoma, ocular hypertension, optic neuropathy, and physiologic cupping (Figure 13–3).

Evaluation

- When taking the **history**, the patient must be asked about systemic diseases, previous eye injuries or surgery, steroid use, and a family history of glaucoma.
- The **eye exam** should pay particular attention to the cornea (central thickness), tonometry (increased IOP), AC (depth), gonioscopy (open angle), iris (normal), lens (normal), and ophthalmoscopy (optic nerve cupping, disc hemorrhage, nerve fiber layer appearance).
- Measure **pachymetry** to determine the central corneal thickness.
- **Visual field** testing must be performed to check for typical defects, including paracentral scotomas (within 10° of fixation), arcuate (Bjerrum) scotomas (isolated, nasal step of Rönne, or Seidel (connected to blind spot)), and temporal wedge scotomas (Figure 13–4). Glaucomatous visual field defects do not respect the vertical meridian, in contrast to neurologic field loss, which does (see Figure 5–4 in Ch. 5). If the visual field does not correlate with the optic nerve appearance, then another cause for the visual field loss must be found (i.e., uncorrected refractive error, poor

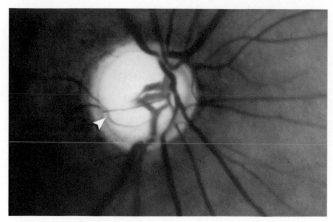

FIGURE 13–1
Optic nerve cupping due to primary open-angle glaucoma. Note the extreme degree of disc excavation and course of the vessels at the poles and temporally as they travel up and over the rim, giving a "bean pot" configuration (arrowhead).

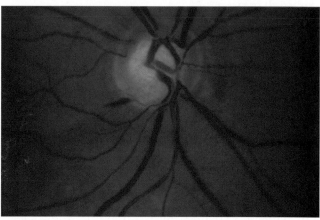

FIGURE 13–2
Optic nerve, demonstrating cupping and splinter hemorrhage.

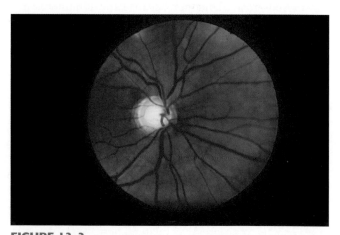

FIGURE 13–3
Physiologic cupping. Although the cup is large, there is a healthy rim of neural tissue 360°.

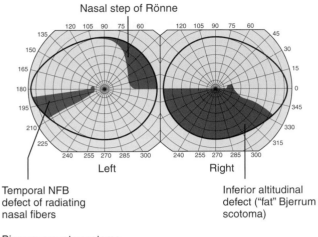

Nasal step of Rönne

Temporal NFB
defect of radiating
nasal fibers

Inferior altitudinal
defect ("fat" Bjerrum
scotoma)

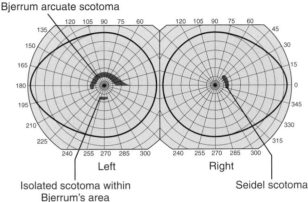

Bjerrum arcuate scotoma

Isolated scotoma within
Bjerrum's area

Seidel scotoma

FIGURE 13–4
Composite diagram depicting different types of field defects.
NFB, nerve fiber bundle.

visual acuity, media opacity, tilted optic nerve head, optic nerve head drusen, retinal lesion).

- Stereoscopic **optic nerve photos** are obtained for comparison at subsequent exams.
- **Optic nerve head analysis** can also be performed. Various methods are available, including confocal scanning laser ophthalmoscopy (HRT, TopSS), optical coherence tomography, scanning laser polarimetry (Nerve Fiber Analyzer, GDx), and optic nerve blood flow measurement (color Doppler imaging and laser Doppler flowmetry).

Management

The primary goal of POAG therapy is to halt or delay progression of the disease in order to prevent the patient from developing blindness. Various treatments exist, but the problem with all of them is that the effect may only be temporary. Typically, therapy is administered in a stepwise fashion beginning with medicine, then laser, and finally surgery. The choice and timing of treatment depend on such factors as the degree of optic nerve damage, level of IOP control, progression of disease, patient's age, and compliance. Specific options are as follows:

- **Observation**: it is recommended that patients with controlled POAG undergo routine monitoring of their IOP every 3–6 months, and gonioscopy, visual field, and optic nerve examinations at least once a year. More frequent evaluation is necessary for uncontrolled disease and when changing treatment.
- **Medical**: numerous ocular hypotensive agents are used in the treatment of POAG. One agent is initially chosen and a monocular trial is performed to make sure the patient is responsive to the medication without adverse affects. Traditionally, topical β-blockers have been the gold standard for first-line therapy; however, the newer topical prostaglandin analogues have replaced the β-blockers as first-line drugs because of better efficacy and side-effect profile. Additional medications are added or substituted as needed to control the IOP adequately (i.e., prevent disease progression). The IOP should be rechecked approximately 3–4 weeks after any medication change to evaluate efficacy. The following medications are used singly or in combination: prostaglandin analogues, β-blockers, α-adrenergic agonists, carbonic anhydrase inhibitors, and miotics (see Ch. 3).
- **Laser**: the mainstay of laser therapy is trabeculoplasty (argon or selective laser trabeculoplasty) to increase trabecular meshwork outflow. In advanced cases, laser treatment can be applied externally at the limbus to destroy the ciliary processes and reduce aqueous production. This is called cyclophotocoagulation.
- **Surgical**: the goal of surgery is to lower the IOP by creating an alternate pathway for aqueous to escape from the eye. The most common procedure is a trabeculectomy, which creates a filtering bleb to allow aqueous to pass from the AC to the subconjunctival space, where it diffuses away (Figure 13–5). Another

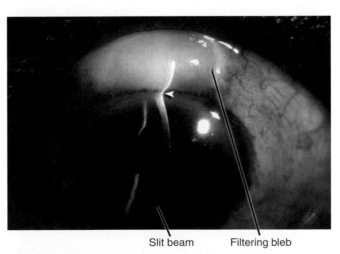

Slit beam   Filtering bleb

FIGURE 13–5
Conjunctival filtering bleb following glaucoma surgery (trabeculectomy), demonstrating typical appearance of a well-functioning, thin, cystic, avascular bleb. Note the curve of the slit beam at the inferior portion of the elevated bleb (arrowhead).

option is a glaucoma drainage implant that enables aqueous to pass directly into an artificial chamber implanted under the conjunctiva.

Prognosis

The prognosis of POAG depends upon the extent of optic nerve damage and the rate of disease progression. It is usually good if the IOP is adequately controlled; however, any visual loss is permanent. African Americans have a worse prognosis because they tend to develop a more severe and aggressive form of the disease. If there is already damage in one eye, the fellow eye has almost a 30% risk over 5 years of developing visual field loss if left untreated.

Secondary Open-Angle Glaucoma

Definition

Secondary open-angle glaucoma refers to open-angle glaucoma with elevated IOP caused by a variety of ocular or systemic disorders.

Etiology

The following conditions can result in secondary open-angle glaucoma: pseudoexfoliation syndrome, pigment dispersion syndrome, drugs, uveitis, lens abnormalities, trauma, and intraocular tumors.

Pseudoexfoliation glaucoma is the most common type of secondary open-angle glaucoma. It is due to uncontrolled increased IOP in pseudoexfoliation syndrome, which causes dispersion of exfoliative basement membrane material (an amyloid-like substance) with subsequent clogging of the trabecular meshwork in individuals >50 years old.

Pigmentary glaucoma is due to uncontrolled increased IOP in patients with pigment dispersion syndrome. In pigment dispersion syndrome, pigment is liberated from the posterior iris surface, with subsequent clogging of the trabecular meshwork by the pigment. It is typically seen in young myopic men. It is an autosomal dominant disease linked to the *GLC1F* gene on chromosome 7q.

Drug-induced glaucoma is most commonly steroid-related. The IOP elevation depends upon the steroid's potency and duration of use. After 4–6 weeks of topical steroid administration, up to 30% of the population may develop increased IOP. Ninety-five percent of patients with POAG are steroid-responders.

Uveitic glaucoma is due to aqueous outflow obstruction from inflammatory cells, trabeculitis (inflammation of the trabecular meshwork), scarring of the trabecular meshwork, and/or increased aqueous viscosity.

Lens-induced glaucoma is due to retained lens material after surgery or trauma (lens particle glaucoma) or lens proteins leaking from a hypermature cataract and clogging the trabecular meshwork (phacolytic glaucoma).

Traumatic glaucoma is due to angle recession, chemical injury, hemorrhage (red blood cells, ghost cells (degenerated red blood cells), or macrophages (that have ingested red blood cells (hemolytic glaucoma)) obstructing the trabecular meshwork), or intraocular foreign-body toxicity (siderosis or chalcosis).

Intraocular tumors can produce secondary open-angle glaucoma by causing angle neovascularization, direct tumor infiltration of the angle, or trabecular meshwork obstruction by tumor, inflammatory cells, or hemorrhage.

Other rarer causes of secondary open-angle glaucoma include elevated episcleral venous pressure (orbital mass, thyroid-related ophthalmopathy, arteriovenous fistulas, orbital varices, superior vena cava syndrome, Sturge–Weber syndrome, idiopathic), retinal disease (retinal detachment, retinitis pigmentosa, Stickler's syndrome), systemic disease (pituitary tumors, Cushing's syndrome, renal disease), postoperative (ocular laser and surgical procedures), and uveitis–glaucoma–hyphema syndrome.

Symptoms

Depending on the underlying etiology and rapidity of IOP rise, patients are asymptomatic, or they may have pain, photophobia, decreased vision, redness, or even systemic symptoms.

Signs

The signs of secondary open-angle glaucoma are the same as for POAG (i.e., elevated IOP, optic nerve cupping, nerve fiber layer defects, characteristic visual field defects, and an open AC angle). Other specific findings depend upon the underlying etiology:

Pseudoexfoliation glaucoma: there is a characteristic target pattern of exfoliative material on the anterior lens capsule consisting of a central disc pattern and a peripheral ring with an intervening clear zone with no exfoliative material (Figures 13–6 and 13–7). In addition, there may be loss of the pupillary ruff, iris rigidity with poor pupillary dilation, increased angle pigmentation anterior to Schwalbe's line (Sampaolesi's line), phacodonesis, and cataract.

Pigmentary glaucoma: there is pigment accumulation on the corneal endothelium (Krukenberg spindle), trabecular meshwork, iris furrows, and anterior lens capsule (Figures 13–8 and 13–9). There are also characteristic radial, mid peripheral slit-like, iris transillumination defects seen on retroillumination at the slit lamp (Figure 13–10).

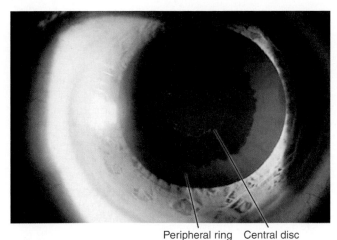

FIGURE 13–6
Exfoliative material on the anterior lens surface in typical pattern of central disc and peripheral ring in a patient with pseudoexfoliation syndrome.

Peripheral ring   Central disc

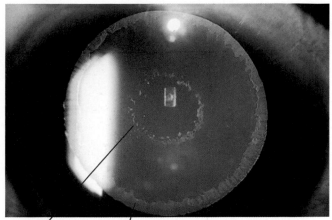

Central disc   Peripheral ring

FIGURE 13–7
Central disc and peripheral ring of exfoliative material as seen with retroillumination.

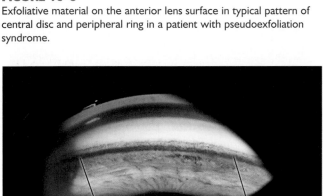

Pigment on TM   Pigment deposition

FIGURE 13–8
Pigment dispersion syndrome demonstrating pigment deposition on the trabecular meshwork (TM) that appears as a dark brown band when viewed with gonioscopy.

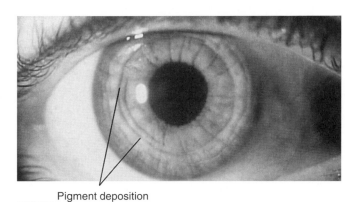

Pigment deposition

FIGURE 13–9
Pigment dispersion syndrome, demonstrating pigment deposition in concentric rings on the iris surface.

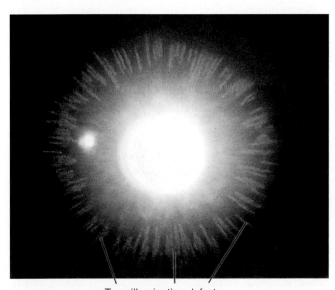

Transillumination defects

FIGURE 13–10
Pigment dispersion syndrome, demonstrating radial, mid peripheral, slit-like iris transillumination defects for 360°.

Uveitic glaucoma: there is usually AC cell and flare from the uveitis. There may also be ciliary injection, keratic precipitates, miotic pupil, synechiae, iris changes, corneal edema, corneal scarring, cataract, and cystoid macular edema.

Lens-induced glaucoma: there is severe AC inflammation and either visible lens fragments (in the AC or vitreous) or a mature, white cataract (Figure 13–11).

Traumatic glaucoma: there may be hyphema, vitreous hemorrhage, angle or iris damage, phacodonesis, cataract, corneal scarring, scleral ischemia, intraocular foreign body, retinal tears, and choroidal rupture.

Tumors: there may be an iris mass, focal iris elevation, hyphema, hypopyon, pseudohypopyon, leukocoria, segmental cataract, invasion of angle by the tumor, extrascleral extension, and sentinel episcleral vessels.

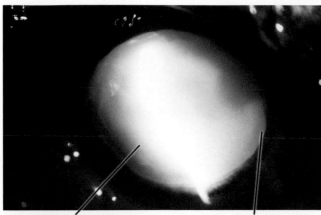

Hypermature cataract   Shallow chamber

FIGURE 13–11
Phacolytic glaucoma, demonstrating mature white cataract with anterior-chamber inflammation.

Evaluation

- A careful **history** should include previous eye diseases, injuries, surgery, and the use of steroids.
- The **eye exam** is performed with attention to the conjunctiva (may have injection, ciliary flush), cornea (may have edema, scarring, keratic precipitates), tonometry (increased IOP), AC (may have cell and flare, hyphema, hypopyon, pseudohypopyon), gonioscopy (open-angle; may have pigmentation, angle recession), iris (may have synechiae, nodules, tears, masses), lens (may have cataract), and ophthalmoscopy (optic nerve cupping, nerve fiber layer appearance).
- **B-scan ultrasonography** is obtained if the fundus cannot be visualized to rule out a mass.
- **Visual field** testing must be performed to check for scotomas.
- Consider **lab tests** for uveitis (see Ch. 12).
- Consider **orbital radiographs** or **computed tomography scan** to rule out an intraocular foreign body.
- **Medical or oncology consultation** for metastatic work-up in cases of tumors.

Management

- Treatment of increased IOP is the same as for POAG (see section on primary open-angle glaucoma, above). Miotics and prostaglandin analogues, both of which can exacerbate inflammation, should be avoided in cases associated with inflammation.
- Laser trabeculoplasty is often quite effective for pseudoexfoliation and pigmentary glaucoma.
- Consider tapering, changing, or discontinuing steroids if a steroid response is suspected.
- Treatment for uveitis may be required, with a topical cycloplegic and steroid.
- Surgery may be required for lens-induced (cataract extraction) and traumatic cases.

- Treatment may be required for a tumor and should be performed by a tumor specialist.

Prognosis

Secondary open-angle glaucoma has a poorer prognosis than POAG because it is more resistant to treatment. Patients with pseudoexfoliation syndrome have an increased incidence of angle closure and a greater risk of complications at cataract surgery due to weak zonules.

Normal (Low)-Tension Glaucoma

Definition

Normal-tension glaucoma is a form of open-angle glaucoma in which the IOP remains in the normal range (<22 mmHg), but optic nerve damage still occurs.

Etiology/mechanism

The etiology of normal-tension glaucoma is unknown, but theories regarding the mechanism of optic nerve damage include:

Nocturnal systemic hypotension: blood pressure follows a diurnal variation similar to IOP. Two-thirds of patients, called "dippers," have a drop in blood pressure >10% during the early morning, and those with systemic hypertension have an even greater blood pressure drop (average of 26%). Furthermore, hypertensive patients on β-blockers can have diastolic pressures <50 mmHg, which may compromise blood supply to the optic nerve.

Autoimmune: patients with normal-tension glaucoma have an increased incidence of autoantibodies and autoimmune disease.

Vasospasm: patients with normal-tension glaucoma also have an increased incidence of vasospastic disorders such as migraine, Raynaud's phenomenon, ischemic vascular disease, and coagulopathies.

Prior hemodynamic crisis: poor optic nerve perfusion can occur with a massive hemorrhage, myocardial infarction, or shock.

Symptoms

Normal-tension glaucoma is asymptomatic. Patients only notice decreased vision or constricted visual fields in late stages of the disease.

Signs

By definition in normal-tension glaucoma, the IOP is normal (≤21 mmHg). Oherwise, the signs of normal-tension glaucoma are the same as for POAG (i.e., optic nerve cupping, nerve fiber layer defects, characteristic visual field defects, and an open AC angle). In normal-tension glaucoma, disc splinter hemorrhages are more common and visual field scotomas tend to be denser and closer to fixation than in POAG. There may be peripapillary atrophy, and the visual acuity is usually normal until the late stages.

Differential diagnosis

Normal-tension glaucoma is a diagnosis of exclusion. Other forms of glaucoma, such as POAG (with undetected increased IOP from large diurnal variations, or a falsely low IOP measurement from a thin central cornea), secondary open-angle glaucoma (steroid-induced, "burned-out" pigmentary, or postuveitic glaucoma), intermittent angle-closure glaucoma, and glaucomatocyclitic crisis (Posner–Schlossman syndrome) may initially be misdiagnosed as normal-tension glaucoma if the pressure reading is not elevated at the time of examination. It is also essential to rule out intracranial processes and other causes of optic nerve damage (i.e., compressive lesions of the chiasm, anterior ischemic optic neuropathy, optic neuritis, and methanol toxicity), which typically cause early loss of central vision and color vision as well as nerve pallor more than optic nerve cupping.

Evaluation

- The **history** should include information regarding autoimmune and vasospastic diseases, hypertension, and the use of β-blockers.
- The **eye exam** must include a careful assessment of the cornea (central thickness), tonometry (normal IOP), AC (depth), gonioscopy (open-angle), iris (normal), lens (normal), and ophthalmoscopy (optic nerve cupping, disc hemorrhage, nerve fiber layer appearance).
- Measure **pachymetry** to determine the central corneal thickness.
- **Visual field** testing must be performed to check for scotomas.
- Consider obtaining a **diurnal IOP curve** (serial IOP measurements q2h for 10–24 hours) to rule out primary or secondary open-angle glaucoma.
- Consider a work-up for other causes of optic neuropathy. This includes color vision, lab tests (complete blood count, erythrocyte sedimentation rate, antinuclear antibody, Venereal Disease Research Laboratory test, and fluorescent treponemal antibody absorption test), **neuroimaging**, and/or a **cardiovascular evaluation** for the following situations: age <60 years old, decreased visual acuity with no apparent cause, atypical visual field defect, visual field and optic nerve appearance do not correlate, nerve pallor greater than cupping, or rapidly progressive, unilateral, or markedly asymmetric disease.

Management

- Treatment of increased IOP is the same as for POAG (see section on primary open-angle glaucoma, above).

- The **Collaborative Normal Tension Glaucoma Study** showed that patients should be monitored every 6 months with a complete eye exam, including visual fields. The treatment goal is a reduction in IOP of 30% from baseline.

Prognosis

Normal-tension glaucoma has a worse prognosis than POAG because it is more difficult to treat.

Primary Angle-Closure Glaucoma

Definition

Primary angle-closure glaucoma refers to glaucoma due to obstruction of the trabecular meshwork by peripheral iris tissue.

Etiology/mechanism

Angle closure is classified as acute, subacute (intermittent), or chronic. It is most commonly caused by pupillary block, but may also occur from plateau iris syndrome.

- **Pupillary block** refers to apposition of the iris to the lens that blocks the flow of aqueous from the posterior chamber through the pupil to the AC in predisposed patients. This situation causes excess fluid to build up in the posterior chamber, causing the peripheral iris to bow forward and occlude the trabecular meshwork when the pupil is in the mid dilated position (i.e., by stress, low light conditions, use of sympathomimetic or anticholinergic medications).
- **Plateau iris syndrome** occurs in the absence of pupillary block, when the peripheral iris tissue occludes the trabecular meshwork in patients with an atypical iris configuration due to anteriorly rotated ciliary processes.

Epidemiology

Approximately 5% of the general population >60 years old have occludable angles, but only 0.5% develop angle closure, often bilaterally, since the risk of fellow eye involvement is 75% within 5 years.

Anatomic factors associated with increased risk of angle closure include a small anterior segment (hyperopia, nanophthalmos, microcornea, microphthalmos), hereditary narrow angle, anterior iris insertion (Eskimos, Asians, and African Americans), and shallow AC (large lens, plateau iris configuration, loose or dislocated lens).

Symptoms

The symptoms at presentation depend on the type of angle closure:

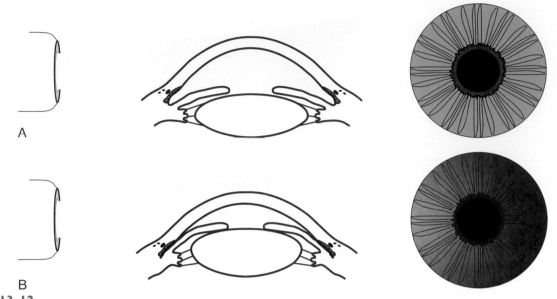

FIGURE 13–12
A penlight shined obliquely on the eye can diagnose a shallow anterior-chamber angle (B) since only a part of the iris is illuminated; the rest has a shadow.

Acute angle closure causes a sudden, extreme elevation in IOP that results in sudden pain, redness, photophobia, blurred vision, halos around lights, headache, nausea, and even emesis.

Subacute angle closure may be asymptomatic or present in a similar manner as the acute form but with less severe symptoms that evolve over the course of days or weeks and resolve spontaneously.

Chronic angle closure is asymptomatic because the gradual occlusion of the angle leads to a slow rise in IOP. In the late stages, patients may notice decreased vision or constricted visual fields.

Signs

Similarly, the exam findings are related to the type of angle closure:

Acute angle closure produces characteristic findings on exam, including decreased visual acuity, severely elevated IOP (up to 70 mmHg), ciliary injection, corneal edema, AC cell and flare, shallow AC (the entire AC is shallow in pupillary block, whereas plateau iris produces a deep central AC and a shallow peripheral AC), closed angles on gonioscopy, and a mid dilated, non-reactive pupil (Figure 13–12 and 13–13).

Patients may also exhibit features of previous attacks, including segmental iris atrophy (due to focal stromal ischemic necrosis), anterior subcapsular lens opacities or **glaukomflecken** (due to lens epithelial cell ischemic necrosis), dilated irregular pupil (due to sphincter and dilator muscle ischemic necrosis), and peripheral anterior synechiae (PAS) (Figure 13–14).

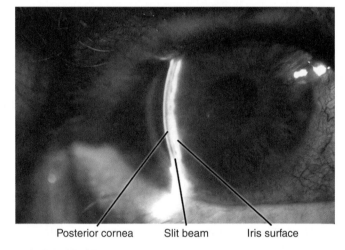

Posterior cornea   Slit beam   Iris surface

FIGURE 13–13
Primary angle-closure glaucoma, demonstrating very shallow anterior chamber and iridocorneal touch (no space between slit beam view of cornea and iris).

Subacute and chronic angle-closure patients have narrow angles with PAS. The IOP is normal or increased, and there may also be glaukomflecken, visual field defects, and optic nerve cupping.

Evaluation

- The **history** should carefully document symptoms of previous angle-closure attacks, especially when the patient is in dim lighting conditions, and the use of sympathomimetic or anticholinergic medications.
- The **eye exam** should focus on the pupils (mid dilated in acute attack), cornea (edema), tonometry (increased IOP), AC (depth), gonioscopy (narrow or occluded

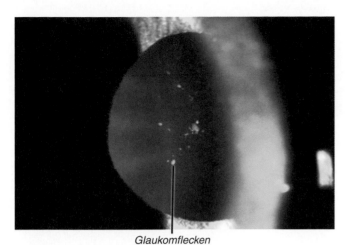

Glaukomflecken

FIGURE 13–14
Dot-like anterior subcapsular lens opacities (glaukomflecken) due to lens epithelial cell ischemia and necrosis from high intraocular pressure.

angles, may have PAS), iris (may have atrophy, plateau configuration), lens (may have glaukomflecken), and ophthalmoscopy (optic nerve cupping, nerve fiber layer appearance).

- **Visual field** testing must be performed to check for scotomas in subacute and chronic angle closure.
- Consider **provocative testing** (prone, dark room, and pharmacologic dilation) to initiate an acute angle-closure attack. An IOP rise >8 mmHg is considered positive.

Management

- **Acute angle closure** is a true *ophthalmic emergency* that requires immediate diagnosis and treatment to minimize optic nerve damage.
  - Topical β-blocker (timolol (Timoptic) 0.5% q15 minutes × 2, then bid), α-agonist (apraclonidine (Iopidine) 1% q15 minutes × 2), and steroid (prednisolone acetate 1% q15 minutes × 4, then q1h).
  - Topical miotic (pilocarpine 1–2% × 1 initially, then qid if effective). Pilocarpine is usually ineffective due to iris sphincter ischemia if the IOP is >40 mmHg, and this drug may actually exacerbate angle closure in 20% of patients due to forward displacement of the lens.
  - Systemic acetazolamide (Diamox 500 mg PO stat, then bid) and hyperosmotic agent (isosorbide up to 2 g/kg PO of 45% solution).
  - Monitor the IOP q30–60 minutes until it has reached a safe level (<30 mmHg).
  - Laser peripheral iridotomy (producing a hole in the iris to prevent pupillary block) with or without iridoplasty (stretching the peripheral iris away from the angle) is the definitive treatment after the acute attack is broken with medical therapy. A prophylactic laser peripheral iridotomy is also performed

in the fellow eye to prevent a future acute angle-closure attack (Figure 13–15).

- **Plateau iris syndrome** may require long-term miotic therapy, peripheral iridotomy, and iridoplasty to reduce the risk of pupillary block.
- **Subacute and chronic angle closure** requires treatment of increased IOP similar to that used in POAG (see section on primary open-angle glaucoma, above). A peripheral iridotomy should be performed if one is not already present.

Prognosis

The prognosis is usually good for acute attacks if treatment is instituted promptly. The outcome is poorer for chronic cases but depends on the extent of optic nerve damage and subsequent IOP control.

Secondary Angle-Closure Glaucoma

Definition

Secondary angle-closure glaucoma refers to angle-closure glaucoma caused by a variety of ocular disorders.

Etiology/mechanism

Similar to primary angle closure, secondary angle closure may be acute or chronic and occur with or without pupillary block.

Pupillary block is caused by disorders that obstruct aqueous from passing through the pupil into the AC. These include lens abnormalities (e.g., phacomorphic (thick cataract), dislocated lens, microspherophakia), seclusio pupillae (pupil completely bound down to the underlying lens by posterior synechiae), and postsurgical states such as aphakia, pseudophakia, and silicone oil in which vitreous, an IOL, or silicone oil, respectively, can block the pupil.

Without pupillary block is due to either a posterior or an anterior process:

- **Posterior mechanism** is caused by "pushing" of the lens and iris forward from:
  - Anterior rotation of the ciliary body due to inflammation (scleritis, uveitis, extensive panretinal photocoagulation), congestion (scleral buckle retinal surgery, nanophthalmos), choroidal effusion (hypotony, uveal effusion), or suprachoroidal hemorrhage.
  - Aqueous misdirection (**malignant glaucoma**).
  - Pressure from a posterior-segment process pushing forward (tumor, expanding intraocular gas after retinal surgery, exudative retinal detachment).

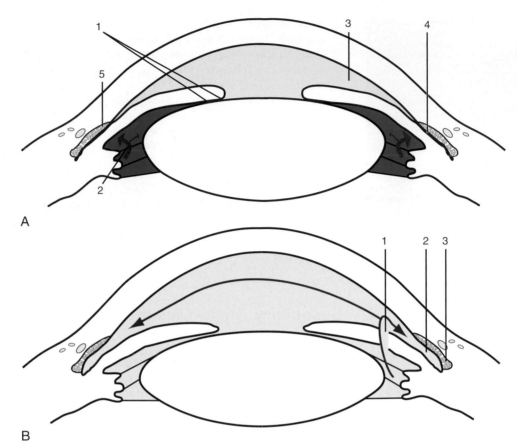

A

B

FIGURE 13-15
(**A**) Schematic illustrating pupillary block. The iris is pressed against the lens (1), blocking aqueous flow through the pupil. Aqueous trapped in the posterior chamber (2), pushes the iris forward, shallowing the anterior chamber (3), closing the angle (4), and blocking aqueous outflow (5).
(**B**) The intraocular pressure is lowered by making a hole in the peripheral iris (laser iridectomy) that enables the trapped aqueous to reach the AC (1), thereby opening the angle (2) and allowing normal aqueous drainage (3).

- Persistent hyperplastic primary vitreous.
- Retinopathy of prematurity.
- **Anterior mechanism** is caused by "pulling" of the iris anteriorly over the trabecular meshwork from:
  - Corneal epithelium due to downgrowth or ingrowth.
  - Corneal endothelium due to iridocorneal endothelial syndrome or posterior polymorphous dystrophy.
  - Neovascularization due to widespread retinal or ocular ischemia (**neovascular glaucoma**).
  - Peripheral anterior synechia due to uveitis or trauma.

Symptoms

Patients present in a similar manner as in primary angle-closure glaucoma:

Acute secondary angle closure causes pain, redness, photophobia, blurred vision, halos around lights, headache, nausea, and even emesis.

Chronic secondary angle closure is asymptomatic until the late stages, when patients may notice decreased vision or constricted visual fields.

Signs

The exam findings are also similar to those encountered in primary angle-closure glaucoma:

Acute secondary angle closure is characterized by decreased visual acuity, extremely high IOP, ciliary injection, corneal edema, AC cell and flare, shallow AC, closed angles on gonioscopy, and a mid dilated, non-reactive pupil. In addition, there are signs of the underlying etiology (see above).

Chronic secondary angle closure is identified by narrow angles with PAS, increased IOP, glaukomflecken, and signs of the underlying etiology (see above). Visual field defects and optic nerve cupping may also be present.

Evaluation

- When taking the **history**, the patient must be asked about previous eye diseases, injuries, and surgery, as well as symptoms of an angle-closure attack.
- The **eye exam** must carefully evaluate the pupils (mid dilated in acute attack), cornea (may have edema, dystrophy, scar tissue), tonometry (increased IOP), AC (depth), gonioscopy (narrow or occluded angles, may have PAS, neovascularization), iris (may have atrophy, scar tissue, neovascularization), lens (presence and position of lens implant, may have glaukomflecken), and ophthalmoscopy (optic nerve cupping, nerve fiber layer appearance, may have retinal or choroidal lesion).
- **Visual field** testing must be performed to check for scotomas.

Management

Treatment of secondary angle-closure glaucoma depends upon the underlying etiology:

- Laser peripheral iridotomy for pupillary block.
- Topical cycloplegic (scopolamine 0.25% qid or atropine 1% bid) for malignant glaucoma, microspherophakia, and after scleral buckling or panretinal photocoagulation. Do *not* use miotics. Refractory cases of malignant glaucoma may require pars plana vitrectomy and lens extraction, or Nd:YAG laser disruption of the anterior vitreous face in pseudophakic and aphakic patients.
- Topical cycloplegic (scopolamine 0.25% qid), steroid (prednisolone acetate 1% qid), and panretinal photocoagulation initially for neovascular glaucoma. Later, filtering surgery, a drainage implant, or a cyclodestructive procedure is often necessary.
- Cataract extraction may be necessary for lens-induced cases.
- Chronic secondary angle closure may require treatment of increased IOP similar to that used in POAG (see section on primary open-angle glaucoma, above).

Prognosis

Secondary angle-closure glaucoma is frequently due to a chronic process, and therefore the prognosis is usually worse than for primary angle closure. However, the outcome depends on the etiology, extent of optic nerve damage, and subsequent IOP control. Neovascular glaucoma has a particularly poor prognosis.

CHAPTER FOURTEEN

Iris

Introduction

The iris is the colored ring of muscular tissue that contains the pupil and regulates the amount of light entering the eye. Abnormalities can therefore affect its size, color, and shape. The most common iris disorders are trauma, heterochromia, neovascularization, and tumors.

Trauma

Blunt trauma to the eye can produce anterior-segment damage involving the iris and ciliary body. If these vascular structures are torn, then bleeding and hyphema occur. Once the hemorrhage resorbs, the type and extent of injury can be assessed with gonioscopy (a special mirrored contact lens that enables inspection of the anterior-chamber angle with the slit lamp),

ANGLE RECESSION

Angle recession is a tear in the ciliary body. The anterior face of the ciliary muscle shears between the longitudinal and circular fibers (Figure 14–1). This is the most common source of intraocular hemorrhage resulting from blunt trauma and is the underlying etiology in >60% of hyphemas.

CYCLODIALYSIS

Cyclodialysis is a separation or disinsertion of the ciliary body from its attachment to the sclera at the scleral spur. This cleft allows aqueous fluid to pass directly into the

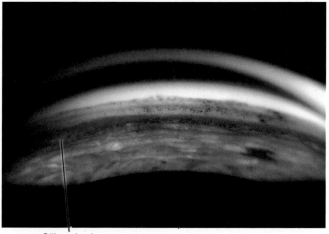

Ciliary body

FIGURE 14–1
Gonioscopic view of angle recession demonstrating deepened angle and blue-gray face of the ciliary body.

suprachoroidal space, and therefore hypotony (low intraocular pressure (IOP)) is a potential complication.

IRIDODIALYSIS

Iridodialysis is a separation or disinsertion of the iris root from its attachment to the ciliary body that appears as a peripheral hole in the iris (Figure 14–2).

SPHINCTER TEARS

Sphincter tears are small radial iris tears at the pupillary margin that look like small V-shaped notches. If the iris sphincter is unable to function properly, the patient

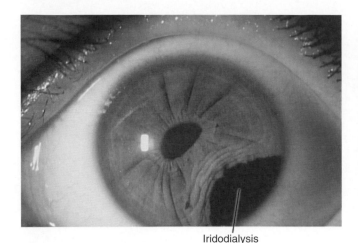

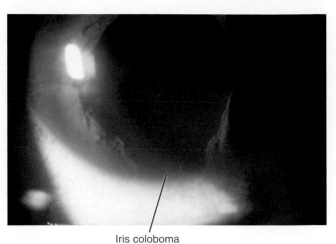

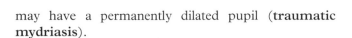

Iridodialysis

Iris coloboma

FIGURE 14–2
Iridodialysis. The iris is disinserted for approximately 90° (from the 3 o'clock to 6 o'clock position).

FIGURE 14–3
Coloboma of inferior iris.

may have a permanently dilated pupil (**traumatic mydriasis**).

Symptoms

Acutely, these injuries can cause pain, redness, and decreased vision. Later, patients may notice photophobia from iridodialysis or traumatic mydriasis, or monocular diplopia/polyopia (double/multiple images) from iridodialysis.

Signs

By definition, iris or ciliary body damage is present. The pathology may initially be obscured by hyphema, and the exact diagnosis may require gonioscopy after the blood clears. Patients may have normal or decreased visual acuity, an unusually deep anterior chamber, abnormal pupil, or iridodonesis (iris looseness, apparent as jiggling movements at the slit lamp). Often the acute findings are conjunctival injection, subconjunctival hemorrhage, altered IOP, anterior-chamber cell and flare, and hyphema. Depending on the mechanism of injury, there may be other evidence of trauma, including lid or orbital damage, dislocated lens, phacodonesis (lens looseness apparent as jiggling movements at the slit lamp), traumatic cataract, vitreous hemorrhage, commotio retinae, retinal tear/detachment, choroidal rupture, and/or optic neuropathy. In chronic cases, signs of glaucoma (i.e., increased IOP, optic nerve cupping, and visual field defects) can be seen.

Differential diagnosis

Other causes of iris defects are iris coloboma (Figure 14–3), essential iris atrophy (Figure 14–4), surgical iridectomy or iridotomy (Figure 14–5), and Reiger's anomaly (Figure 14–6).

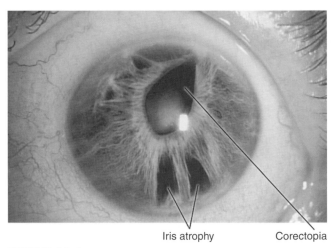

Iris atrophy   Corectopia

FIGURE 14–4
Essential iris atrophy, demonstrating iris atrophy and corectopia (displaced pupil).

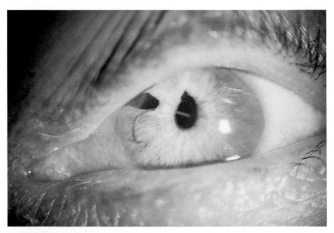

FIGURE 14–5
A surgical iridectomy. Note that a haptic of the posterior chamber intraocular lens is dislocated through the iridectomy.

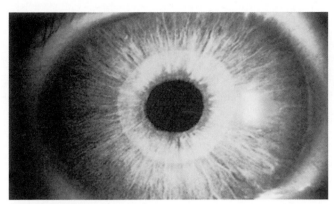

FIGURE 14–6
Reiger's anomaly with iris stromal hypoplasia. Holes in the iris eventually develop.

Evaluation

- Take a careful **history** to document previous eye injuries and surgery, with particular attention to the mechanism of any trauma.
- The **eye exam** must rule out an open globe and intraocular foreign body (see Ch. 10) in acute cases. **Gonioscopy** and **scleral depression** are essential in order to diagnose angle trauma and peripheral retinal trauma, respectively, when the globe is intact and there is no hyphema. The remainder of the exam focuses on tonometry (may have increased IOP or hypotony), anterior chamber (cell and flare, hyphema, depth), iris (tears, may have iridodonesis), lens (may have cataract, phacodonesis), and ophthalmoscopy (may have posterior-segment damage, optic nerve cupping).
- **B-scan ultrasonography** if the fundus cannot be adequately visualized.

Management

Treatment depends on the type of injury:

- **Angle recession**: observe for angle recession glaucoma by monitoring the IOP and optic nerve appearance.
- **Cyclodialysis**: consider surgical or laser reattachment of the cleft if hypotony unresponsive to treatment with topical atropine is present.
- **Iridodialysis**: consider a cosmetic contact lens or surgical repair for disabling glare or monocular diplopia/polyopia.
- **Sphincter tears**: consider a cosmetic contact lens or surgical repair for a dilated, non-reactive pupil.
- All forms may require treatment of increased IOP (see Ch. 13) or other ocular injuries.

Prognosis

The prognosis depends on the type and extent of iris damage. Up to 10% of patients with angle recession involving more than two-thirds of the angle will eventually develop glaucoma. The outcome is poor for angle recession glaucoma or chronic hypotony.

Heterochromia

Definition

Iris heterochromia means iris of different colors. This condition may be unilateral (**heterochromia iridis**) or bilateral (**heterochromia iridum**), congenital or acquired.

Heterochromia iridis occurs when one iris is two different colors (iris bicolor).

Heterochromia iridum occurs when the two irises are different colors (e.g., one blue, one brown) (Figure 14–7).

Etiology

Heterochromia iridum has numerous causes and is generally classified according to which iris is the abnormal one.

CONGENITAL

- **Hypochromic** (involved iris is lighter): is due to congenital Horner's syndrome, Waardenburg's syndrome, Hirschsprung's disease, and Parry–Romberg hemifacial atrophy.
- **Hyperchromic** (involved iris is darker): is due to ocular or oculodermal melanocytosis, and iris pigment epithelium hamartoma.

ACQUIRED

- **Hypochromic**: is due to acquired Horner's syndrome, Fuchs' heterochromic iridocyclitis, iris stromal atrophy, juvenile xanthogranuloma, and metastatic carcinoma.
- **Hyperchromic**: is due to medication (topical prostaglandin analogues), intraocular foreign body (siderosis, hemosiderosis, chalcosis), iris tumor (nevus, melanoma), and iris neovascularization.

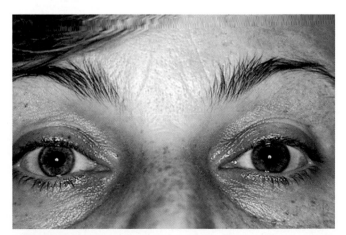

FIGURE 14–7
Heterochromia iridum. The patient's right iris is blue and the left iris is hazel.

Symptoms

Patients are aware of the difference in iris color but are otherwise usually asymptomatic. However, depending on the etiology, they may have other ocular or systemic symptoms.

Signs

By definition, iris heterochromia is apparent. Other findings depend on the etiology:

- Ptosis, miosis, and anhidrosis in Horner's syndrome.
- White forelock, premature graying, leucism (cutaneous hypopigmentation), facial anomalies, dystopia canthorum, and deafness in Waardenburg's syndrome.
- Skin, scleral, and choroidal pigmentation in ocular or oculodermal melanocytosis.
- Anterior-chamber cell and flare, keratic precipitates, and increased IOP in uveitis, siderosis, and chalcosis.
- May have an intraocular foreign body (siderosis, chalcosis), old hemorrhage (hemosiderosis), or tumor.

Evaluation

- The **history** should include systemic disorders, eye diseases, and injuries.
- The **eye exam** must specifically rule out a tumor or intraocular foreign body. In addition, the examination should concentrate on the lids (may have ptosis, pigmentation), pupils (may have miosis), sclera (may have pigmentation), tonometry (may have increased IOP), anterior chamber (may have cell and flare), iris (color, may have atrophy, tumor, neovascularization), and ophthalmoscopy (may have retinal or choroidal lesion).
- Consider **B-scan ultrasonography** if the fundus cannot be adequately visualized.
- Consider **orbital radiographs** or **computed tomography scan** to rule out an intraocular foreign body.
- Consider an **electroretinogram** to evaluate retinal function in siderosis, hemosiderosis, and chalcosis.
- Consider a **medical consultation**.

Management

- Iris heterochromia is usually benign and does not require treatment.
- Treatment may be necessary for active uveitis (see Ch. 12), increased IOP (see Ch. 13), or malignancy (see section on tumors, below).
- Surgical removal may be required for an intraocular foreign body or tumor.

Prognosis

The heterochromia is benign, but the prognosis depends on the etiology.

Rubeosis Iridis

Definition

Neovascularization of the iris is called rubeosis iridis and may involve the angle.

Etiology

Neovascularization is caused by ocular ischemia, which most commonly occurs in proliferative diabetic retinopathy, central retinal vein occlusion, and carotid occlusive disease. It is also associated with anterior-segment ischemia, sickle-cell retinopathy, central retinal artery occlusion, chronic retinal detachment, tumors, and chronic inflammation.

Symptoms

Patients are often asymptomatic, but decreased vision or angle-closure symptoms (see Ch. 13) may occur.

Signs

The hallmark of rubeosis is the presence of fine, lacy blood vessels on the anterior iris surface, particularly at the pupillary margin and around iridectomies (Figure 14–8). Gonioscopy is necessary to evaluate angle involvement. The abnormal vessels are fragile and may bleed, causing a spontaneous hyphema. Depending on the underlying etiology, there may be decreased visual acuity, retinal lesions, and signs of angle closure or neovascular glaucoma (i.e., increased IOP, peripheral anterior synchiae, shallow anterior chamber, optic nerve cupping, and visual field defects).

Evaluation

- The **history** must note systemic disorders, eye diseases, and any symptoms of angle closure.

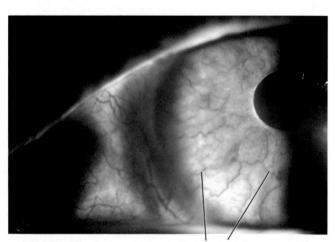

Rubeosis iridis

FIGURE 14–8

Rubeosis iridis, demonstrating florid neovascularization of the iris with large branching vessels.

- The **eye exam** must include pupillary response (may have a positive relative afferent pupillary defect), tonometry (may have increased IOP), gonioscopy (neovascularization, may have peripheral anterior synechiae, narrow or occluded angle), iris (neovascularization), and ophthalmoscopy (may have retinal lesion, optic nerve cupping).
- Consider **fluorescein angiogram** to determine the cause of ocular ischemia if it is not apparent on direct examination.
- Consider **medical consultation** for systemic diseases, including duplex and Doppler scans of the carotid arteries to rule out carotid occlusive disease.

Management

- Topical steroid (prednisolone acetate 1% qid) and cycloplegic (atropine 1% bid) for inflammation.
- Laser photocoagulation or peripheral cryotherapy for retinal ischemia.
- Treatment of increased IOP and neovascular glaucoma may be required (see Ch. 13); therefore observe patients by monitoring the IOP and optic nerve appearance.

Prognosis

Despite regression of the rubeotic vessels with appropriate therapy, the prognosis is poor because most causes of neovascularization are chronic progressive diseases.

Tumors

Various benign and malignant tumors can involve the iris. These masses may arise from the iris stroma or pigment epithelium. They are usually categorized by their cell of origin.

IRIS CYST

A cyst can develop anywhere in the iris. Primary cysts, the most common form, arise from either the stroma (may be congenital from sequestration of epithelium during fetal development) or the iris pigment epithelium (due to spontaneous separation of pigmented and non-pigmented epithelium). Secondary cysts are stromal and usually result from trauma or surgery, but they may also occur from chronic use of strong topical miotic drops, which cause cysts at the pupillary border.

On examination, transillumination with a thin slit beam is used to differentiate a cyst from a solid tumor. Cysts may cause segmental elevation of the iris, angle closure, distortion of the pupil, and occlusion of the visual axis (Figure 14–9). Surgical excision is considered if the vision is affected or secondary glaucoma occurs.

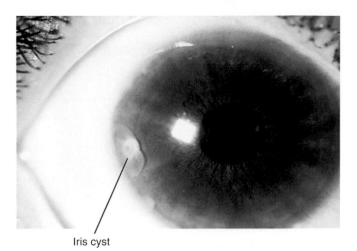

Iris cyst

FIGURE 14–9
Peripheral iris cyst seen as a translucent round lesion at the iris periphery.

IRIS NEVUS

An iris nevus is a flat, variably pigmented, benign lesion of the iris stroma that obscures the underlying crypts (Figure 14–10). It can be either focal or diffuse. These pigmented spots or iris "freckles" occur in 50% of the population, but are rare before 12 years of age. An iris nevus is differentiated from a malignant melanoma by size (<3 mm in diameter), thickness (<1 mm thick), and the absence of vascularity, ectropion uveae, cataract, secondary glaucoma, and enlargement over time. Iris nevi must be monitored for growth and suspicious lesions should be followed with serial photographs. There is a small risk of malignant transformation into melanoma.

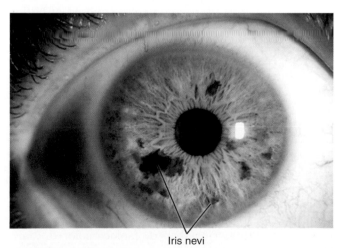

Iris nevi

FIGURE 14–10
Variably pigmented, small, flat iris nevi are seen diffusely scattered over the anterior iris surface.

IRIS NODULES

Nodules are collections of cells on the iris surface.

Brushfield spots

Brushfield spots are small peripheral areas of focal iris hyperplasia that appear as a ring of elevated white-gray spots (Figure 14–11). They are associated with Down syndrome (85%), but may also occur in 24% of normal individuals (Kunkmann–Wolffian bodies).

Lisch nodules

Lisch nodules are bilateral tan melanocytic hamartomas associated with neurofibromatosis type 1 (92%) (Figure 14–12). They usually involve the lower half of the iris and may become more abundant with age.

Inflammatory nodules

Inflammatory nodules are composed of inflammatory cells and debris from granulomatous uveitis. They are distinguished by location: **Busacca** nodules occur on the anterior iris surface, while **Koeppe** nodules are found at the pupillary border (see Figures 12–11 and 12–12).

IRIS PIGMENT EPITHELIUM ADENOMAS AND ADENOCARCINOMAS

Iris pigment epithelium adenomas (benign) and adeno-carcinomas (malignant) are very rare. They present as a darkly pigmented, well-circumscribed or multinodular mass. Secondary glaucoma can occur and is caused by tumor involvement of the angle. The treatment, which should be performed by a tumor specialist, is with chemotherapy, radiation, and surgical excision.

JUVENILE XANTHOGRANULOMA

Juvenile xanthogranuloma is a systemic disease characterized by multiple orange nodules composed of histiocytes (Figure 14–13). These lesions can involve the iris and may bleed, producing a spontaneous hyphema. They appear prior to age 1 year old and often regress by age 5. If necessary, the iris nodules can be treated with steroids, radiation, and excision.

MALIGNANT MELANOMA

Malignant melanoma is a pigmented or amelanotic, elevated, vascular mass that destroys the iris stroma (Figures 14–14 and 14–15). Up to 3% of uveal melanomas involve the iris and are more common in Caucasians, especially with light iris color. The tumor may be localized, ring-shaped, tapioca-colored (dark tapioca appearance), or diffuse (appearing as iris heterochromia) and associated with secondary glaucoma. Many patients report a history of an iris nevus that has

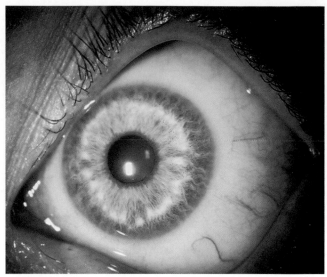

FIGURE 14–11
Brushfield spots in a patient with Down syndrome, demonstrating a ring of white spots in the iris stroma.

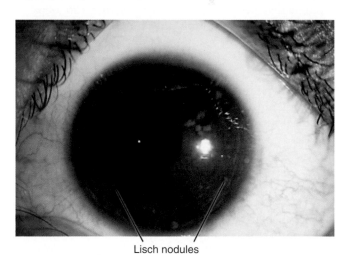

Lisch nodules

FIGURE 14–12
In a patient with neurofibromatosis, Lisch nodules appear as small, round, lightly colored nodules.

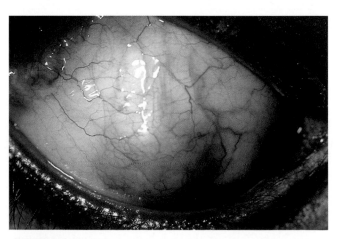

FIGURE 14–13
Superior limbal epibulbar orange mass in patient with juvenile xanthogranuloma.

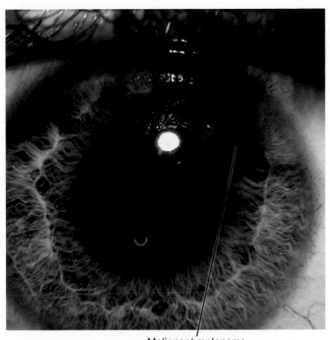

Malignant melanoma

FIGURE 14–14
Malignant melanoma is seen as a hazy brown confluent patch on this blue iris.

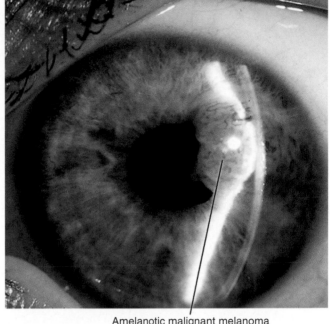

Amelanotic malignant melanoma

FIGURE 14–15
Amelanotic melanoma is visible as a large, pedunculated, vascular mass with obvious elevation, as depicted by the bowed appearance of the slit-beam light over the iris surface.

enlarged over time. Other findings include feeder vessels, spontaneous hyphema, sectoral cataract, invasion of angle structures, increased IOP, and ectropion uveae.

B-scan ultrasonography may be necessary to rule out ciliary body involvement. Treatments, which should be performed by a tumor specialist, include chemotherapy, radiation, surgical excision, and sometimes enucleation. Patients who require management of increased IOP (see Ch. 13) should not undergo filtering surgery. Metastasis occurs in 14% of patients and is associated with tumor extension into the trabecular meshwork, poorly defined margins, glaucoma, and older age. Malignant melanoma has a mortality rate of 4–10%.

METASTATIC TUMORS

Metastatic tumors to the iris are rare. They usually originate from breast, lung, and prostate carcinomas, and appear as a fluffy, friable, amelanotic mass (Figure 14–16). Other findings that may be present are pseudohypoyon of tumor cells, anterior uveitis, hyphema, rubeosis, and glaucoma. Lymphoma and leukemia can also affect the iris. Leukemic involvement produces nodular or diffuse milky lesions with intense hyperemia, iris thickening, and loss of the normal crypts. Iris hetero-

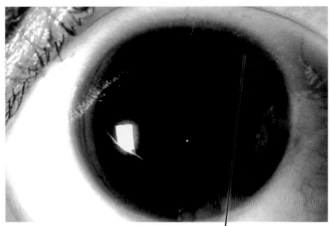

Metastatic carcinoid

FIGURE 14–16
Metastatic carcinoid appearing as an orange-brown peripheral iris lesion.

chromia and pseudohypopyon may also occur. Metastatic lesions should be treated by a tumor specialist with chemotherapy, radiation, and surgical excision. Patients may also require treatment of increased IOP (see Ch. 13), but glaucoma filtering surgery is not recommended.

CHAPTER FIFTEEN

Lens

Introduction

The crystalline lens helps focus images on the retina. It is the structure responsible for the eye's fine focusing ability, which enables sharp vision at all distances. Abnormalities that affect lens position, shape, clarity, or flexibility can impair vision. Conditions that cannot be adequately corrected with glasses or contact lenses often require surgery. If lens abnormalities occur in children and are not corrected as early as possible, then amblyopia may result. For adults, the timing of treatment is less important.

Dislocated Lens (Ectopia Lentis)

Definition

Ectopia lentis refers to displacement of the lens from its normal position in the eye. The displacement may be partial (**subluxation**) or complete (**luxation**). A subluxated lens remains partly in the pupillary axis behind the iris, while a luxated lens is entirely displaced from the pupillary space into the anterior chamber or vitreous cavity. In some luxated cases, the lens may actually rest on the retina.

Etiology

Lens dislocation is caused by defective zonules, the fine fibers that support the lens from the ciliary body. Lens dislocation can occur in many congenital, developmental, and acquired conditions:

- **Simple ectopia lentis**: condition with a small, spherical lens that is often displaced up and out at birth.

- **Ectopia lentis et pupillae**: condition with oval or slit-like pupils pointed in the opposite direction from the displaced lens.
- **Homocystinuria**: disorder of methionine metabolism with elevated levels of homocystine and methionine that causes a progressive lens dislocation down and inward. Also associated with seizures, osteoporosis, mental retardation, and thromboembolism.
- **Hyperlysinemia**: disorder of lysine metabolism that leads to lens subluxation, muscular hypotony, and mental retardation.
- **Sulfite oxidase deficiency**: disorder of sulfur metabolism with ectopia lentis, seizures, and mental retardation.
- **Marfan's syndrome**: disorder with long extremities, arachnodactyly, joint laxity, pectus deformities, scoliosis, dilated ascending aorta, aortic insufficiency, and lens displacement up and outward.
- **Stickler's syndrome**: progressive arthro-ophthalmopathy with Marfanoid features, retinal detachment, cataract, glaucoma, and ectopia lentis.
- **Microspherophakia**: small spherical lens occurring in isolation or as part of various syndromes (dominant spherophakia, Weill–Marchesani syndrome, Lowe's syndrome).
- **Ehlers–Danlos syndrome**: disorder of type 3 collagen with ectopia lentis, keratoconus, angioid streaks, blue sclera, hyperextensible joints, and elastic skin.
- **Pseudoexfoliation syndrome**: ocular disorder with weak zonules, ectopia lentis, and increased risk of glaucoma.
- **Aniridia** (see Ch. 6).
- **Megalocornea**: congenital disorder with enlarged corneas, ectopia lentis, glaucoma, and cataracts.
- **Congenital glaucoma** (see Ch. 6).

- **Trauma**.
- **Tertiary syphilis**.

Epidemiology

Trauma is the most common cause of a dislocated lens, accounting for up to 50% of cases. The most frequent cause of heritable lens dislocation is Marfan's syndrome.

Symptoms

Symptoms depend on the amount of lens displacement. Patients may be asymptomatic with minimal subluxation or have decreased vision, monocular diplopia, or symptoms of angle closure if the lens causes pupillary block (see Ch. 13). In some patients, the vision may vary as the lens moves into and out of the visual axis.

Signs

By definition, the lens is displaced anteriorly, posteriorly, or laterally from its normal position behind the iris (Figures 15–1–15–4). The iris and lens demonstrate iridodonesis and phacodonesis, respectively (looseness apparent as jiggling movements at the slit lamp). Additional findings may include variable decreased visual acuity, astigmatism, increased intraocular pressure (IOP) if the angle is closed, anterior-chamber cell and flare, vitreous in the anterior chamber or around the subluxated lens, cataract, and signs of ocular trauma.

Evaluation

- The **history** should concentrate specifically on systemic diseases, eye diseases, injuries or surgery, and the characteristics of any visual changes, especially monocular diplopia and variable decreased acuity.
- The **eye exam** is performed with attention to vision (distance and near acuity, pinhole, refraction), cornea (may have large diameter), tonometry (may have increased IOP), gonioscopy (angle appearance), iris (iridodonesis), and lens (position, phacodonesis, may

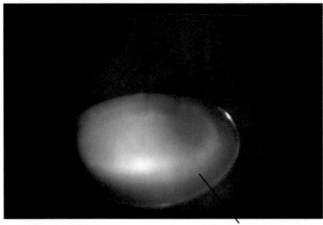

FIGURE 15–1
Dislocated crystalline lens resting on the retina.

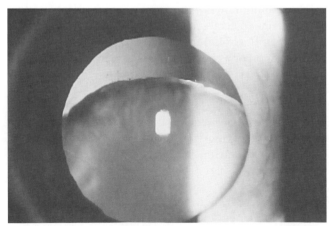
Dislocated crystalline lens

FIGURE 15–3
Lens subluxed (downward) due to trauma.

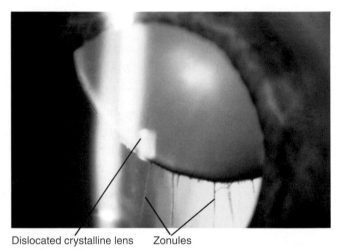
Dislocated crystalline lens   Zonules

FIGURE 15–2
Subluxed lens (up and out) due to trauma. The broken inferior zonular fibers are visible.

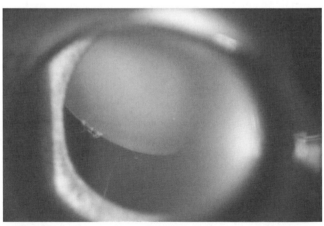

FIGURE 15–4
Lens subluxed (upward) in a patient with Marfan's syndrome.

have exfoliative material). In cases of trauma, a complete eye examination with ophthalmoscopy should be performed to rule out other traumatic injuries.

- **Lab tests** include Venereal Disease Research Laboratory test, fluorescent treponemal antibody absorption test, and lumbar puncture if syphilis is suspected.
- **Medical consultation** for systemic diseases if no other causes can be determined.

Management

- Small lens displacements can be observed and managed with correction of any induced refractive error.
- Progressive and large dislocations are treated with lens extraction and insertion of an intraocular lens (IOL) implant.
- Treatment of angle closure may be required (see Ch. 13). Miotics should be avoided since they may exacerbate pupillary block. Microspherophakia causing pupillary block is treated with a cycloplegic (scopolamine 0.25% tid or atropine 1% bid) and may require laser iridotomy.
- Treat any underlying disorder (e.g., dietary restriction for homocystinuria, penicillin for syphilis).

Prognosis

In most cases, the lens displacement is correctable, but the prognosis depends on the underlying etiology. In general, it is good.

Acquired Cataracts

Definition

An acquired cataract is an acquired opacity of the crystalline lens (see Ch. 6 for discussion of congenital cataracts).

Etiology

Cataracts are typically classified by location:

Cortical cataracts are caused by swelling, degeneration, and liquefaction of the younger outer (cortical) fibers. These types of cataract include:

- **Spokes and vacuoles**: radial line and punctate dot opacities (Figure 15–5).
- **Mature cataract**: completely white lens with no red reflex visible from the fundus (Figure 15–6).
- **Morgagnian cataract**: white liquefied cortex in which the dense, inner, brown nucleus has sunken inferiorly.
- **Hypermature cataract**: the stage following a morgagnian cataract, in which the lens shrinks, the capsule wrinkles, calcium deposits form, and proteins can leak into the anterior chamber (Figure 15–7).

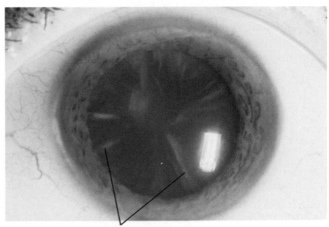

Cortical spokes

FIGURE 15–5
Cortical cataract, demonstrating white cortical spoking.

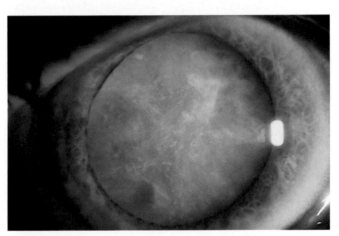

FIGURE 15–6
Mature cataract with white, liquefied cortex.

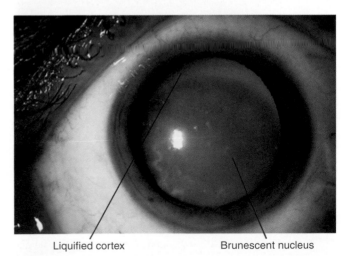

Liquified cortex   Brunescent nucleus

FIGURE 15–7
Morgagnian cataract, demonstrating a dense, brown nucleus sinking inferiorly in a white, liquefied cortex.

Nuclear sclerotic cataracts are due to diffuse lens hardening and discoloration (yellow, green, white, or brown) from deterioration of the older central (nuclear) fibers (Figures 15–8 and 15–9). This increases the index of refraction, often resulting in myopia, commonly known as "second sight" in presbyopic individuals who are once again able to read without glasses when their cataract progresses. Eventually, however, the second sight is overshadowed by the decreased vision from the cataract. Extreme nuclear sclerosis may produce a dark mahogany-colored, almost black, lens (cataract nigrans).

Subcapsular cataracts occur just beneath the lens capsule:

- **Anterior subcapsular (ASC) cataract**: fibrous plaque from metaplasia of the central anterior lens epithelial cells.
- **Posterior subcapsular (PSC) cataract**: granular opacity from posterior migration and swelling of epithelial cells (Figures 15–10 and 15–11).

Cataracts may also be categorized by etiology:

Senile: all forms of cataracts are most commonly due to aging changes. They are related in part to ultraviolet B radiation from chronic sun exposure.

Systemic diseases can produce characteristic cataracts: diabetes mellitus (cortical or PSC cataract), hypocalcemia (white dots or flakes in the lens), myotonic dystrophy (central, polychromatic,

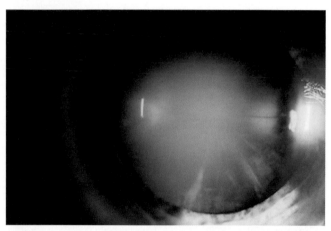

FIGURE 15–8
Cataract with 2+ yellow-brown nuclear sclerosis.

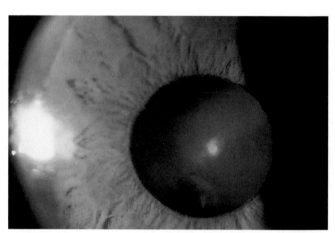

FIGURE 15–9
Brunescent nuclear sclerotic cataract.

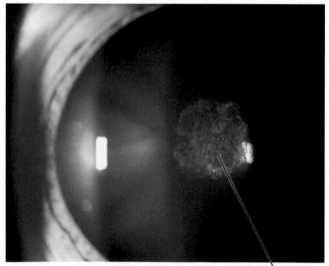

Posterior subcapsular cataract

FIGURE 15–10
Posterior subcapsular cataract, demonstrating typical white, hazy appearance.

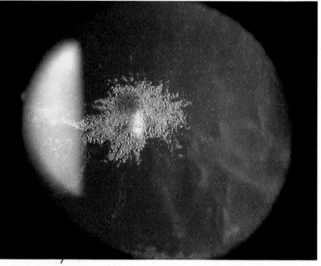

Posterior subcapsular cataract

FIGURE 15–11
Posterior subcapsular cataract due to topical steroid use, as viewed with retroillumination.

iridescent, cortical crystals that have the appearance of a "Christmas tree"), Wilson's disease ("sunflower cataract" (chalcosis lentis)), Fabry's disease, atopic dermatitis (PSC cataract), neurofibromatosis type 2 (PSC cataract), and ectodermal dysplasia (Figures 15–12–15–14).

Eye diseases: uveitis (ASC or PSC cataract), angle-closure glaucoma (glaukomflecken), intraocular tumors (sector cataract near the tumor), retinitis pigmentosa (PSC cataract), Stickler's syndrome (cortical cataract), and phthisis bulbi.

Toxicity: medications are the primary cause of toxic cataracts and include steroids (PSC cataract), miotics (ASC cataract), phenothiazines (ASC cataract), amiodarone (ASC cataract), and busulfan (PSC cataract) (Figure 15–15). Toxic cataracts also result from radiation (ionizing (PSC cataract), infrared (anterior capsule exfoliation), ultraviolet, argon laser (nuclear sclerotic cataract), microwave, and short-wave), electricity (cortical cataract), and chemicals (i.e., mercury) (Figure 15–16).

Trauma: blunt trauma often results in a cortical rosette-pattern cataract, penetrating trauma leads to a cataract if the lens capsule is perforated due to hydration of the lens, and an intraocular foreign body can produce a distinctive cataract if it contains iron (orange ASC deposits) or copper (green lens capsule and cortical petaloid pattern) (Figures 15–17 and 15–18).

Postoperative: after almost any intraocular surgery there is an increased risk of cataract. This is especially true if intraocular gas is used in retinal surgery.

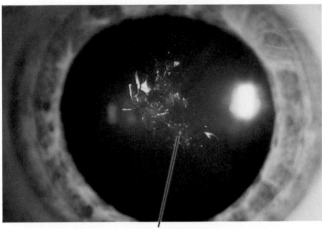

"Christmas tree" cholesterol cataract

FIGURE 15–12
Polychromatic, refractile cholesterol deposits within the crystalline lens.

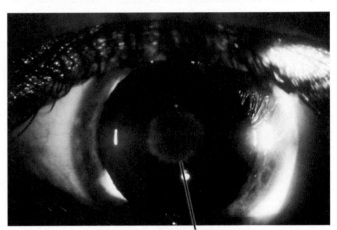

Sunflower cataract

FIGURE 15–13
Sunflower cataract in a patient with Wilson's disease.

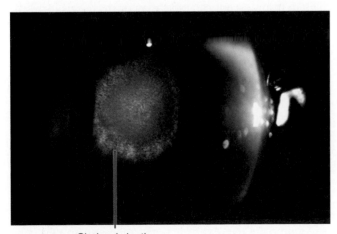

Chalcosis lentis

FIGURE 15–14
Sunflower cataract (chalcosis lentis) with green-brown central opacities in the lens.

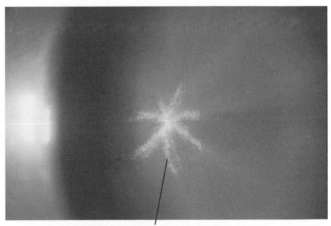

Anterior subcapsular cataract

FIGURE 15–15
Anterior subcapsular star-pattern cataract due to phenothiazine use.

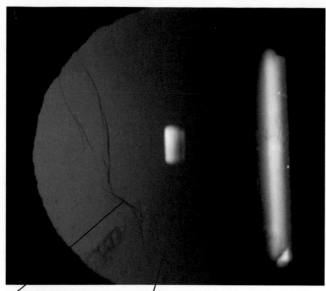

Lens capsule exfoliation   Capsular edge

FIGURE 15–16
Lens capsule exfoliation from infrared radiation.

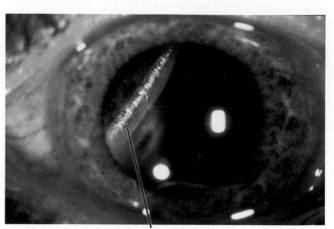

Intralenticular foreign body

FIGURE 15–18
Intralenticular foreign body.

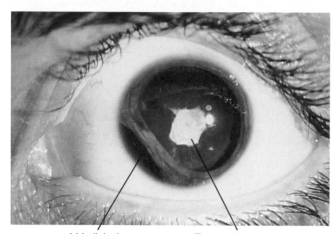

Iridodialysis   Traumatic cataract

FIGURE 15–17
Dense white central cataract due to trauma. There is also an iridodialysis (arrow).

Epidemiology

Cataracts are the leading cause of blindness worldwide. In the Framingham Eye Study, the prevalence of senile cataracts was approximately 42% in adults 52–64 years old, 73% in those 65–74 years old, and 91% in individuals 75–85 years old. African Americans are at increased risk of developing cataracts in every age group. Smoking is also a risk factor for nuclear sclerotic cataracts.

Symptoms

With early cataracts, the vision may be unchanged. Over time, patients experience painless progressive blurring of vision, dimmer vision with the need for more light to see clearly, glare from bright light sources, and occasionally monocular diplopia. If left untreated, cataracts can lead to blindness.

Signs

The exam is notable for decreased visual acuity, contrast sensitivity, and color vision (especially blue discrimination). Characteristically, nuclear sclerosis affects distance vision more than near vision, often by inducing myopia, whereas PSC cataracts reduce near vision more than distance vision and also result in visual deterioration with glare testing. The lens opacification is seen as focal or diffuse discoloration, usually best appreciated with retroillumination at the slit lamp and with the pupil dilated. Intumescent cataracts may push the iris forward, leading to angle closure, and hypermature cataracts may leak lens proteins, causing phacolytic glaucoma (see Ch. 13).

Evaluation

- The **history** should include any systemic diseases, medications (especially prior use of steroids), ocular trauma or surgery, radiation exposure, and other ocular diseases. It is also important to characterize the patient's visual changes, inquire about the functional difficulties they cause, and note any exacerbating factors (e.g., near versus distance, at night, with bright lights).
- A complete **eye exam** is performed and should concentrate on quantifying the decreased vision (distance and near acuity, pinhole, refraction, glare testing, contrast sensitivity, color vision) and documenting

the appearance of the cataract (type, size, density, and location). It is important to rule out other causes of poor vision, so attention must also be directed to the cornea (for central staining, edema, or scarring), tonometry (for increased IOP), gonioscopy, and ophthalmoscopy (for macular pathology).

- Consider **potential acuity meter testing**, which is a device that attaches to the slit lamp and shines a small illuminated eyechart directly on to the retina in order to estimate the patient's visual potential, especially when there is coexisting posterior-segment pathology.
- **B-scan ultrasonography** if the fundus cannot be adequately visualized through the cataract to make sure that there are no posterior-segment problems.
- **Keratometry** and **A-scan biometry** must be performed to calculate the intraocular lens (IOL) implant power before cataract surgery. Other tests to consider prior to cataract extraction are **specular microscopy** and **pachymetry** if corneal edema is suspected or evident.

Management

- Initially, vision may be improved satisfactorily with new glasses or contact lenses, but definitive treatment is surgical. The indications for cataract extraction and insertion of an IOL are: visual symptoms that interfere with specific activities and the patient desires improved visual function, a cataract that causes other ocular diseases (e.g., secondary glaucoma or uveitis), or a cataract that prevents adequate examination or treatment of a pre-existing posterior-segment condition (e.g., diabetic retinopathy, age-related macular degeneration, or glaucoma).
- Pupillary dilation (tropicamide 1% (Mydriacyl) ± phenylephrine 2.5% (Mydfrin) tid) may, in rare cases, enable a patient to see around a central cataract when he/she cannot undergo or refuses surgery.

Prognosis

Cataracts cause significant visual morbidity; however, they are a treatable condition. The success rate for routine cataract surgery is >98%, and the prognosis is excellent. Complications are rare but include ptosis, corneal edema or burn, hyphema, iris damage, secondary glaucoma, retained lens material, retinal detachment, cystoid macular edema (CME), choroidal effusion, suprachoroidal hemorrhage, and endophthalmitis.

Posterior Capsular Opacification

Definition

Posterior capsular opacification (PCO) refers to clouding of the normally clear posterior lens capsule after cataract surgery.

Etiology

PCO is due to capsular fibrosis and proliferation of residual lens epithelial cells along the posterior capsule (Elschnig's pearls). PCO is sometimes referred to as a "secondary cataract" since the vision becomes cloudy and symptoms of a cataract return again after successful cataract surgery.

Epidemiology

PCO is the most common sequela of cataract surgery, affecting up to 50% of patients. Improvements in IOL material (acrylic) and design (square edge) have decreased the incidence to <10%. However, the incidence approaches 100% in children and patients with uveitis.

Symptoms

Mild PCO is usually asymptomatic. The symptoms of a significant PCO are decreased vision, glare, or streaks radiating from lights.

Signs

PCO is evident on slit-lamp examination as whitening and/or wrinkling of the posterior capsule, usually best appreciated with the pupil dilated (Figure 15–19). The patient may have decreased visual acuity and will usually be pseudophakic, but can be aphakic.

Evaluation

- The **history** should document when the previous cataract surgery was performed.
- A complete **eye exam** must be done with particular attention to the vision (distance and near acuity, pinhole, refraction) and posterior capsule (size, density,

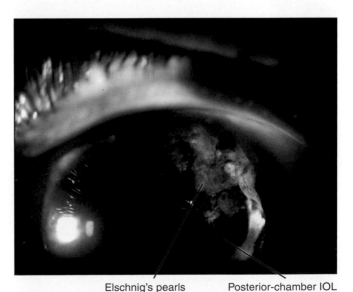

Elschnig's pearls   Posterior-chamber IOL

FIGURE 15–19
Secondary cataract composed of Elschnig's pearls.

and location of the opacity). It is also necessary to rule out other causes of decreased vision with careful inspection of the cornea (for central staining, edema, or scarring), IOL (presence, position, and stability), and ophthalmoscopy (for macular pathology).

Management

- The treatment for a visually significant PCO is to create a central opening in the capsule (posterior capsulotomy). This is accomplished by using a Nd:YAG laser with a slit-lamp delivery system (Figure 15–20).
- In young children, a primary posterior capsulotomy and anterior vitrectomy are performed at the time of cataract surgery.

Prognosis

PCO is a treatable condition with an excellent prognosis. The complications of laser capsulotomy are rare, but increased IOP, IOL damage or dislocation, corneal burn, retinal detachment, and CME may occur.

Aphakia

Definition

Aphakia means absence of the crystalline lens.

Etiology

This condition is most commonly caused by surgical lens removal, but can very rarely be congenital. Total

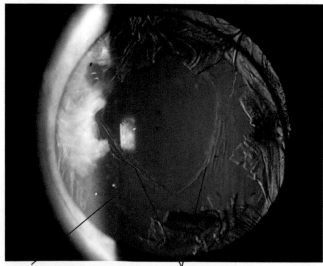

Posterior-chamber IOL   Capsular opening

FIGURE 15–20
Posterior capsule opening following Nd:YAG laser capsulotomy when viewed with retroillumination. Jagged edges or leaflets of the larger anterior capsulotomy are visible, as is the superior edge of the intraocular lens optic from the 12 o'clock to 3 o'clock position.

dislocation of the crystalline lens (usually from trauma, see section on dislocated lens (ectopia lentis), above) produces a functional aphakia since the lens can no longer perform its job.

Symptoms

Aphakia causes decreased uncorrected vision and a total loss of accommodation (ability to focus) since the lens is absent.

Signs

By definition, there is no lens. As a result, the patient has decreased uncorrected visual acuity (usually very high hyperopia) that can be corrected with a plus lens, and the iris demonstrates iridodonesis (jiggling movements at the slit lamp due to lack of support by a lens). There is usually a visible surgical wound. Other possible findings include vitreous in the anterior chamber, complications from surgery (i.e., corneal edema, increased IOP, iritis, iris damage, CME), or evidence of trauma or other disorders that can cause lens dislocation.

Evaluation

- The **history** should note if and when previous cataract surgery was performed. If the aphakia is due to a dislocated lens, then the appropriate information should be recorded (see section on dislocated lens (ectopia lentis), above).
- The **eye exam** should focus on the vision (distance and near acuity, refraction), confirm the absence of the lens, and rule out any complications. It is therefore important to assess the cornea (for edema), tonometry (for increased IOP), anterior chamber (for cell and flare, presence of vitreous), iris (for an iridectomy), and ophthalmoscopy (for CME).
- Consider **specular microscopy** and **pachymetry** if corneal edema is suspected or evident.

Management

- Aphakia can be corrected with contact lenses, glasses, or surgery. Aphakic glasses can only be used if the condition is bilateral, otherwise the image size disparity between the two eyes (aniseikonia) will be too great to allow binocular vision. If the patient is unable or prefers not to wear a contact lens or glasses, then consider secondary IOL implantation to make the patient pseudophakic.
- Treatment of complications may be required.

Prognosis

The prognosis for aphakia is typically good, unless there are complications (i.e., corneal edema, secondary glaucoma, CME). However, aphakia increases the risk of retinal detachment, especially in high myopes and if the posterior capsule is not intact.

Pseudophakia

Definition

Pseudophakia refers to the presence of an IOL implant. The IOL may be inserted primarily at the time of surgical crystalline lens removal or secondarily as a separate procedure to correct aphakia. The IOL may be placed in the anterior chamber (anterior-chamber IOL) or posterior chamber (posterior-chamber IOL).

Symptoms

Pseudophakia is generally asymptomatic. Patients with monofocal implants experience a loss of accommodation and can only see clearly at one distance without correction. Most lenses can cause positive (bright) or negative (dark) visual phenomena (dysphotopsias) from internal reflections within the IOL that occur in certain lighting conditions. If the IOL becomes decentered, then patients may report blurred vision or monocular diplopia/polyopia (double/multiple images).

Signs

By definition, there is an IOL implant, which can be located in the anterior chamber, iris plane, capsular bag, or ciliary sulcus with or without suture fixation to the iris or sclera (Figures 15–21 and 15–22). There is usually a visible surgical wound in the cornea or sclera near the limbus. Other possible findings include a peripheral iridectomy or complications from surgery (i.e., corneal edema, decentered IOL, iris capture of the IOL, increased IOP, iritis, hyphema, PCO, vitreous in the anterior chamber, CME).

Evaluation

- The **history** should document when the previous cataract surgery was performed and if any complications occurred.
- The **eye exam** must assess the vision (distance and near acuity, refraction), cornea (for edema), tonometry (for increased IOP), anterior chamber (for cell and flare, presence of vitreous), gonioscopy, iris (for an iridectomy), IOL (position and stability), posterior capsule (integrity and clarity), and ophthalmoscopy (for CME).

Management

- No treatment is usually required.
- Pseudophakic patients may require correction of a residual refractive error, but often only reading glasses are necessary.
- Treatment of complications may be required.

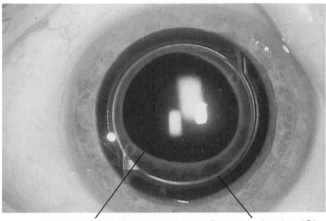

Anterior capsulorhexis   Posterior-chamber IOL

FIGURE 15–21
Pseudophakia demonstrating posterior-chamber intraocular lens (IOL) well centered in the capsular bag. The anterior capsulorhexis edge has fibrosed and is visible as a white circle overlying the IOL optic; the edges of the IOL haptics where they insert into the optic are also seen.

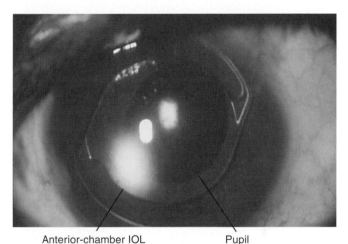

Anterior-chamber IOL   Pupil

FIGURE 15–22
Pseudophakia demonstrating anterior-chamber intraocular lens in good position above the iris.

Prognosis

Pseudophakia is a very common condition in elderly individuals. It is benign, but does increase the risk of retinal detachment, especially in high myopes and if the posterior capsule is not intact.

CHAPTER SIXTEEN

Vitreous

Introduction

The vitreous humor is the clear, gel-like substance that occupies almost 80% of the volume of the eye, and is composed of 99% water, collagen fibers, mucopolysaccharide, and hyaluronic acid. It has two main structures: the central core vitreous, and the peripheral cortical vitreous, which is firmly adherent to the peripheral retina in a 6 mm-wide area known as the vitreous base. The vitreous also has attachments at the macula, optic nerve, and retinal blood vessels. Therefore, changes in the vitreous from aging, trauma, and inflammation may have affects on the retina as well as the patient's vision.

Posterior Vitreous Detachment

Definition

A PVD refers to the dehiscence of the posterior vitreous surface from the retina.

Etiology

Liquefaction (syneresis) of the vitreous gel causes separation of the posterior hyaloid (posterior aspect of the vitreous humor that is in contact with the retina) from the retina and collapse of the vitreous away from the macula and optic disc towards the center of the eye.

Epidemiology

The risk of a PVD increases with age. By the age of 50 years old, 53% of patients will have a PVD, 65% by 65 years old, and by age 70, the majority of patients will have vitreous that is liquefied (synchysis senilis). PVDs can occur earlier after trauma, vitritis, cataract surgery, Nd:YAG laser posterior capsulotomy, and in patients with myopia, diabetes mellitus, hereditary vitreoretinal degenerations, and retinitis pigmentosa.

Symptoms

When the vitreous liquefies, patients generally notice the acute appearance of gray/black "floaters" which are described as lines, spots, hairs, or cobwebs suspended or moving in the visual field. Occasionally, patients will also notice photopsias (flashes of light), especially with eye movement. This is due to vitreous traction on the retina. In general, the flashes will improve over time; however, the floaters may remain indefinitely. In some cases, the floaters of a PVD can affect visual acuity, especially when located over the macula.

Signs

The signs of a PVD are only visible on fundus examination and include a circular or oval condensation within the vitreous that appears to float over the optic disc (**Weiss ring**), vitreous opacities, vitreous pigment cells ("tobacco dust," best seen on narrow slit-beam examination), and focal retinal hemorrhages (Figures 16–1 and 16–2). There may be a vitreous hemorrhage and/or a retinal tear.

Differential diagnosis

The acute onset of a PVD rules out most other diseases in the differential diagnosis; however, patients with vitreous hemorrhage from other causes and vitritis may be difficult to differentiate from a PVD.

Evaluation

- The **history** should document any previous ocular injuries, surgery, or laser procedures, and the

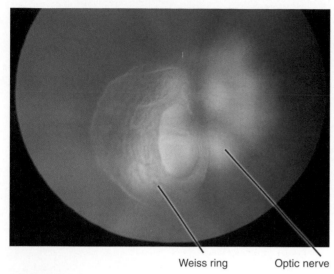

Weiss ring   Optic nerve

FIGURE 16–1
Circular Weiss ring seen over the optic nerve in the mid vitreous cavity.

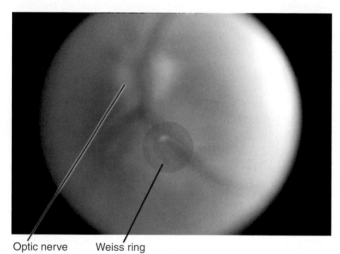

Optic nerve   Weiss ring

FIGURE 16–2
Horseshoe-shaped posterior vitreous detachment seen over the optic nerve in the mid vitreous cavity.

characteristics of any visual changes, including the presence of photopsias.

- The **eye exam** is performed with attention to ophthalmoscopy (Weiss ring, may have anterior vitreous cells, vitreous hemorrhage, retinal hemorrhages). The fundus examination should be performed with a careful dilated, depressed peripheral retinal examination to identify any retinal tears, holes, or detachments.

Management

- No treatment is generally needed for a PVD; however, given the risk of a retinal tear or retinal detachment, patients should be instructed about the warning signs for retinal tear/detachment, including photopsias,

increased floaters, and the sudden appearance of a shadow or web in their visual field.
- Patients should return immediately if any of the retinal tear/detachment warning signs occur, to rule out retinal tear or detachment.
- Repeat dilated retinal exam 1–3 months after acute PVD to rule out asymptomatic retinal tear or detachment.
- Treatment of complications may be required, in particular, laser or cryotherapy for retinal tears and surgery for retinal detachments.

Prognosis

The prognosis for a PVD is excellent. However, retinal tears occur in 10–15% of acute, symptomatic PVDs. In patients with a PVD and vitreous hemorrhage, the risk of a retinal tear increases to almost 70%.

Vitreous Hemorrhage

Definition

Vitreous hemorrhage is blood in the vitreous space.

Etiology

There are multiple causes of vitreous hemorrhage, including retinal break, PVD avulsing a retinal vessel, ruptured retinal arterial macroaneurysm, juvenile retinoschisis, familial exudative vitreoretinopathy, Terson's syndrome (blood from subarachnoid hemorrhage travels along the optic nerve and into the eye), trauma, retinal angioma, retinopathy of blood disorders, Valsalva retinopathy, and neovascularization from various disorders, including diabetic retinopathy, Eales' disease, hypertensive retinopathy, radiation retinopathy, sickle-cell retinopathy, and retinopathy of prematurity.

The most common cause of vitreous hemorrhage in adults is diabetic retinopathy. In children, consider child abuse, pars planitis, and juvenile retinoschisis.

Symptoms

Patients usually notice the sudden onset of floaters and decreased vision.

Signs

The exam is significant for decreased visual acuity and blood in the vitreous cavity that makes viewing the retina difficult (Figure 16–3). In severe cases, there may be no view of the retina, and the red reflex may be poor or even absent. Old vitreous hemorrhage appears gray-white (**ochre membrane**).

Differential Diagnosis

Vitreous hemorrhage is obvious when red blood cells are present; however, it may be difficult to differentiate the

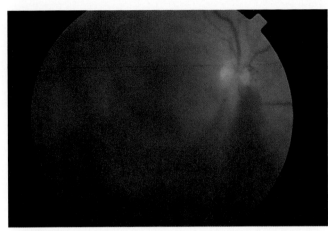

FIGURE 16–3
Vitreous hemorrhage obscures the view of the retina in this diabetic patient. Gravity has layered the blood inferiorly.

blood from other material (white blood cells, calcium particles, or pigment cells) due to vitritis, pars planitis, or asteroid hyalosis.

Evaluation

- The **history** should concentrate specifically on systemic diseases, eye diseases, and ocular injuries or surgery.
- The **eye exam** is performed with attention to visual acuity (decreased), tonometry (may have increased intraocular pressure (IOP)), and ophthalmoscopy (vitreous hemorrhage, may be difficult to see retinal details).
- **B-scan ultrasonography** is performed to rule out a retinal detachment if the fundus cannot be adequately visualized.

Management

- Most cases of vitreous hemorrhage respond to conservative treatment, so patients can be followed for resolution of the hemorrhage.
- Bedrest and elevation of the head may settle blood inferiorly to allow visualization of the fundus and speed visual recovery.
- Avoid aspirin and aspirin-containing products (and other anticoagulants).
- Consider pars plana vitrectomy by a vitreoretinal specialist if there is persistent vitreous hemorrhage,

intractable increased IOP, decreased vision in the fellow eye, or retinal detachment.
- Treat any underlying medical conditions.

Prognosis

The prognosis for a vitreous hemorrhage is usually good.

Asteroid Hyalosis

Asteroid hyalosis is refractive particles of calcium phosphate soaps suspended in the vitreous framework. On examination, the asteroids appear as multiple, yellow-white, round, birefringent crystals floating in the vitreous space (Figure 16–4). Asteroid hyalosis is a common degenerative process seen in elderly patients over 60 years of age (0.5% of the population) and in patients with diabetes mellitus (30% of diabetics). Most cases are unilateral (75%). Surprisingly, it is usually asymptomatic, and does not cause floaters or interfere with vision. However, the particles can interfere with the examiner's view of the retina. The prognosis is good and in general no treatment is recommended. In rare circumstances, a pars plana vitrectomy is performed if the asteroids become so severe that they affect vision or interfere with the diagnosis or treatment of retinal disorders.

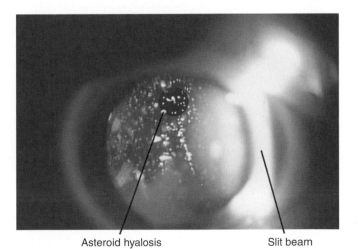

Asteroid hyalosis   Slit beam

FIGURE 16–4
The yellow-white particles of asteroid hyalosis are seen in the anterior vitreous cavity behind the lens. They are best seen using a fine slit beam at an oblique angle.

CHAPTER SEVENTEEN

Retina

Introduction

The retina is the inner neurosensory tissue of the eye that receives images from the world around us, thereby acting like film in a camera. This delicate multilayered array of cells is responsible for converting these images into information that can be interpreted by the brain. Because of its vital function, the retina is the most protected ocular structure and receives the greatest blood supply. Nevertheless, many systemic and ocular conditions are characterized by retinal involvement and can result in profound, often permanent, visual disturbances.

Trauma

Blunt and penetrating trauma can produce considerable retinal injury. Most blunt trauma can be observed; however, careful examination for retinal tears and breaks should always be performed.

CHOROIDAL RUPTURE

A choroidal rupture is a tear in the choroid, Bruch's membrane, and retinal pigment epithelium (RPE) that results most commonly from blunt ocular trauma. Anterior ruptures are usually parallel to the ora serrata; posterior ruptures are usually crescent-shaped and concentric to the optic nerve. Patients may have normal vision or dramatically decreased vision if commotio retinae (see below) or subretinal hemorrhage is present, or if the rupture is located in the macula (Figure 17–1). No treatment is required and patients should be observed. Because of the defect in Bruch's membrane there is an increased risk of developing a choroidal neovascular

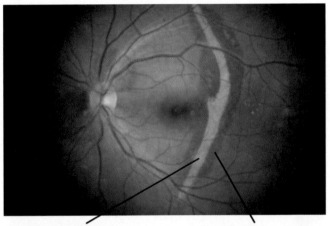

Choroidal rupture   Subretinal hemorrhage

FIGURE 17–1
Crescent-shaped, choroidal rupture that is concentric to the optic nerve with surrounding subretinal hemorrhage.

membrane (CNV) through the rupture site. In general, the prognosis is good if the macula is not involved.

COMMOTIO RETINAE

Commotio retinae is a gray-white discoloration of the retina due to photoreceptor outer-segment disruption following blunt ocular trauma. Commotio can affect any area of the retina and may be accompanied by hemorrhages or choroidal rupture (Figures 17–2 and 17–3). Depending on the location of the commotio retinae, vision can be normal, acutely decreased if the macula is involved, or permanently reduced if the fovea is damaged. Patients should be observed for resolution of the retinal discoloration, when vision usually improves. No other treatment is effective.

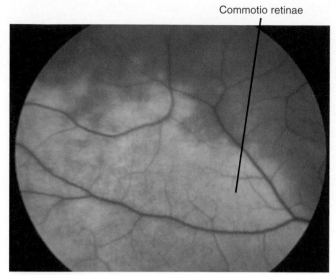

Commotio retinae

FIGURE 17–2
Gray-white discoloration of the outer retina in a patient with commotio retinae.

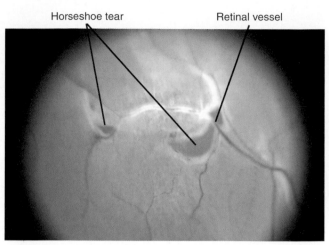

Horseshoe tear   Retinal vessel

FIGURE 17–4
Two horseshoe-shaped retinal tears with a bridging retinal vessel seen across the larger tear.

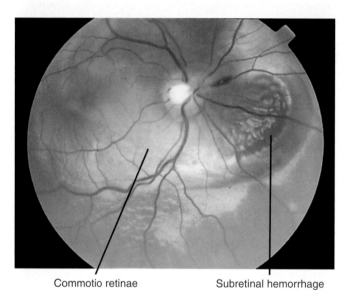

Commotio retinae   Subretinal hemorrhage

FIGURE 17–3
Commotio retinae following blunt trauma, demonstrating retinal whitening; note subretinal hemorrhage from underlying choroidal rupture.

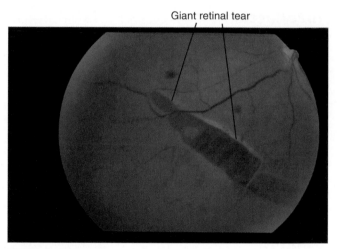

Giant retinal tear

FIGURE 17–5
Very posterior giant retinal tear that extends for more than 3 clock hours.

RETINAL BREAK

A retinal break is a full-thickness tear in the retina. It is often horseshoe-shaped, and usually occurs at areas with strong vitreoretinal adhesions, such as the vitreous base, posterior border of lattice degeneration, or at cystic retinal tufts (Figure 17–4). Other more specific forms of retinal break common after trauma are **giant retinal tears** (span >90° or 3 clock hours in circumferential extent) (Figure 17–5), **avulsion of the vitreous base**, and **retinal dialysis** (separation of the retina at the ora

serrata). On slit-lamp examination, retinal breaks are associated with pigmented cells ("tobacco dust") in the anterior vitreous that are best seen with a narrow slit beam, mild vitreous hemorrhages, and posterior vitreous detachment. Patients may be asymptomatic, but usually report photopsias (flashes of light) and floaters, especially with eye movement. Symptomatic retinal breaks often require immediate attention since liquefied vitreous can pass through the break into the subretinal space, causing a rhegmatogenous retinal detachment. Breaks are treated with cryopexy (freezing treatment) along the edge of the tear or two to three rows of laser photocoagulation around the tear. Asymptomatic retinal holes and chronic breaks may be observed, especially when signs of chronicity, such as pigment around the hole, are present.

Vascular disorders

HEMORRHAGES

Retinal hemorrhages can be located under, within, and over the retina. In addition, there are several patterns of hemorrhage that can help determine the etiology. All three types of hemorrhage may occur together in age-related macular degeneration (AMD), acquired retinal macroaneurysms, Eales' disease, Valsalva retinopathy, and capillary hemangioma.

Preretinal hemorrhage

Preretinal hemorrhage is located between the retina and posterior vitreous face (subhyaloid) or under the internal limiting membrane of the retina. It has an amorphous or boat shape with a flat upper border and curved lower border that obscures the underlying retina and retinal vessels (Figures 17–6 and 17–7).

Causes of preretinal hemorrhage include trauma, retinal neovascularization (diabetic retinopathy, radiation retinopathy, vascular occlusion), breakthrough bleeding from a CNV, hypertensive retinopathy, Valsalva retinopathy, posterior vitreous detachment, shaken-baby syndrome, and retinopathy of blood disorders.

Intraretinal hemorrhage

There are several different types of intraretinal hemorrhage (Figures 17–8 and 17–9). The pattern – flame-shaped, dot/blot, or Roth spot – is characteristic of the level of the hemorrhage. Bilateral intraretinal hemorrhages are usually associated with systemic disorders (e.g., diabetes mellitus and hypertension).

- **Flame-shaped intraretinal hemorrhages** have feathery borders and are located in the superficial retina where they are oriented with the nerve fiber layer. They are usually seen in hypertensive retinopathy and venous occlusion.
- **Dot/blot intraretinal hemorrhages** appear as round dots or larger blots and are located in the outer plexiform layer. They are usually seen in diabetic retinopathy.

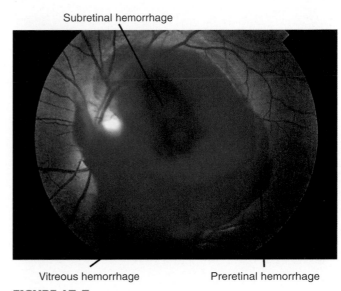

Subretinal hemorrhage

Vitreous hemorrhage   Preretinal hemorrhage

FIGURE 17–7
Valsalva retinopathy, demonstrating vitreous, preretinal, and subretinal hemorrhages.

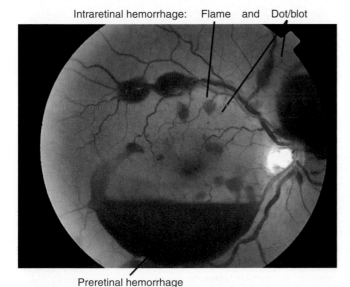

Intraretinal hemorrhage: Flame   and   Dot/blot

Preretinal hemorrhage

FIGURE 17–6
Diabetic retinopathy, demonstrating intraretinal and preretinal (boat-shaped configuration due to attached hyaloid containing the blood) hemorrhages.

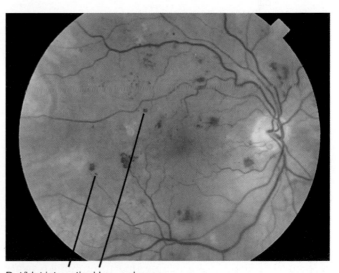

Dot/blot intraretinal hemorrhages

FIGURE 17–8
Intraretinal dot and blot hemorrhages in a patient with non-proliferative diabetic retinopathy.

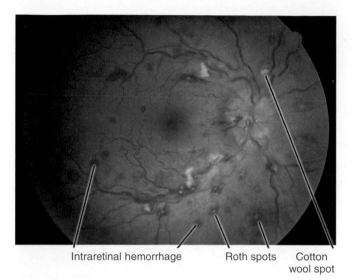

Intraretinal hemorrhage   Roth spots   Cotton wool spot

FIGURE 17–9
Retinopathy of anemia, demonstrating intraretinal hemorrhage, cotton wool spots, and Roth spots.

- **Roth spots** are rare intraretinal hemorrhages with a white center that represents an embolus with lymphocytic infiltration. They are classically associated with subacute bacterial endocarditis (seen in 1–5% of such patients), but also occur in leukemia, severe anemia, sickle-cell disease, collagen vascular diseases, diabetes mellitus, multiple myeloma, and acquired immunodeficiency syndrome (AIDS).

Subretinal hemorrhage

Subretinal hemorrhage appears dark and is deep to the retinal vessels since it is located under the neurosensory retina or RPE (see Figures 17–3 and 17–7). This type of hemorrhage is usually associated with trauma, CNV, and macroaneurysms.

ARTERY OCCLUSIONS

Definition

Artery occlusions are disruptions of vascular perfusion in a branch of the central retinal artery (BRAO), leading to focal retinal ischemia, or the central retinal artery (CRAO), leading to complete retinal ischemia and profound loss of vision.

Etiology

In BRAO, the site of the obstruction is usually at the bifurcation of retinal arteries. CRAO is usually due to emboli or thrombus at the level of the lamina cribrosa.

Artery occlusions are mainly due to embolism from cholesterol (Hollenhorst plaques), calcifications (heart valves), or platelet fibrin plugs (ulcerated atheromatous plaques due to arteriosclerosis). In rare cases the emboli are due to leukoemboli (vasculitis, Purtscher's retin-

opathy, collagen vascular diseases), fat emboli (long bone fractures), thrombus (mitral valve prolapse), amniotic fluid emboli, tumor emboli (atrial myxoma), septic emboli (heart valve vegetations seen in bacterial endocarditis or intravenous (IV) drug abuse), or particles (talc from IV drug abuse). In very rare cases, the occlusion is not embolic, but due to temporal arteritis, vasospasm (migraine), compression of the artery, or systemic coagulopathies.

Epidemiology

Artery occlusions usually occur in elderly patients and are associated with hypertension (67%), carotid occlusive disease (25%), diabetes mellitus (33%), and cardiac valvular disease (25%). CRAO is more common than BRAO.

Symptoms

The hallmark of an artery occlusion is sudden, unilateral, painless, loss of vision, with a visual field defect. BRAO produces a visual field defect that corresponds to the area of occlusion. CRAO produces diffuse loss of vision. Patients often have a prior history of cerebrovascular accident (CVA) or transient ischemic attacks (TIAs), especially amaurosis fugax (transient unilateral visual loss).

Signs

BRAO produces a focal, wedge-shaped area of retinal whitening within the distribution of a branch arteriole that resolves over several weeks. Emboli are sometimes visible (Figures 17–10 and 17–11). Vision may be decreased depending on the location of the involved vessel.

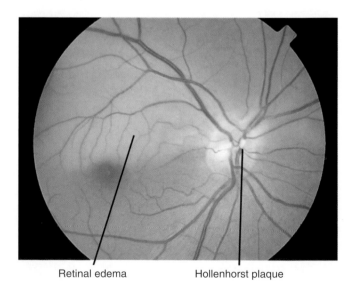

Retinal edema   Hollenhorst plaque

FIGURE 17–10
Superior branch artery occlusion with retinal edema extending in a wedge-shaped pattern from the artery occluded by the Hollenhorst plaque.

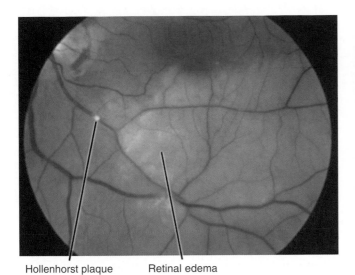

Hollenhorst plaque   Retinal edema

FIGURE 17–11
Inferior branch retinal artery occlusion with Hollenhorst plaque and wedge-shaped retinal edema.

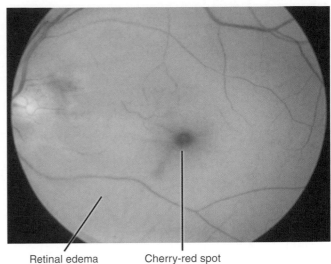

Retinal edema   Cherry-red spot

FIGURE 17–13
Central retinal artery occlusion with cherry-red spot.

Patients with a CRAO present with profound loss of vision in the counting fingers (CF) to light perception (LP) range and have a marked positive relative afferent pupillary defect (RAPD). There is diffuse retinal whitening of almost the entire retina, arteriole constriction with segmentation ("boxcarring") of blood flow, and in acute stages a cherry-red spot in the macula because the thin fovea allows visualization of the underlying choroidal circulation that appears red (Figures 17–12 and 17–13). Over time, the retinal whitening fades. In 25% of patients, a ciliary retinal artery is present and allows sparing of a small wedge-shaped area of perfused retina that appears normal just temporal to the optic disc, extending into the fovea (Figures 17–14 and 17–15).

Differential diagnosis

The appearance of a BRAO is very specific, but can be confused with the retinal whitening of commotio retinae. Similarly, the cherry-red spot seen in acute CRAO can be confused with inherited metabolic or lysosomal storage diseases (i.e., Tay–Sachs disease; see Ch. 6). Ophthalmic artery obstructions can have diffuse retinal whitening,

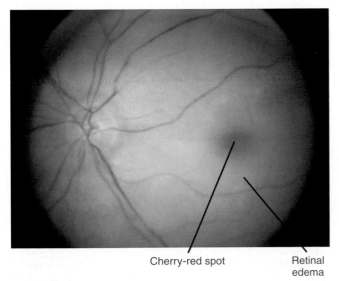

Cherry-red spot   Retinal edema

FIGURE 17–12
Central retinal artery occlusion with cherry-red spot in the fovea and surrounding retinal edema.

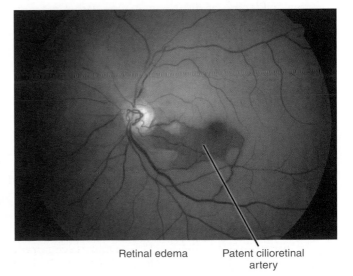

Retinal edema   Patent cilioretinal artery

FIGURE 17–14
Cilioretinal artery-sparing central retinal artery occlusion with patent cilioretinal artery allowing perfusion (thus no edema) in a small section of the macula.

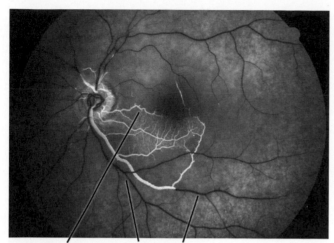

Patent cilioretinal artery   Absent flow

FIGURE 17–15
Fluorescein angiogram of same patient as in Figure 17–14, demonstrating no filling of retinal vessels except in cilioretinal artery and surrounding branches.

but usually do not produce a cherry-red spot because the underlying choroid is also ischemic. The hemorrhages that accompany a central retinal vein occlusion (CRVO) are often sufficient to differentiate between these two entities that both produce sudden loss of vision.

Evaluation

- The **history** should concentrate on any systemic diseases, previous episodes of visual loss, CVA, or TIAs.
- The **eye exam** is performed with attention to visual acuity (often profoundly decreased), pupillary response (positive RAPD), and ophthalmoscopy (focal area of retinal whitening or diffuse whitening with a red spot in the fovea; may have visible emboli in the retinal arteries).
- **Lab tests** include fasting blood glucose and complete blood count (CBC) with differential. Also consider platelets, prothrombin time/partial thromboplastin time (PT/PTT), protein C, protein S, antithrombin III, homocystine, antinuclear antibody (ANA), rheumatoid factor (RF), antiphospholipid antibody, serum protein electrophoresis, hemoglobin electrophoresis, Venereal Disease Research Laboratory (VDRL) test, and fluorescent treponemal antibody absorption (FTA-ABS) test. In patients >50 years old, check erythrocyte sedimentation rate (ESR) to rule out temporal arteritis. If positive, start temporal arteritis treatment immediately (see Ch. 5, section on anterior ischemic optic neuropathy).
- A **fluorescein angiogram** should be performed to evaluate for delayed or absent retinal arterial filling in a branch or the central retinal artery. Capillary non-perfusion in a wedge-shaped area supplied by the

branch artery is seen in BRAO, and global ischemia is the hallmark of CRAO.
- Consider **B-scan ultrasonography** or **orbital computed tomography (CT) scan** to rule out a compressive lesion if the history is suggestive of compression.
- Consider **electrophysiologic testing** in CRAO which shows reduced b-wave amplitude with normal a wave on the electroretinogram.
- Consider **medical consultation** for complete cardiovascular evaluation, including blood pressure, electrocardiogram, echocardiogram, and carotid Doppler studies.

Management

Treatment of artery occlusions remains controversial due to the questionable benefit of therapy. In BRAO, since the prognosis is good, most patients are observed. However, if the foveal circulation is affected, or in cases of CRAO, patients should be treated immediately before starting the work-up (if the patient presents within 24 hours of visual loss) with a variety of methods aimed at dislodging the vascular obstruction:

- Rapidly reduce the intraocular pressure with systemic acetazolamide (Diamox 500 mg IV or PO), topical ocular hypotensive drops (i.e., timolol 0.5%, Iopidine, and/or Xalatan 1 gtt q15min × 2, repeat as necessary), and anterior-chamber paracentesis.
- Digital ocular massage and rebreathing into a paper bag can be implemented while the necessary medications and equipment are being obtained.
- Consider hospital admission for carbogen treatment (95% oxygen–5% carbon dioxide for 10 minutes q2h for 24–48 hours) to attempt to increase oxygenation and induce vasodilation.
- Unproven treatments include hyperbaric oxygen, antifibrinolytic drugs, retrobulbar vasodilators, and sublingual nitroglycerine.
- If arteritic ischemic optic neuropathy is suspected, then start systemic steroids (methylprednisolone 1 g IV qd in divided doses for 3 days, then prednisone 60–100 mg PO qd with a slow taper; decrease by no more than 2.5–5.0 mg/week).

Prognosis

The prognosis for BRAO is generally good, with fading of the retinal edema and restoration of circulation over the ensuing weeks. If the fovea is spared, vision usually returns, with 80% of patients having better than 20/40 vision, but most will have some degree of permanent visual field loss. In contrast, the prognosis for CRAO is poor, with most patients having persistent severe visual loss with constricted retinal arterioles, optic atrophy, and positive RAPD, even though the retinal edema fades over time.

VEIN OCCLUSIONS

Definition

Venous occlusions are due to blockage of vascular perfusion in a branch of the central retinal vein (BRVO) or in the central retinal vein (CRVO). In patients where the superior and inferior retinal drainage does not merge into a central retinal vein, a hemiretinal vein occlusion (HRVO) can occur.

Etiology

BRVO is usually caused by a thrombus at an arteriovenous crossing where a thickened artery compresses the underlying venous wall, while a CRVO is usually caused by a thrombus in the area of the lamina cribrosa.

Vein occlusions are associated with hypertension, coronary artery disease, diabetes mellitus, and peripheral vascular disease. They are rarely associated with hypercoagulable states (e.g., macroglobulinemia, cryoglobulinemia), hyperviscosity states (polycythemia vera, Waldenström's macroglobulinemia), systemic lupus erythematosus, syphilis, sarcoidosis, homocystinuria, malignancies (e.g., multiple myeloma, polycythemia vera, leukemia), optic nerve drusen, and external compression. In younger patients, there is an association with oral contraceptive pills, collagen vascular disease, AIDS, protein S/protein C/antithrombin III deficiency, factor XII (Hageman factor) deficiency, antiphospholipid antibody syndrome, or activated protein C resistance.

Epidemiology

Venous occlusion is the second most common retinal vascular disease after diabetic retinopathy. It is usually seen in elderly patients, 60–70 years old. Venous occlusion is associated with hypertension (50–70%), cardiovascular disease, diabetes mellitus, increased body mass index, and open-angle glaucoma with a slight male and hyperopic predilection.

There are two types: **non-ischemic** (two-thirds) and **ischemic** (one-third), distinguished by the amount of capillary non-perfusion on fluorescein angiography. The ischemic form is more common in patients with cardiovascular disease.

Symptoms

Venous occlusion usually causes a sudden, unilateral, painless, loss of vision. The visual loss is variable, and some patients may have normal vision, especially when the macula is not involved.

Signs

BRVO produces a quadrantic visual field defect with dilated, tortuous retinal veins, superficial, retinal hemorrhages, and cotton wool spots in a wedge-shaped area radiating from an arteriovenous crossing (usually arterial over-crossing, where an arteriole and venule share a common vascular sheath) (Figures 17–16 and 17–17). Vision is variably decreased depending on the amount of retinal edema and ischemia. The closer the obstruction is to the optic disc, the greater the area of retina involved and the more serious the complications.

Vision is also variably decreased in CRVO depending on the amount of retinal edema and ischemia. Characteristic findings include dilated, tortuous retinal veins

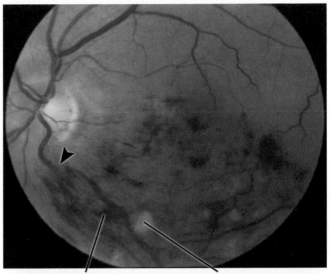

Intraretinal hemorrhage   Cotton wool spots

FIGURE 17–16
Inferior branch retinal vein occlusion, demonstrating wedge-shaped area of intraretinal hemorrhages and cotton wool spots.

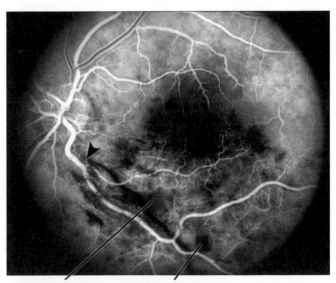

Cotton wool spots   Intraretinal hemorrhage

FIGURE 17–17
Fluorescein angiogram of same patient as in Figure 17–16, demonstrating lack of perfusion in inferior retinal vein with blocking defects from the intraretinal hemorrhages. Arrowhead indicates site of occlusion.

with superficial, retinal hemorrhages, and cotton wool spots in all four quadrants extending to the periphery (Figures 17–18–17–21). Macular edema is common. The optic disc is often hyperemic and edematous. A positive RAPD correlates with the amount of ischemia. Collateral optociliary shunt vessels between retinal and ciliary circulations (50%) occur late (Figure 17–22).

Both BRVO and CRVO can produce neovascularization, especially in ischemic cases in which rubeosis (20% in CRVO, rare in BRVO), disc neovascularization, retinal neovascularization (at the border of perfused and non-perfused retina), neovascular glaucoma, and vitreous hemorrhages can occur.

Differential diagnosis

The intraretinal hemorrhages seen in venous occlusion can mimic venous stasis retinopathy, ocular ischemic syndrome, hypertensive retinopathy, leukemic retinopathy, retinopathy of anemia, diabetic retinopathy, papilledema, and papillophlebitis (benign inflammatory condition in young patients).

Evaluation

• The **history** should concentrate on any systemic diseases with particular attention to hypertension, cardiovascular disease, and diabetes mellitus.

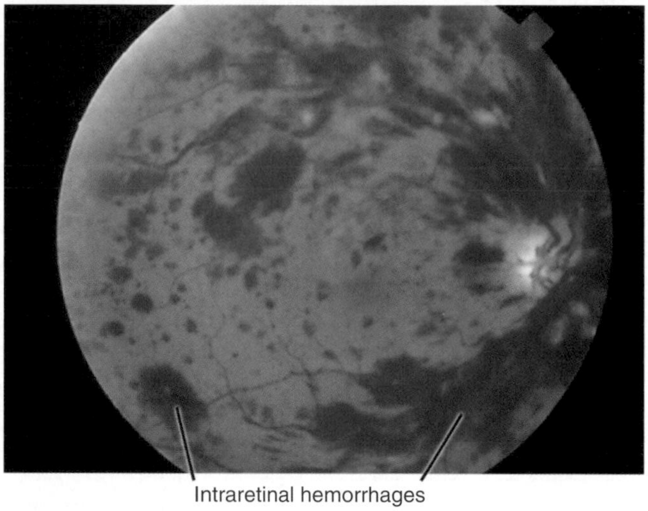

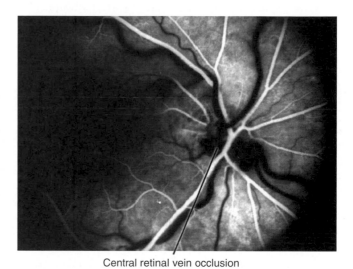

Central retinal vein occlusion

FIGURE 17–20
Fluorescein angiogram, demonstrating no filling of the central retinal vein.

Intraretinal hemorrhages

FIGURE 17–18
Central retinal vein occlusion demonstrating hemorrhages in all four quadrants.

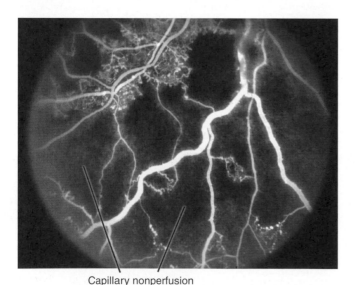

Capillary nonperfusion

FIGURE 17–19
Fluorescein angiogram of a patient with a retinal vein occlusion, demonstrating peripheral capillary non-perfusion.

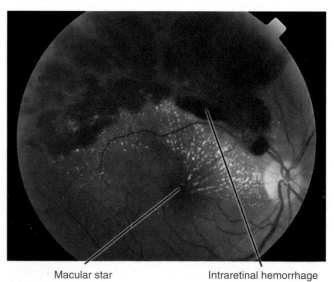

Macular star   Intraretinal hemorrhage

FIGURE 17–21
Hemiretinal vein occlusion with exudates forming partial macular star.

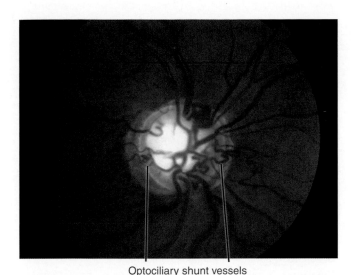

Optociliary shunt vessels

FIGURE 17–22
Optociliary shunt vessels in a patient with an old central retinal vein occlusion.

- The **eye exam** must evaluate the visual acuity (variably decreased, worse than 20/400 is likely ischemic), pupillary response (may have a positive RAPD in ischemic CRVO), visual field testing (defect in ischemic), tonometry (may have increased intra-ocular pressure), gonioscopy (may have rubeosis, especially in ischemic), and ophthalmoscopy (intra-retinal hemorrhages, cotton wool spots, may have macular edema, disc edema, neovascularization, and optociliary shunt vessels).
- **Lab tests** to consider include fasting blood glucose, glycosylated hemoglobin, CBC with differential, platelets, PT/PTT, ANA, RF, angiotensin-converting enzyme (ACE), ESR, serum protein electrophoresis, lipid profile, hemoglobin electrophoresis, VDRL, and FTA-ABS, depending on the clinical situation. In a patient <40 years old suspected of having a hyper-coagulable state, check human immunodeficiency virus (HIV) status, functional protein S assay, functional protein C assay, functional antithrombin III assay (type II heparin-binding mutation), antiphospholipid antibody titer, lupus anticoagulant, anticardiolipin antibody titer (immunoglobulin G (IgG) and IgM), homocystine level (if elevated, then also test for folate, vitamin B_{12}, and creatinine), factor XII (Hageman factor) levels, and factor V Leiden mutation poly-merase chain reaction assay (for activated protein C resistance). If these tests are normal, then also check plasminogen antigen assay, heparin cofactor II assay, thrombin time, reptilase time, and fibrinogen func-tional assay.
- A **fluorescein angiogram** is very helpful in the evaluation of venous occlusion. It shows delayed retinal venous filling in a branch of the central retinal vein, increased transit time in the affected venous

distribution, blocked fluorescence in areas of retinal hemorrhages, and capillary non-perfusion (ischemic defined as ≥5 disc areas of capillary non-perfusion) in the area supplied by the involved retinal vein in BRVO. In CRVO, there is delayed retinal venous filling, increased transit time (>20 seconds increases the risk of developing rubeosis), extensive capillary non-perfusion (ischemic defined as ≥10 disc areas of capillary non-perfusion), staining of vascular walls, and blocking defects due to retinal hemorrhages.
- Consider **electrophysiologic testing** which may show reduced b-wave amplitude, reduced b:a-wave ratio, and prolonged b-wave implicit time on the electroretinogram.
- Consider **medical consultation** for complete cardio-vascular evaluation.

Management

- Macular grid/focal laser photocoagulation when macular edema lasts more than 3 months and vision is worse than 20/40 in patients with BRVO. Focal laser treatment is not effective in CRVO.
- Experimental options to treat macular edema include intravitreal triamcinolone acetonide (Kenalog), pegaptnib (Macugen), bevacizumab (Avastin), or ranibizumab (Lucentis).
- Quadrantic scatter laser photocoagulation in BRVO and panretinal laser photocoagulation (PRP) in CRVO when rubeosis (≥2 clock hours of iris or any angle neovascularization), disc or retinal neovascularization, or neovascular glaucoma develops. Prophylactic laser is not beneficial.
- Discontinue oral contraceptives.
- Consider aspirin (80–325 mg PO qd).
- Treat any underlying medical condition.

Prognosis

The prognosis is good for BRVO, with 50% having better than 20/40 vision unless foveal ischemia or chronic macular edema is present. The risk of another BRVO in the same eye is 3% and in the fellow eye is 12%. For CRVO, the prognosis depends on the amount of ischemia, since this determines the risk of developing neovascular complications. Two-thirds of patients with ischemic disease develop neovascular complications. The non-ischemic form has a better prognosis, with complete resolution in 10% of cases; however, one-third of these patients develop ischemic disease, especially older patients.

VENOUS STASIS RETINOPATHY

Venous stasis retinopathy is a milder form of non-ischemic CRVO, representing patients with better per-fusion. It is associated with hyperviscosity syndromes, including polycythemia vera, multiple myeloma, and

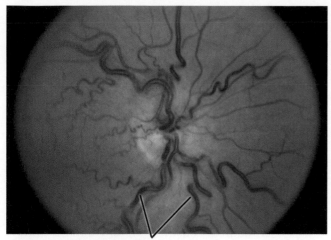

Dilated, tortuous vasculature

FIGURE 17–23
Dilated tortuous retinal vessels in a patient with hyperviscosity syndrome.

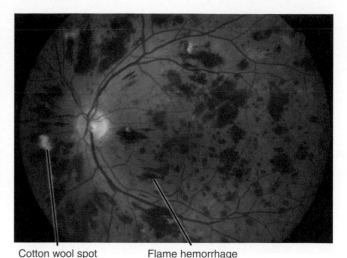

Cotton wool spot   Flame hemorrhage

FIGURE 17–25
Retinopathy of anemia, demonstrating intraretinal hemorrhage and cotton wool spots.

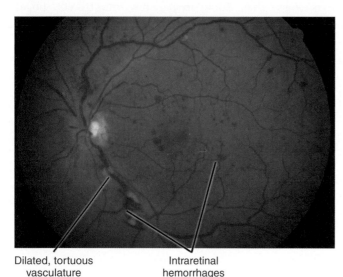

Dilated, tortuous   Intraretinal
vasculature   hemorrhages

FIGURE 17–24
Intraretinal hemorrhages in a patient with venous stasis retinopathy.

Waldenström's macroglobulinemia. The fundus examination reveals dot/blot and flame-shaped hemorrhages in all four quadrants with dilated and tortuous vasculature (Figures 17–23 and 17–24). The course is more benign than CRVO.

Retinopathies Associated with Systemic Disease

BLOOD ABNORMALITIES

Retinopathy of anemia

In patients with anemia, a distinct retinopathy characterized by superficial, flame-shaped, intraretinal,

hemorrhages, cotton wool spots, and, rarely, retinal exudates, retinal edema, and vitreous hemorrhage can occur (Figure 17–25). It is seen in patients with hemoglobin <8 g/100 ml, and is worse when associated with thrombocytopenia. Roth spots occur in pernicious anemia and aplastic anemia. No treatment is required. If patients do not have an underlying known hematologic disorder, then medical or hematology consultation should be obtained.

Leukemic retinopathy

Ocular involvement in leukemia is common, with up to 80% of patients developing some signs. Although most patients are usually asymptomatic, retinal examination reveals superficial, flame-shaped, intraretinal hemorrhages (24%), microaneurysms, Roth spots (11%), cotton wool spots (16%), dilated/tortuous vessels, perivascular sheathing, and disc edema (Figures 17–26 and 17–27). Most of the complications are related to the associated hematologic abnormalities, including anemia, thrombocytopenia, and hyperviscosity, and only rarely are direct leukemic retinal infiltrates (3%) or choroidal involvement with choroidal thickening and overlying serous retinal detachments seen. Most cases resolve with treatment of the underlying hematologic abnormality. Direct leukemic infiltrates are treated with systemic chemotherapy and/or ocular radiation therapy if systemic therapy fails. Opportunistic infections also occur in patients with leukemia, but are not considered part of leukemic retinopathy.

Sickle-cell retinopathy

The sickling hemoglobinopathies can produce a retinopathy due to poor flow through capillaries from the altered hemoglobin conformation and rigid erythrocytes.

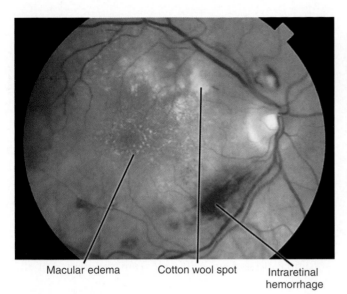

Macular edema   Cotton wool spot   Intraretinal
                                     hemorrhage

FIGURE 17-26
Leukemic retinopathy with macular edema, cotton wool spots, and intraretinal hemorrhages.

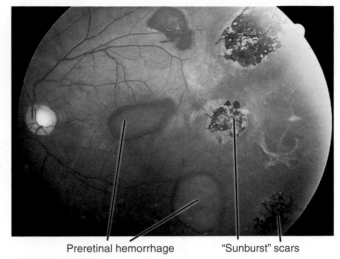

Preretinal hemorrhage   "Sunburst" scars

FIGURE 17-28
Non-proliferative sickle-cell retinopathy, demonstrating salmon-patch hemorrhages, iridescent spots, and black sunbursts.

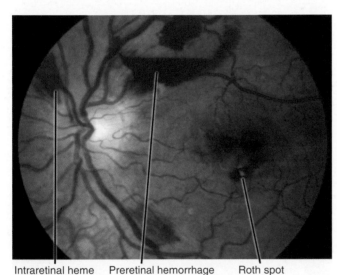

Intraretinal heme   Preretinal hemorrhage   Roth spot

FIGURE 17-27
Leukemic retinopathy with intraretinal and preretinal hemorrhages, cotton wool spots, and Roth spots.

They are more common in people of African and Mediterranean descent. Neovascularization in response to retinal ischemia is more common with Hb SC (most severe) and Hb SThal variants, while Hb AS and Hb AC mutations rarely cause ocular manifestations. Patients who do not carry a diagnosis should be evaluated with a sickle-cell prep and hemoglobin electrophoresis because those with hemoglobin C disease and sickle-cell trait may have a negative sickle-cell prep. Most patients are asymptomatic, but some may have decreased vision, visual field defects, floaters, photopsias, scotomas, and dyschromatopsia (altered color perception). Patients

can be observed unless signs of active peripheral neovascularization develop; in such cases, scatter laser photocoagulation to non-perfused retina should be performed.

The retinopathy follows an orderly progression:

- **Stage I:** Background (non-proliferative) stage consisting of venous tortuosity, "salmon-patch" hemorrhages (pink intraretinal hemorrhages), iridescent spots (schisis cavity with refractile elements), cotton wool spots, hairpin vascular loops, macular infarction, angioid streaks, black "sunburst" chorioretinal scars, comma-shaped conjunctival and optic nerve head vessels, and peripheral arteriole occlusions (Figure 17–28).
- **Stage II:** Arteriovenous anastomosis stage in which peripheral "silver-wire" vessels and shunt vessels between arterioles and medium-sized veins at the border of perfused and non-perfused retina are found.
- **Stage III:** Neovascular (proliferative) stage characterized by sea-fan peripheral neovascularization that grows along the retinal surface in a circumferential pattern and has a predilection for the superotemporal quadrant. Neovascularization can spontaneously regress in 60% of cases due to autoinfarction (Figure 17–29).
- **Stage IV:** Vitreous hemorrhage stage due to contraction around the sea-fan peripheral neovascularization (most common in SC variant (21–23%); SS (2–3%)). Patients with non-clearing vitreous hemorrhage may require surgery.
- **Stage V:** Retinal detachment stage with traction and rhegmatogenous retinal detachments from contraction of vitreous bands. These patients usually undergo surgical repair of the retinal detachments.

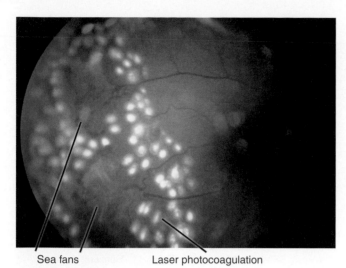

Sea fans   Laser photocoagulation

FIGURE 17–29
Proliferative sickle-cell retinopathy, demonstrating sea-fans and laser treatment.

DIABETIC RETINOPATHY

Definition

Retinal vascular complications of diabetes mellitus are classified into **non-proliferative** (NPDR) and **proliferative** (PDR) forms depending on the absence or presence of neovascularization, respectively.

Epidemiology

Diabetic retinopathy is the leading cause of blindness in the US population aged 20–64 years old. The risk of diabetic retinopathy increases with concomitant hypertension, chronic hyperglycemia, renal disease, hyperlipidemia, and pregnancy.

Insulin-dependent diabetes (IDDM, type I): Type I diabetes is usually juvenile-onset and occurs before 30 years of age. Most patients are free of retinopathy during the first 5 years after diagnosis, but 95% of patients with IDDM develop diabetic retinopathy after 15 years. Seventy-two percent of patients will develop PDR and 42% will develop clinically significant macular edema (CSME). The severity of retinopathy worsens with increasing duration of diabetes mellitus.

Non-insulin-dependent diabetes (NIDDM, type II): Type II or adult-onset diabetes is usually diagnosed after 30 years of age and is the more common form (90%). Most patients have optimal glucose control without insulin. At the time of diagnosis, retinopathy exists in 30% of patients with NIDDM and 3% have PDR or CSME. Sixty percent of patients will have retinopathy in 5 years and 80% in 15 years.

Symptoms

Diabetic retinopathy is often asymptomatic, especially early in the course of the disease. As the retinopathy worsens, patients may have decreased or fluctuating vision. Advanced retinopathy can result in complete blindness.

Signs

Non-proliferative diabetic retinopathy

NPDR is characterized in early stages by bilateral dot/blot intraretinal hemorrhages, hard and soft exudates, microaneurysms, and cotton wool spots. As the retinopathy worsens, venous beading and loops and intraretinal microvascular abnormalities can be seen (Figures 17–30–17–33). Visual loss is related to macular ischemia and macular edema, which is considered CSME if one of the following conditions are present:

- Retinal thickening <500 μm from the center of the fovea *or*
- Hard exudates < 500 μm from the center of the fovea with adjacent thickening *or*
- Retinal thickening >1 disc size in area <1 disc diameter from the center of the fovea.

Proliferative diabetic retinopathy

The hallmark of proliferative disease is the presence of neovascularization. This can manifest as neovascularization of the disc (NVD) or elsewhere in the retina (NVE), preretinal and vitreous hemorrhages, fibrovascular proliferation on the posterior vitreous surface or extending into the vitreous cavity, and traction retinal detachments (TRDs) (Figures 17–34–17–37). Patients may also develop neovascularization of the iris (NVI) and subsequent neovascular glaucoma (NVG). PDR

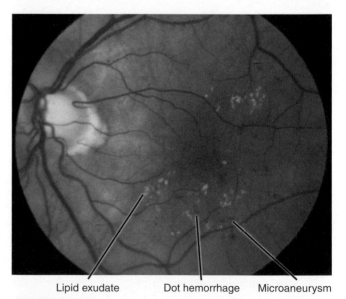

Lipid exudate   Dot hemorrhage   Microaneurysm

FIGURE 17–30
Moderate non-proliferative diabetic retinopathy with intraretinal hemorrhages, microaneurysms, and lipid exudate.

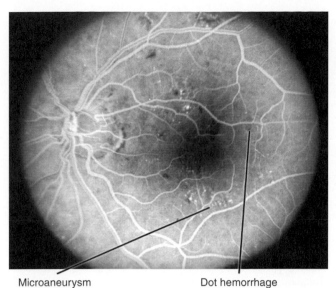

Microaneurysm   Dot hemorrhage

FIGURE 17–31
Fluorescein angiogram of the same patient as in Figure 17–30, demonstrating tiny blocking defects from the intraretinal hemorrhages and spots of hyperfluorescence due to microaneurysms.

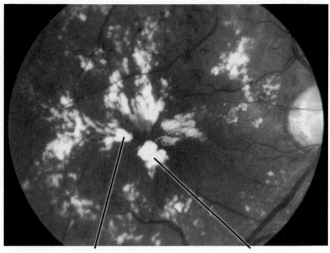

Diffuse macular edema and exudate

FIGURE 17–33
Severe non-proliferative diabetic retinopathy with diffuse macular edema and lipid exudate.

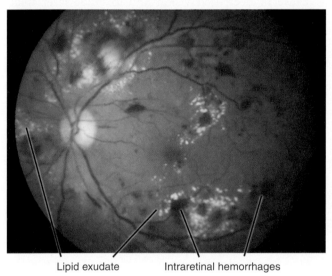
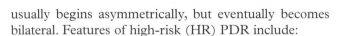

Lipid exudate   Intraretinal hemorrhages

FIGURE 17–32
Severe non-proliferative diabetic retinopathy with extensive hemorrhages, microaneurysms, and exudates.

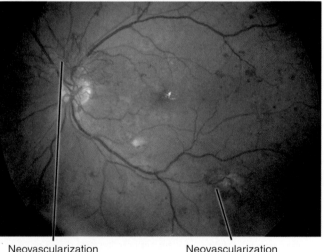

Neovascularization   Neovascularization
of the disc   elsewhere

FIGURE 17–34
Proliferative diabetic retinopathy, demonstrating florid neovascularization of the disc and elsewhere.

usually begins asymmetrically, but eventually becomes bilateral. Features of high-risk (HR) PDR include:

- NVD > one-quarter to one-third disc area *or*
- Any NVD and vitreous hemorrhage or preretinal hemorrhage *or*
- NVE > one-half disc area and vitreous hemorrhage or preretinal hemorrhage.

Differential diagnosis

The hemorrhages and exudates seen in diabetic retinopathy can look like hypertensive retinopathy, CRVO, BRVO, ocular ischemic syndrome, radiation retinopathy,

retinopathy associated with blood disorders, and Eales' disease.

Evaluation

- When obtaining the **history**, it is important to inquire about concomitant systemic diseases, glucose control, and blood pressure control.
- The **eye exam** should focus on the visual acuity (normal or decreased), tonometry (may have increased IOP), gonioscopy (may have rubeosis, NVG), iris (may have NVI), lens (may have posterior subcapsular cataract), ophthalmoscopy (intraretinal hemorrhages,

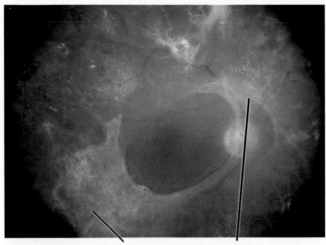

Traction retinal detachment

FIGURE 17-35

Proliferative diabetic retinopathy, demonstrating neovascularization, fibrosis, and traction retinal detachment.

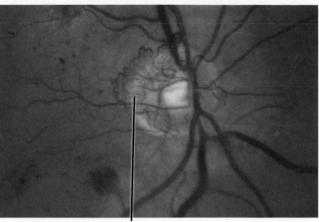

Neovascularization of the disc

FIGURE 17-37

Proliferative diabetic retinopathy, demonstrating neovascularization of the disc.

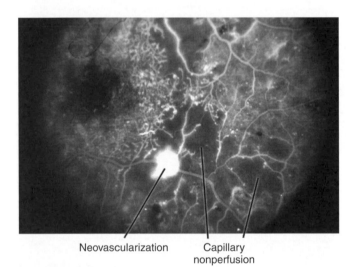

Neovascularization   Capillary
nonperfusion

FIGURE 17-36

Fluorescein angiogram of a patient with proliferative diabetic retinopathy, showing extensive capillary non-perfusion, neovascularization elsewhere, and vascular leakage.

exudates, vascular abnormalities, and cotton wool spots, may have vitreous hemorrhage, cystoid macular edema (CME), NVD, NVE, TRD) using the following schedule:

- **IDDM (type I)**: examine 5 years after onset of diabetes mellitus, then annually if no retinopathy is present.
- **NIDDM (type II)**: examine at diagnosis of diabetes mellitus, then annually if no retinopathy is present.
- **During pregnancy**: examine before pregnancy, each trimester, and 3–6 months after delivery.
- **Lab tests** to consider include fasting blood glucose, hemoglobin A1c, blood urea nitrogen, and creatinine.

- A **fluorescein angiogram** is useful to establish the cause of decreased vision and to guide laser treatment. Findings include capillary non-perfusion, microaneurysms, macular edema, and disc/retinal neovascularization.
- In cases of macular edema, **optical coherence tomography** can offer assistance in management decisions and can illustrate increased retinal thickness, subretinal fluid, CME, and posterior hyaloidal traction.
- **B-scan ultrasonography** can be used to rule out a TRD when the fundus cannot be adequately visualized (i.e., in eyes with dense vitreous hemorrhage or other media opacities).
- Consider **medical consultation** with attention to blood pressure, cardiovascular system, renal status, and glycemic control.

Management

- Tight blood glucose control (**Diabetes Control and Complications Trial (DCCT)** conclusion for type I diabetics and **United Kingdom Prospective Diabetes Study (UKPDS)** conclusion for type II diabetics).
- Tight control of blood pressure (**UKPDS** conclusion for type II diabetics).
- Laser photocoagulation with transpupillary delivery of argon green (focal and panretinal photocoagulation (PRP)) or krypton red laser (panretinal photocoagulation when vitreous hemorrhage or cataract is present), depending on the stage of diabetic retinopathy:
  - **CSME**: perform macular grid photocoagulation to areas of diffuse leakage and focal treatment to focal leaks regardless of visual acuity (**Early Treatment Diabetic Retinopathy Study (ETDRS)** conclusion). If there is enlargement of the foveal avascular zone (FAZ) on the fluorescein angiogram,

then consider low-energy treatment away from the foveal ischemia.

- **HR PDR**: perform scatter PRP in two to three sessions (**Diabetic Retinopathy Study (DRS)** conclusion). The inferior and nasal quadrants are treated first to allow further treatment in case of vitreous hemorrhage during treatment and to avoid worsening macular edema.
- Additional indications for PRP include rubeosis, NVG, widespread retinal ischemia on fluorescein angiogram, NVE alone in type I IDDM, poor patient compliance, severe NPDR in the fellow eye, and a poor outcome in the first eye.
- Consider surgery by a retina specialist in patients with non-clearing vitreous hemorrhage, monocular patient with vitreous hemorrhage, bilateral vitreous hemorrhage, diabetic macular edema due to posterior hyaloidal traction, TRD with rhegmatogenous component, TRD involving macula, progressive fibrovascular proliferation despite complete PRP, dense premacular hemorrhage, or if the ocular media are not clear enough to perform PRP adequately.
- Experimental pharmaceutical treatments for refractory, diffuse macular edema include posterior subTenon's injection of 40 mg triamcinolone acetonide, intravitreal 4 mg triamcinolone acetonide, Retisert sustained-release implant with fluocinolone acetonide, Occulex biodegradable dexamethasone implant, protein kinase beta inhibitors, and intravitreal antivascular endothelial growth factor (VEGF) injections with pegaptanib (Macugen), bevacizumab (Avastin), or ranibizumab (Lucentis).

Prognosis

The prognosis is good for NPDR without CSME but poorer for patients with CSME or PDR. After adequate treatment, diabetic retinopathy often becomes quiescent for extended periods of time.

HYPERTENSIVE RETINOPATHY

Definition

Hypertensive retinopathy refers to retinal vascular changes due to chronic or acutely (malignant) elevated systemic blood pressure.

Epidemiology

Hypertension, defined as blood pressure >140/90 mmHg, occurs in over 60 million Americans. It is more prevalent in African Americans.

Symptoms

Hypertensive retinopathy is usually asymptomatic, and only rarely leads to decreased vision in late stages. However, maglinant hypertension can cause sudden blurry vision.

Signs

The characteristic retinal findings include retinal arteriole narrowing and straightening, copper or silver-wire arteriole changes due to arteriolosclerosis, arteriovenous crossing changes (nicking), cotton wool spots, microaneurysms, flame-shaped hemorrhages, hard exudates (may be in a circinate or macular star pattern), Elschnig spots (yellow (early) or hyperpigmented (late) patches of RPE overlying infarcted choriocapillaris lobules), Siegrist streaks (linear hyperpigmented areas of RPE over choroidal vessels), arterial macroaneurysms, and disc hyperemia or edema with dilated tortuous vessels (in malignant hypertension) (Figures 17–38 and 17–39).

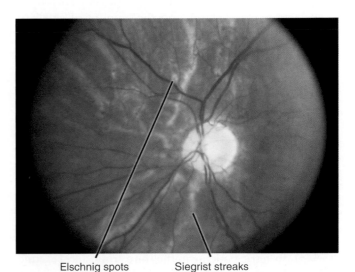

Elschnig spots   Siegrist streaks

FIGURE 17–38
Hypertensive retinopathy, demonstrating attenuated arterioles, choroidal ischemia, Elschnig spots, and Siegrist streaks.

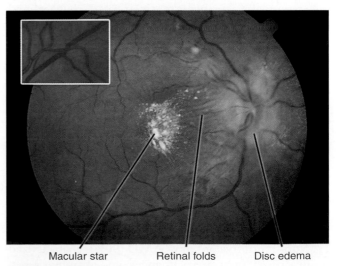

Macular star   Retinal folds   Disc edema

FIGURE 17–39
Hypertensive retinopathy with disc edema, macular star, and retinal folds in a patient with acute malignant hypertension. Inset shows arteriovenous nicking.

Differential diagnosis

The hemorrhages and exudates seen in hypertensive retinopathy can look like diabetic retinopathy, radiation retinopathy, CRVO, BRVO, leukemic retinopathy, retinopathy of anemia, or collagen vascular disease.

Evaluation

- The **history** must include concomitant systemic diseases, blood pressure control, and cardiovascular risk factors.
- The **eye exam** concentrates on ophthalmoscopy (changes in retinal vasculature and arteriovenous crossings, may have hemorrhages, exudates, cotton wool spots, RPE changes, and disc edema).
- A **fluorescein angiogram** can be considered to evaluate macular status and the amount of capillary non-perfusion and macular edema.
- Consider **medical consultation** to evaluate the cardiovascular and cerebrovascular systems.

Management

- Control blood pressure.

Prognosis

The prognosis is usually good.

TOXEMIA OF PREGNANCY

Toxemia with severe hypertension, proteinuria, edema (pre-eclampsia), and seizures (eclampsia) is seen in 2–5% of obstetric patients in the third trimester. Toxemic patients can develop focal arteriolar narrowing, cotton wool spots, retinal hemorrhages, hard exudates, Elschnig spots (RPE changes from choroidal infarction), bullous exudative retinal detachments, neovascularization, and disc edema (Figure 17–40). All the findings that occur in this retinopathy are hypertensive-related changes, and resolve without sequelae after treating the hypertension and delivery.

Macular Disorders

AGE-RELATED MACULAR DEGENERATION

Definition

AMD is a progressive degenerative disease of the RPE, Bruch's membrane, and choriocapillaris. It is typically classified into two types:

1. **Non-exudative** or "dry" **AMD** (90%): characterized by drusen, pigmentary changes, and atrophy.
2. **Exudative** or "wet" **AMD** (10%): characterized by CNV and subsequent disciform scarring.

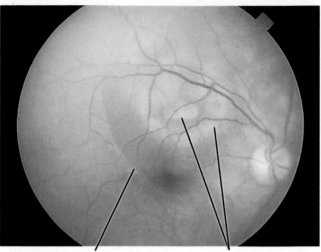

Serous retinal detachment   Exudates

FIGURE 17–40
Toxemia of pregnancy with serous retinal detachment and yellow-white patches.

Epidemiology

AMD is the leading cause of blindness in the US population aged >65 years old, as well as the most common cause of blindness in the western world. In the Framingham Eye Study, AMD was seen in 6.4% of patients 65–74 years old and 19.7% of patients >75 years old. AMD is more common in Caucasians, and there is a slight female predilection. Risk factors for AMD include increasing age (>75 years old), positive family history, cigarette smoking, hyperopia, light iris color, hypertension, hypercholesterolemia, female gender, and cardiovascular disease. There is also a genetic component to AMD.

Non-exudative (dry) macular degeneration

Symptoms

Most patients with non-exudative AMD are asymptomatic. Those with atrophy may notice metamorphopsia (visual distortion) and central or paracentral scotomas.

Signs

Non-exudative AMD in early stages is characterized by small, hard drusen and pigmentary changes. In later stages, larger, soft drusen and geographic atrophy of the RPE can occur. The **Age Related Eye Disease Study (AREDS)** categorized AMD as follows:

- **Category 1**: fewer than five small (<63 μm) drusen.
- **Category 2 (mild AMD)**: multiple small drusen or single or non-extensive intermediate (63–124 μm) drusen; or pigment abnormalities.
- **Category 3 (intermediate AMD)**: extensive intermediate-size drusen or one or more large

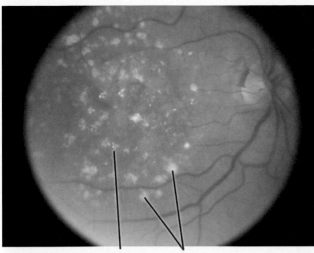

Hard drusen Soft drusen

FIGURE 17–41
Dry, age-related macular degeneration demonstrating drusen and pigmentary changes (category 3).

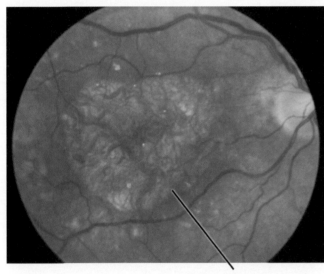

Geographic atrophy

FIGURE 17–42
Advanced atrophic, non-exudative, age-related macular degeneration, demonstrating subfoveal geographic atrophy (category 4).

(>125 μm) drusen; or non-central geographic atrophy (Figure 17–41).

- **Category 4 (advanced AMD)**: vision loss (<20/32) due to AMD in one eye (due to either central/subfoveal geographic atrophy or exudative macular degeneration) (Figure 17–42).

Differential diagnosis

Drusen and pigmentary changes can also occur in dominant drusen, pattern dystrophy, Best's disease, Stargardt's disease, cone dystrophy, and drug toxicities.

Evaluation

- The **history** should concentrate on AMD risk factors, including family history, cigarette smoking, hypertension, hypercholesterolemia, vitamin use, and cardiovascular disease.
- The **eye exam** is performed with attention to visual acuity (normal or decreased), Amsler grid (to evaluate for metamorphopsia and scotoma), and ophthalmoscopy (drusen, RPE changes, geographic atrophy).
- A **fluorescein angiogram** or **optical coherence tomography** should be performed to rule out CNV.

Management

- Patients with non-exudative AMD should check an Amsler grid daily to monitor their vision. If they notice a change in vision, metamorphopsia, or change in Amsler grid, they should be re-examined promptly.
- Vitamin supplemention with high-dose antioxidants and vitamins (vitamin C, 500 mg; vitamin E, 400 IU; beta-carotene, 15 mg; zinc, 80 mg; and copper, 2 mg) should be prescribed for patients with category 3 or 4 disease. *Warning*: smokers should not take beta-carotene at such high doses because of an increased risk of lung cancer (**AREDS** conclusion).
- Consider supplements with lower-dose antioxidants (e.g. Centrum Silver, iCaps, Occuvite) for patients with category 1, category 2, and strong family history.
- Supplementation with other vitamins, including lutein and bilberry, is still unproven.

Prognosis

Non-exudative AMD usually has a good prognosis unless patients develop central geographic atrophy or exudative AMD. The presence of large, soft drusen and focal RPE hyperpigmentation increases the risk of developing exudative AMD. The risk of advanced AMD over 5 years varies depending on AREDS category: category 1 and 2 (1.8%), category 3 (18%), category 4 (43%).

Exudative (wet) macular degeneration

Symptoms

Patients with exudative AMD report a sudden onset of decreased vision, metamorphopsia, and central scotoma.

Signs

A CNV is the hallmark of exudative AMD. The CNV produces the other findings of this disease, including lipid exudates, subretinal or intraretinal hemorrhage/fluid, pigment epithelial detachment, retinal pigment epithelial tears, and in late stages a disciform scar (Figures 17–43–17–46).

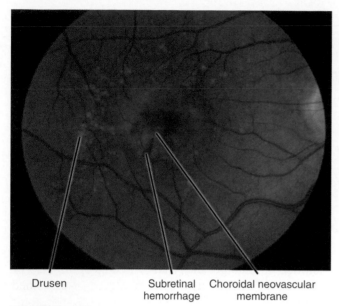

Drusen   Subretinal   Choroidal neovascular
           hemorrhage   membrane

FIGURE 17–43
Exudative age-related macular degeneration, demonstrating
subretinal hemorrhage from classic choroidal neovascular membrane.

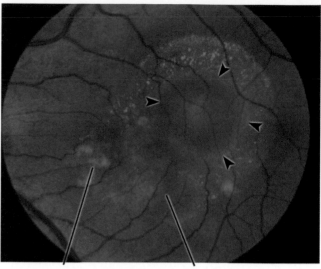

Drusen   Choroidal neovascular membrane

FIGURE 17–45
Exudative age-related macular degeneration, demonstrating drusen,
pigmentary changes, and an occult choroidal neovascular membrane
with associated serous pigment epithelial detachment (arrowheads).

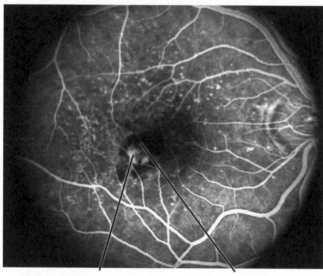

Choroidal neovascular membrane   Hemorrhage

FIGURE 17–44
Fluorescein angiogram of same patient as in Figure 17–43,
demonstrating leakage from the choroidal neovascular membrane
and blocking from the surrounding subretinal blood.

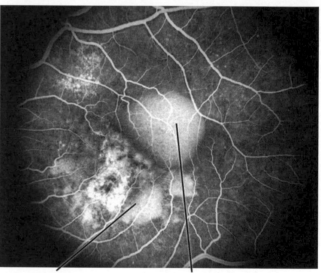

Choroidal neovascular   Serous pigment
membrane   epithelial detachment

FIGURE 17–46
Fluorescein angiogram of the same patient as in Figure 17–45,
demonstrating hyperfluorescent staining of pigmentary changes and
drusen, leakage from the choroidal neovascular membrane, and
pooling of fluorescein dye within the serous pigment epithelial
detachment.

Differential diagnosis

CNV can occur in other diseases, including presumed
ocular histoplasmosis syndrome, angioid streaks, myopic
degeneration, traumatic choroidal rupture, retinal
dystrophies, inflammatory choroidopathies, and optic
nerve drusen.

Evaluation

- The **history** should contain AMD risk factors,
  including family history, cigarette smoking, hypertension, hypercholesterolemia, vitamin use, and
  cardiovascular disease.
- The **eye exam** must pay particular attention to
  ophthalmoscopy (drusen, intraretinal hemorrhage,

subretinal hemorrhage, exudates, pigment epithelial detachment).

- A **fluorescein angiogram** is required to diagnose a CNV definitively. The CNV will leak on the fluorescein angiogram in two forms:
  1. **Classic leakage**: bright fluorescence that increases throughout the angiogram and late leakage.
  2. **Occult leakage**: non-homogeneous persistent hyperfluorescence (type 1) or late leakage of undetermined origin (type 2) with no early leakage but hyperfluorescent stippling later.
- Consider an **indocyanine green angiogram** when the CNV is poorly demarcated or obscured by hemorrhage on fluorescein angiogram or if a fibrovascular pigment epithelial detachment is present (to identify areas of focal neovascularization).
- **Optical coherence tomography** is useful to verify the diagnosis of CNV and to delineate the presence and extent of intraretinal and subretinal fluid, as well as the presence of a pigment epithelial detachment to determine treatment.

Management

- Focal laser photocoagulation by a retina specialist for classic, well-defined CNV using argon green/yellow or krypton red laser and a transpupillary delivery system to form confluent white burns over the entire CNV, depending on size, location, and visual acuity based on the results of the **Macular Photocoagulation Study (MPS)** if the lesion is extra- or juxtafoveal.
  - **Extrafoveal** (200–2500 μm from center of FAZ): treat the entire CNV and 100 μm beyond all boundaries.
  - **Juxtafoveal** (1–199 μm from center of FAZ or CNV 200–2500 μm from center of FAZ with blood or blocked fluorescence within 1–199 μm of FAZ center): treat the entire CNV and 100 μm beyond on the non-foveal side, and up to the CNV border on the foveal side.
- **Subfoveal** (under geometric center of FAZ): although laser photocoagulation is beneficial, its use to treat subfoveal lesions has been replaced by photodynamic therapy (PDT) with verteporfin (Visudyne) and anti-VEGF therapy. PDT prevents visual loss in subfoveal, predominantly classic lesions (>50% of the entire lesion is composed of classic CNV) (**Treatment of AMD with Photodynamic Therapy Study (TAP)** conclusion). PDT retreatment is applied as often as every 3 months if fluorescein leakage is found from the CNV. Patients should avoid direct sunlight or bright indoor light for a minimum of 48 hours after each treatment (drug labeling states 5 days).
- Alternatively, intravitreal pegaptanib (Macugen) injections can be performed for all lesion compositions at 6-week intervals, or intravitreal ranibizumab (Lucentis) for all lesion compositions at 4-week intervals.
- Low-vision aids and registration with blind services is recommended for patients who are legally blind (<20/200 best corrected visual acuity or <20° visual field in better-seeing eye).

Prognosis

Exudative AMD usually has a poor prognosis, although newer anti-VEGF therapies such as ranibizumab (Lucentis) can improve vision in a significant number of patients. The risk of the fellow eye developing CNV is 4–12% annually.

MYOPIC DEGENERATION

High myopia (≥–6.00 D or axial length >26.5 mm) and pathologic myopia (≥–8.00 D or axial length >32.5 mm) can produce a progressive retinal degeneration that causes scleral thinning, posterior staphyloma, lacquer cracks (irregular, yellow streaks), peripapillary atrophic crescent, tilted optic disc, Fuchs' spots (dark spots in the macula due to RPE hyperplasia), "tigroid" fundus due to thinning of the RPE allowing visualization of larger choroidal vessels, and chorioretinal atrophy (Figures 17–47 and 17–48). These individuals have an increased incidence of posterior vitreous detachment, premature cataract formation, glaucoma, lattice degeneration, giant retinal tears, retinal breaks, rhegmatogenous retinal detachments, macular hole, subretinal hemorrhage (especially near lacquer cracks), and CNV (Figure 17–49). No treatment will prevent this progressive degeneration. Patients should wear polycarbonate safety glasses for sports due to the increased risk of choroidal rupture with minor trauma.

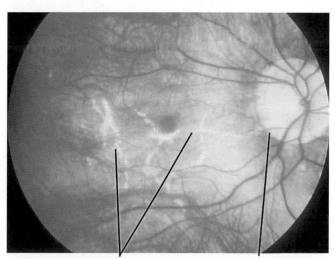

Lacquer cracks   Peripapillary atrophy

FIGURE 17–47
Myopic degeneration with lacquer cracks.

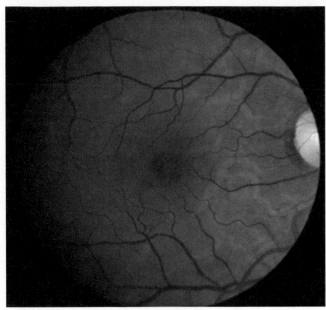

Tigroid fundus

FIGURE 17–48
"Tigroid" fundus due to thinning of retinal pigment epithelium, allowing visualization of larger choroidal vessels.

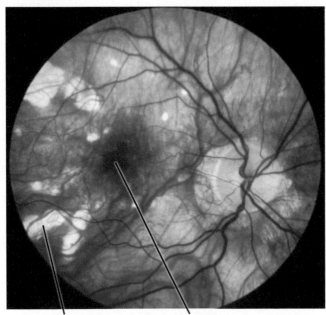

Chorioretinal atrophy   Subretinal hemorrhage

FIGURE 17–49
Myopic degeneration with peripapillary and chorioretinal atrophy, and subretinal hemorrhage from choroidal neovascular membrane.

CENTRAL SEROUS CHORIORETINOPATHY

Definition

Central serous chorioretinopathy (CSR) refers to idiopathic leakage of fluid from the choroid into the subretinal space (94%), under the RPE (3%), or both (3%) presumably from RPE or choroidal dysfunction.

Epidemiology

CSR usually occurs in males (10:1) aged 20–50 years old. It is more common in Caucasians, Hispanics, and Asians, while rare in African Americans. CSR is associated with type A personality, stress, hypochondriasis, pregnancy, steroid use, hypertension, Cushing's syndrome, systemic lupus erythematosus, and organ transplantation.

Symptoms

Patients may be asymptomatic, or note a unilateral decrease in vision, micropsia (objects appear smaller), metamorphopsia, central scotoma, and mild dyschromatopsia.

Signs

The retinal exam reveals single or multiple round or oval-shaped shallow, serous retinal detachments or pigment epithelial detachments that are deep yellow spots at the level of the RPE (Figures 17–50 and 17–51). In general, the vision is only mildly reduced and can be improved with a pinhole or plus lens due to the induced hyperopia by the fluid. Patients may have an abnormal Amsler grid. Areas of RPE atrophy may be seen at sites of previous episodes.

Differential diagnosis

Subretinal fluid accumulation is also seen in exudative AMD (especially in patients >50 years old), Vogt–Koyanagi–Harada syndrome or other inflammatory choroidal disorders, uveal effusion syndrome, toxemia of pregnancy, optic nerve pit, choroidal tumors, vitelliform macular dystrophy, and pigment epithelial detachment from other causes of neovascular membranes.

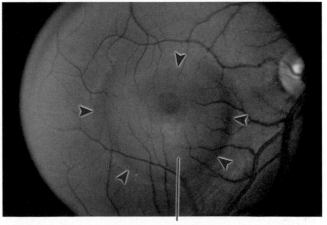

Pigment epithelial detachment

FIGURE 17–50
Idiopathic central serous retinopathy with large serous retinal detachment.

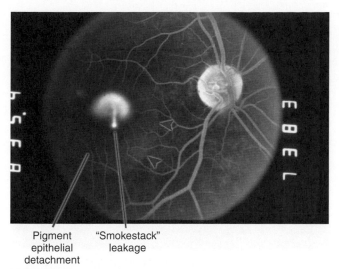

Pigment epithelial detachment   "Smokestack" leakage

FIGURE 17–51

Fluorescein angiogram of the same patient as shown in Figure 17–50, demonstrating classic smokestack appearance.

Evaluation

- The **history** should include possible risk factors such as stress, steroid use (including inhaled steroids), and systemic diseases.
- The **eye exam** is performed with attention to visual acuity (decreased), refraction (hyperopic shift), Amsler grid (central distortion), and ophthalmoscopy (serous retinal detachments or pigment epithelial detachments).
- A **fluorescein angiogram** can be performed to verify the diagnosis. This shows either a focal dot of early hyperfluorescence that leaks in a characteristic smokestack pattern (10%) in late views or gradually pools into a pigment epithelial detachment (90%). More than one site of leakage may be present.
- Consider **optical coherence tomography** in equivocal cases or in younger patients in whom exudative AMD is not being considered. The optical coherence tomography shows subretinal fluid and/or a pigment epithelial detachment.

Management

- No treatment is required in most cases because CSR usually resolves spontaneously over 6 weeks.
- Focal laser photocoagulation is considered for patients who require quicker visual rehabilitation for occupational reasons (monocular, pilots, etc.); have poor vision in their fellow eye due to central serous retinopathy; have no resolution of fluid after 4–6 months; have recurrent episodes with poor vision; or have severe forms of central serous retinopathy known to carry a poor prognosis. Laser shortens the duration of symptoms, but has no effect on the final visual acuity. It is debatable whether photocoagulation reduces the recurrence rate.

- PDT may have some benefit but is experimental.
- Discontinue or reduce risk factors if possible.

Prognosis

The prognosis is good, with 94% of patients regaining better than 20/30 acuity, and 95% of pigment epithelial detachments resolving spontaneously in 3–4 months. Recurrences are common (45%) and usually occur within a year. The prognosis is worse in patients with recurrent disease, multiple areas of detachment, or a chronic course.

CYSTOID MACULAR EDEMA

Definition

CME is accumulation of extracellular fluid in the macular region with characteristic cystoid spaces forming in the outer plexiform layer.

Etiology

CME results from intraocular surgery (especially in older patients and if the posterior lens capsule is violated with vitreous loss; CME following cataract surgery is called **Irvine–Gass syndrome**), after laser treatment (Nd:YAG laser capsulotomy, especially if performed within 3 months of cataract surgery), uveitis, diabetic retinopathy, juxtafoveal retinal telangiectasia, vein occlusions, retinal vasculitis, epiretinal membrane, hereditary retinal dystrophies (dominant CME, retinitis pigmentosa), drug toxicity (epinephrine in aphakic patients, dipivefrin, and prostaglandin analogues), hypertensive retinopathy, AMD, intraocular tumors, collagen vascular diseases, hypotony, and chronic inflammation.

Symptoms

Patients may be asymptomatic or have decreased or faded, "washed-out" vision.

Signs

CME is difficult to visualize on retinal exam unless the intraretinal cystoid spaces are large. Findings that suggest the presence of CME include loss of the foveal reflex, thickened fovea, and foveal folds (Figures 17–52–17–54). Other clues that CME may exist are signs of causes of CME such as uveitis or surgical complications, including open posterior capsule, vitreous to the wound, peaked pupil, and iris incarceration in the wound.

Differential diagnosis

Intraretinal cystoid spaces can appear similar to an early macular hole (stage 1), foveal retinoschisis, central serous retinopathy, CNV, pseudocystoid macular edema (due to juvenile retinoschisis, nicotinic acid (niacin) maculopathy, Goldmann–Favre disease, and some forms

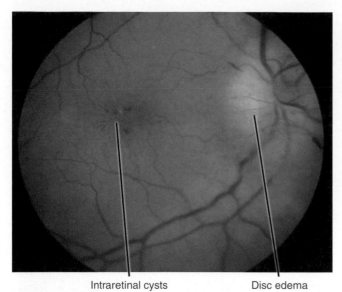

Intraretinal cysts   Disc edema

FIGURE 17–52
Cystoid macular edema with decreased foveal reflex, cystic changes in fovea, and intraretinal hemorrhages.

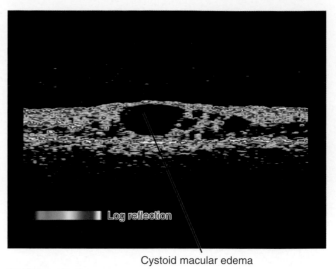

Cystoid macular edema

FIGURE 17–54
Optical coherence tomography of cystoid macular edema, demonstrating intraretinal cystoid spaces and dome-shaped configuration of fovea.

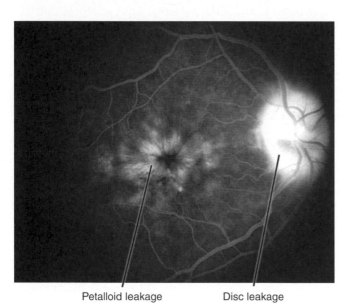

Petalloid leakage   Disc leakage

FIGURE 17–53
Fluorescein angiogram of same patient as shown in Figure 17–52, demonstrating characteristic petalloid appearance and optic nerve leakage.

of retinitis pigmentosa, but there is no leakage on the fluorescein angiogram).

Evaluation

- The **history** should document possible risk factors, including previous ocular surgery and systemic diseases.
- The **eye exam** must evaluate the cornea (for signs of previous surgery), anterior chamber (for cell and flare or vitreous), iris (for signs of previous surgery), lens (may be pseudophakic or aphakic), and ophthalmoscopy (intraretinal cystoid spaces).
- A **fluorescein angiogram** shows early, perifoveal, punctate hyperfluorescence and characteristic late leakage in a petalloid pattern.
- **Optical coherence tomography** shows increased retinal thickness with cystoid spaces and loss of the normal foveal contour with or without subretinal fluid. An optical coherence tomography exam will always show CME and is all that is necessary for diagnosis; however, a fluorescein angiogram is usually added to evaluate the etiology and to aid in management.

Management

- The mainstay of management is a topical non-steroidal anti-inflammatory (NSAID: such as Voltaren or Acular qid, Nevanac tid, or Xibrom bid) and a topical steroid (prednisolone acetate 1% qid) for 1 month, then taper slowly.
- Consider a posterior subTenon's steroid injection (triamcinolone acetonide 40 mg/ml) in patients who do not respond to topical medications.
- In refractory cases, consider an intravitreal steroid injection (triamcinolone acetonide (Kenalog) 4 mg).
- If vitreous is present to the wound and vision is <20/80, consider an Nd:YAG laser vitreolysis or perform a pars plana vitrectomy with peeling of the posterior hyaloid (**Vitrectomy-Aphakic Cystoid Macular Edema Study** conclusion).
- Discontinue topical epinephrine, dipvefrin, or prostaglandin analogue drops, and nicotinic acid-containing medications. Rarely, diuretics and oral contraceptive

pills can cause an atypical CME that resolves on discontinuing the medication.

- Treat the underlying disorder if possible. Focal laser treatment may be required (i.e., CME due to diabetic retinopathy or BRVO).

Prognosis

The prognosis is usually good, with spontaneous resolution over weeks to months for post-surgical CME. The prognosis is poorer for chronic CME (>6 months).

MACULAR HOLE

Definition

A macular hole is a full-thickness hole in the retina located in the fovea.

Etiology

Most macular holes are idiopathic, but other risk factors include CME, vitreomacular traction, inflammation, trauma, ocular surgery, and laser treatment.

Epidemiology

Idiopathic macular holes (83%) usually occur in women (3:1) aged 60–80 years old.

Symptoms

Patients have a sudden onset of decreased vision, metamorphopsia, and, less commonly, a central scotoma.

Signs

The level of decreased visual acuity depends on the stage of the hole and ranges from 20/40 in stage 1 to 20/200 in stages 3 and 4. The fundus findings can be classified into four stages:

- **Stage 1**: Premacular hole (impending hole) with foveal detachment, absent foveal reflex, macular cyst (1A = yellow spot, 100–200 μm in diameter; 1B = yellow ring, 200–300 μm in diameter).
  Stage 2: Early, small, full-thickness hole either centrally within the ring or eccentrically at the ring's margin.
- **Stage 3**: Full-thickness hole (≥400 μm in diameter) with yellow deposits at the level of the RPE (Klein's tags), operculum (the retinal tissue fragment in the overlying vitreous), cuff of subretinal fluid, CME, absence of a Weiss ring, and positive Watzke–Allen sign (subjective interruption of the slit beam on biomicroscopy) (Figure 17–55).
- **Stage 4**: Stage 3 hole plus a complete posterior vitreous detachment (Figure 17–56).

Differential diagnosis

Central defects and a pseudo-hole appearance can be seen with epiretinal membrane, solar retinopathy, central

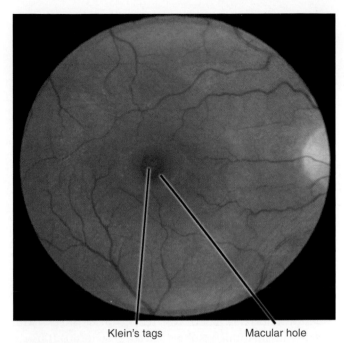

Klein's tags   Macular hole

FIGURE 17–55
Macular hole with multiple yellow spots (Klein's tags) at the base of the hole.

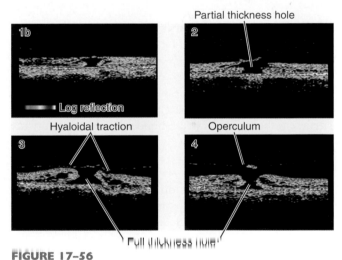

FIGURE 17–56
Optical coherence tomography scans demonstrating cross-sectional image of all stages of macular hole formation and the full-thickness retinal defect characteristic of stages 3 and 4 holes.

serous retinopathy, AMD, vitreomacular traction syndrome, CME, solitary drusen, macular cyst, and lamellar hole.

Evaluation

- The **history** should note possible risk factors, including previous ocular surgery, trauma, and inflammation.
- The **eye exam** should concentrate on the visual acuity (decreased), Amsler grid (central scotoma), and ophthalmoscopy (macular hole, positive Watzke–Allen sign).

- **Optical coherence tomography** is very useful for staging holes and to differentiate macular holes from other diseases in the differential diagnosis, especially pseudo-holes, lamellar holes, and cysts. The OCT demonstrates the full-thickness retinal defect with or without traction on the edges of the hole.

Management

- No treatment is recommended for stage 1 holes because spontaneous closure can occur.
- No medical therapy can successfully close a macular hole; therefore, surgery by a retina specialist should be performed for stage 2–4 holes of recent onset (<1 year) and reduced visual acuity in the range of 20/60 to 20/400. Surgery consists of a pars plana vitrectomy, membrane peel, gas fluid exchange, and gas injection with 7–14 days of prone positioning.

Prognosis

The prognosis is good for recent-onset holes, with successful anatomic results after surgery in 60–100% of patients, depending on the duration of the hole. Most patients will have improved acuity. The prognosis for holes >1 year's duration is worse.

EPIRETINAL MEMBRANE

Definition

An epiretinal membrane is cellular proliferation along the internal limiting membrane and retinal surface of the macula. Contraction of this membrane causes the retinal surface to become wrinkled, hence giving this entity the name "macular pucker" or "cellophane maculopathy."

Etiology

An epiretinal membrane is often idiopathic, but can also result from prior retinal surgery, intraocular inflammation, retinal vascular occlusions, sickle-cell retinopathy, vitreous hemorrhage, trauma, retinal breaks, macular holes, intraocular tumors (i.e., angiomas and hamartomas), telangiectasis, retinal arteriolar macroaneurysms, retinitis pigmentosa, laser photocoagulation, and cryotherapy.

Epidemiology

The incidence of epiretinal membrane formation increases with increasing age. It occurs in 2% of the population >50 years old and in 20% >75 years old. There is a slight female predilection (3:2). Most cases are unilateral, but 20–30% are bilateral and asymmetric.

Symptoms

An epiretinal membrane is usually asymptomatic with normal or near-normal vision. As more contraction occurs, mild metamorphopsia or blurred vision begins.

Less commonly, macropsia (objects appear larger), central photopsia, or monocular diplopia can occur with significant macular pucker.

Signs

An epiretinal membrane appears as a thin, translucent membrane on the retinal surface. It can range from a mild sheen (cellophane) to a considerable membrane that may produce dragged or tortuous retinal vessels, retinal striae, pseudo-holes, foveal ectopia, and CME (Figures 17–57 and 17–58).

Differential diagnosis

The traction produced by an epiretinal membrane is usually easy to differentiate from other traction maculopathies, including TRD from diabetic retinopathy,

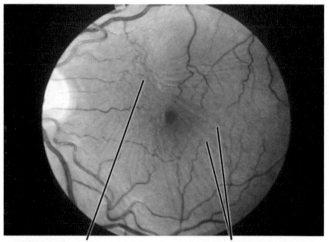

Cellophane membrane   Retinal striae

FIGURE 17–57
Cellophane epiretinal membrane and macular pucker with retinal striae.

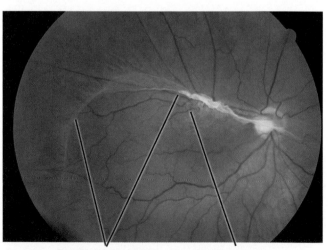

Epiretinal membrane   Dragged vessels

FIGURE 17–58
Epiretinal membrane with macular pucker and dragged vessels.

sickle-cell retinopathy, or radiation retinopathy, or the corrugations seen with choroidal folds.

Evaluation

- The **history** should note possible risk factors, including previous ocular surgery and systemic diseases.
- The **eye exam** must evaluate visual acuity (may be decreased), Amsler grid (central distortion), and ophthalmoscopy (epiretinal membrane).
- **Optical coherence tomography** is very useful for evaluating an epiretinal membrane and its effect on the retina and to differentiate it from other diseases in the differential diagnosis, especially pseudo-holes, lamellar holes, and macular holes. The optical coherence tomography demonstrates the increased retinal thickening and the traction on the retina due to the epiretinal membrane.

Management

- There is no medical treatment for an epiretinal membrane.
- In patients with reduced acuity (e.g., <20/50) or intractable symptoms, surgery consisting of a pars plana vitrectomy and membrane peel can be performed by a retina specialist.

Prognosis

The prognosis is usually good, with over 75% of patients having an improvement in symptoms and vision after surgery.

TOXIC MACULOPATHIES

Systemic medications can produce retinal toxicity.

Canthaxanthine

This oral tanning agent produces characteristic refractile yellow spots in a wreath-like pattern around the fovea (gold-dust retinopathy) (Figure 17–59). It is usually asymptomatic or produces mild metamorphopsia and decreased vision. When the retinopathy occurs, with cumulative doses >35 g, patients should decrease or discontinue the medication.

Chloroquine (Aralen)/hydroxychloroquine (Plaquenil)

Initially used as antimalarial agents, these drugs are now used to treat systemic lupus erythematosus, rheumatoid arthritis, short-term pulse treatment for graft-versus-host disease, and amoebiasis. Early retinal changes, including loss of the foveal reflex and abnormal macular pigmentation, are reversible. However, with continued administration, a "bull's-eye" maculopathy, peripheral bone spicules, vasculature attenuation, and disc pallor appear, and these conditions are usually not reversible (Figure 17–60). In very late stages chloroquine retin-

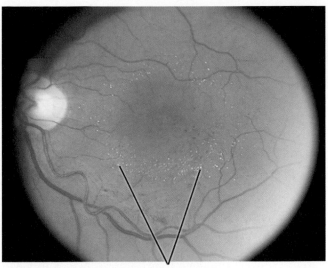

Refractile crystals

FIGURE 17–59
Crystalline maculopathy due to canthaxanthine.

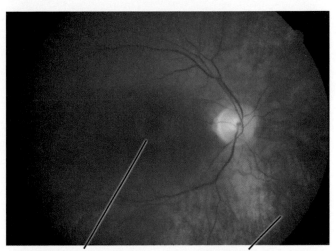

Bull's-eye maculopathy   Peripheral atrophy

FIGURE 17–60
"Bull's-eye" maculopathy due to chloroquine toxicity.

opathy looks similar to end-stage retinitis pigmentosa. Patients may also develop eyelash whitening (poliosis) and whorl-like subepithelial corneal deposits (cornea verticillata, vortex keratopathy). Early stages are often asymptomatic, but continued toxicity can produce central or paracentral scotomas, blurry vision, nyctalopia, photopsias, dyschromatopsia, photophobia, and in late stages constriction of the visual field, loss of color vision, decreased vision, and absolute scotomas. The retinopathy is seen with doses >3.5 mg/kg per day or 300 g total (chloroquine), and >6.5 mg/kg per day (<400 mg/day appears safe) or 700 g total (hydroxychloroquine). The total daily dose seems more critical than total cumulative dose. The medication should be decreased or discontinued if toxicity develops; however, the retinopathy often progresses even after discontinuation because the drug concentrates in the eye. Since these medications often cannot be stopped, examination of visual acuity, red Amsler grid, and visual fields (central 10° with red test object) at baseline and every 6 months (chloroquine) or 12 months (hydroxychloroquine) is recommended while the patient is taking the medication. Hydroxychloroquine is safer since it does not cross the blood–retinal barrier as readily (toxicity is rarely seen with usage of <7 years).

Niacin

Niacin, which is used to treat hypercholesterolemia, can cause pseudocystoid macular edema with decreased vision. This appears clinically as CME and is only distinguished by fluorescein angiography, which shows early perifoveal punctate hyperfluorescence as in CME but without leakage. If toxicity develops, then the medication should be decreased or discontinued.

Talc

Refractive yellow deposits near or in retinal arterioles due to talc are seen in IV drug abusers. A similar picture is seen in IV drug abusers who inject suspensions of crushed methylphenidate (Ritalin) tablets. There is no effective treatment.

Tamoxifen

Tamoxifen, which is used to treat breast carcinoma, causes a characteristic retinopathy with refractile yellow-white crystals scattered throughout the posterior pole in a donut-shaped pattern, and mild CME. Later, retinal pigmentary changes that produce a mild decrease in vision can occur. Patients may develop whorl-like, white, subepithelial corneal deposits. The toxicity is observed with doses >30 mg/day. Crystals often occur at the initial higher dosage levels, but can resolve with lowering the dose.

Sildenafil (Viagra)/Vardenafil (Levitra)/Tadalafil (Cialis)

These medications, which are phosphodiesterase-5 inhibitors used to treat male erectile dysfunction, can produce transient changes in color perception, including a blue or blue-green tint or central haze of vision (may be pink or yellow); changes in light perception, including darker colors appearing darker and increased awareness of brightness; and flashing lights within 15–30 minutes after drug ingestion and peaking within 1–2 hours. The visual symptoms resolve for Viagra within 1 hour at doses <50 mg, 2 hours with 100 mg, and 4–6 hours for 200 mg. The visual phenomenon is thought to be secondary to the drug modifying the transduction cascade in photoreceptors (blocks phosphodiesterase-5 10× more than phosphodiesterase-6, leading to interference in cyclic guanosine monophosphate). Thus, these drugs should

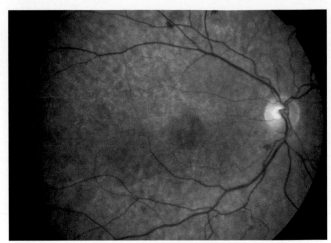

FIGURE 17–61
Diffuse pigmentary retinopathy in end-stage thioridazine toxicity.

be used with extreme caution in patients with retinitis pigmentosa and congenital stationary night blindness. The visual effects of Viagra occur in 3% of patients taking a dose of 25–50 mg; 11% of patients taking 100 mg dose, and in 40–50% taking >100 mg. There may be a possible, rare association with non-arteritic anterior ischemic optic neuropathy with permanent visual loss.

Thioridazine (Mellaril)

Thioridazine, used to treat psychoses, produces nyctalopia, decreased vision, ring or paracentral scotomas, and brown discoloration of vision. On retinal exam, pigment granularity and clumping in the midperiphery appear first and are reversible. These changes progress and coalesce into large areas of pigmentation (salt-and-pepper pigment retinopathy) or chorioretinal atrophy with short-term, high-dose use (Figure 17–61). A variant, known as **nummular retinopathy**, consisting of chorioretinal atrophy posterior to the equator occurs with chronic use. In late stages, the appearance may be similar to retinitis pigmentosa. Doses >800 mg/day (300 mg is the recommended) can produce the toxic retinopathy. The total daily dose seems to be more critical than the total cumulative dose. Patients should decrease or discontinue the medication if toxicity develops; however, the changes may progress after the medication is withdrawn because the drug is stored in the eye. Patients should have vision, color vision, and visual fields tested every 6 months while on the medication.

Retinal Detachment

A retinal detachment is the separation of the neurosensory retina from the RPE. There are several different types of retinal detachment: rhegmatogenous, serous, and traction.

RHEGMATOGENOUS RETINAL DETACHMENT

Definition

Rhegmatogenous is derived from the Greek word *rhegma* or rent. A rhegmatogenous retinal detachment is a retinal detachment due to a full-thickness retinal break (tear, hole, or dialysis) that allows vitreous fluid access to the subretinal space.

Etiology

Lattice degeneration (30%), posterior vitreous detachment (especially with vitreous hemorrhage), myopia, trauma (5–10%, particularly retinal dialysis and giant retinal tears (>3 clock hours in extent)), and previous ocular surgery (especially with vitreous loss) all increase the risk of rhegmatogenous retinal detachment.

Symptoms

A rhegmatogenous retinal detachment causes the acute onset of photopsias (flashes of light), floaters (often described as "spots" or "cobwebs"), shadow or curtain across the visual field, and decreased vision. Rarely, a detachment that is in the periphery may be asymptomatic or produce a peripheral visual field defect.

Signs

In patients with a rhegmatogenous retinal detachment, the retina appears as an undulating mobile convex tissue with corrugated folds (Figure 17–62). By definition, one or more retinal breaks are present (Figure 17–63). Examination of the anterior vitreous may reveal "tobacco dust" (pigment cells in the vitreous). Depending on the size of the detachment, there may be lower intraocular

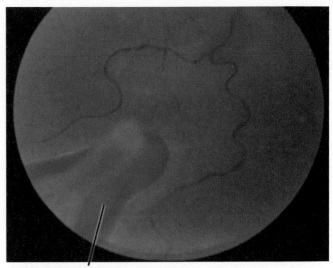

Horseshoe retinal tear within detachment

FIGURE 17–63
Same patient as shown in Figure 17–62, demonstrating peripheral horseshoe tear that caused the rhegmatogenous retinal detachment.

pressure in the affected eye. There may be a positive RAPD. Chronic rhegmatogenous retinal detachments may have pigmented demarcation lines, intraretinal cysts, fixed folds, or subretinal precipitates. The configuration of detachment helps localize the retinal break:

- **Superotemporal or superonasal detachment**: break within 1–1.5 clock hours of the highest border.
- **Superior detachment that straddles 12 o'clock**: break between 11 and 1 o'clock.
- **Inferior detachment with one higher side**: break within 1–1.5 clock hours of the highest border.
- **Inferior detachment equally high on either side**: break between 5 and 7 o'clock.

Differential diagnosis

A rhegmatogenous retinal detachment can look like retinoschisis, choroidal detachment, and serous retinal detachment.

Evaluation

- The **history** should note risk factors, especially previous ocular surgery and trauma, and the timing and onset of symptoms.
- The **eye exam** is performed with attention to visual acuity (decreased), pupillary response (positive RAPD), intraocular pressure (may be decreased), ophthalmoscopy (retinal detachment; depressed peripheral retinal exam to identify any retinal breaks).
- If the fundus cannot be visualized, then **B-scan ultrasonography** should be performed and shows the smooth, convex freely mobile retina that appears as a highly reflective echo in the vitreous cavity that

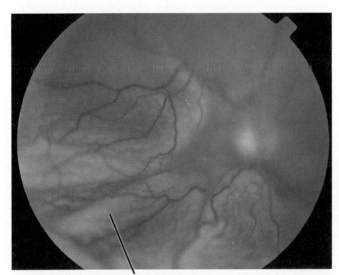

Rhegmatogenous retinal detachment

FIGURE 17–62
Rhegmatogenous retinal detachment, demonstrating corrugated folds.

is attached at the optic nerve head and ora serrata. Sometimes, retinal tears can be visualized in the periphery.

Management

- A rhegmatogenous retinal detachment needs to be treated immediately with surgery by a retina specialist. A macular threatening ("mac on") rhegmatogenous retinal detachment is a true *ophthalmic emergency* that requires treatment within 24 hours. If the macula is already detached ("mac off"), then treat urgently (within 48–96 hours).

Prognosis

The prognosis is variable and depends on the type of break and extent and duration of the detachment, especially whether or not the macula is involved. After rhegmatogenous retinal detachment repair, 5–10% of patients develop proliferative vitreoretinopathy (preretinal or subretinal fibrotic membranes that contract and pull on the retinal surface 6–8 weeks after surgery).

SEROUS/EXUDATIVE RETINAL DETACHMENT

Definition

A serous retinal detachment is a non-rhegmatogenous retinal detachment (not secondary to a retinal break) caused by subretinal transudation of fluid from a tumor, inflammatory process, vascular lesion, or degenerative lesion.

Etiology

Serous retinal detachments are due to Vogt–Koyanagi–Harada syndrome, Harada's disease, idiopathic uveal effusion syndrome, choroidal tumors, central serous retinopathy, posterior scleritis, hypertensive retinopathy, Coats' disease, optic nerve pit, retinal coloboma, and toxemia of pregnancy.

Symptoms

A serous retinal detachment is usually asymptomatic until it involves the macula, producing photopsias, floaters, a shadow across the visual field, or decreased vision.

Signs

A serous retinal detachment appears as a smooth elevation of the retina (Figure 17–64). The key feature is that the subretinal fluid shifts with changing head position. By definition, there are no retinal breaks. Patients may also demonstrate a mild positive RAPD.

Differential diagnosis

A serous retinal detachment can look like retinoschisis, choroidal detachment, and rhegmatogenous retinal detachment.

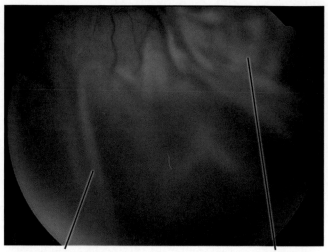
Serous retinal detachment   Melanoma
FIGURE 17–64
Exudative retinal detachment secondary to malignant melanoma.

Evaluation

- The **history** should document other ocular conditions and systemic diseases.
- The **eye exam** should concentrate on visual acuity (may be decreased), pupillary response (may have a mild positive RAPD), and ophthalmoscopy (serous detachment; depressed peripheral retinal exam to rule out any retinal breaks).
- If the fundus cannot be visualized, then **B-scan ultrasonography** should be performed and shows a smooth, convex, freely mobile echo that shifts with changing head position. The retina appears as a highly reflective echo in the vitreous cavity that is attached at the optic nerve head and ora serrata.

Management

- Treat the underlying condition.
- A serous retinal detachment rarely requires surgical intervention.

Prognosis

The prognosis is variable and depends on the underlying condition.

TRACTION RETINAL DETACHMENT

Definition

A TRD is a non-rhegmatogenous retinal detachment (not secondary to a retinal break) caused by fibrovascular or fibrotic proliferation and subsequent contraction that pulls the retina off.

Etiology

TRDs are usually due to diabetic retinopathy, sickle-cell retinopathy, retinopathy of prematurity, venous occlusions, proliferative vitreoretinopathy, toxocariasis, and familial exudative vitreoretinopathy.

Symptoms

A TRD may be asymptomatic if it does not involve the macula. When the macula is involved, then patients notice decreased vision and a shadow across the visual field.

Signs

A TRD appears as a concave, usually localized detachment with fibrovascular proliferation or fibrosis (Figure 17–65). It does not extend to the ora serrata. Occasionally, retinal holes can form, causing a combined traction–rhegmatogenous detachment that progresses more rapidly than a TRD alone. If a retinal tear develops, then the detachment may become convex. Patients may also demonstrate a mild positive RAPD.

Differential diagnosis

A TRD can look like retinoschisis, choroidal detachment, or rhegmatogenous retinal detachment.

Evaluation

- The **history** should record possible risk factors, including previous ocular surgery and systemic diseases.
- The **eye exam** should focus on visual acuity (decreased), pupillary response (may have a mild positive RAPD), and ophthalmoscopy (traction detachment that does not extend to the ora serrata, fibrosis, fibrovascular proliferation; depressed peripheral retinal exam to identify any concomitant retinal breaks).
- If the fundus cannot be visualized, then **B-scan ultrasonography** should be performed and usually

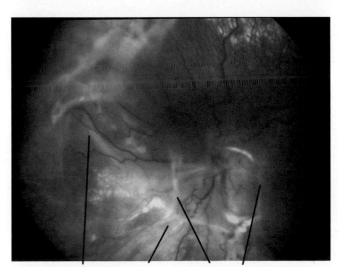

Retinal detachment   Preretinal traction

FIGURE 17–65

Traction retinal detachment due to proliferative vitreoretinopathy following penetrating ocular trauma.

shows a tented appearance with vitreous adhesions. The retina appears as a highly reflective echo in the vitreous cavity that is attached at the optic nerve head and ora serrata.

Management

- Management is by observation, unless the TRD threatens the macula or becomes a combined traction–rhegmatogenous detachment.
- Depending on the clinical situation, surgery can be performed by a retina specialist to release the traction.

Prognosis

The prognosis is variable and depends on the underlying condition.

Retinitis Pigmentosa

Definition

Retinitis pigmentosa is a term that describes a group of hereditary, progressive retinal degenerations (rod–cone dystrophies) that result from abnormal production of photoreceptor proteins. There are more than 29 genetic loci associated with various types of retinitis pigmentosa.

ATYPICAL FORMS OF RETINITIS PIGMENTOSA

Retinitis pigmentosa inversus primarily involves the macula and posterior pole, and therefore it can appear similar to hereditary macular disorders. Visual acuity and color vision are reduced early.

Retinitis pigmentosa sine pigmento refers to a form of retinitis pigmentosa in which patients have symptoms of retinitis pigmentosa but do not show pigmentary retinal changes. It may occur in as many as 20% of cases and causes more marked cone dysfunction.

Retinitis punctata albescens (autosomal recessive) is characterized by multiple small punctate white spots scattered in the mid peripheral retina at the level of the RPE as well as attenuated vessels and bone spicules.

Sector retinitis pigmentosa is a type of retinitis pigmentosa in which the pigmentary changes are limited to one retinal area, usually in the inferonasal quadrant. The electroretinogram responses are relatively good.

FORMS OF RETINITIS PIGMENTOSA ASSOCIATED WITH SYSTEMIC ABNORMALITIES

Bassen–Kornzweig syndrome (abetalipoproteinemia (autosomal recessive)) is a lack of serum beta-

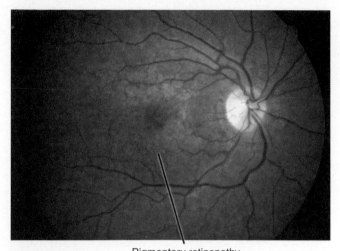

Pigmentary retinopathy

FIGURE 17–66
Kearns–Sayre syndrome with pigmentary retinopathy.

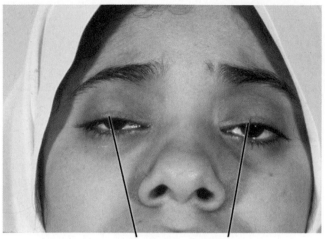

Ptosis due to CPEO

FIGURE 17–67
Same patient as shown in Figure 17–66, demonstrating chronic progressive external ophthalmoplegia (CPEO) with ptosis. This patient could not move her eyes.

lipoprotein that results in intestinal malabsorption of fat-soluble vitamins (A, D, E, and K), triglycerides, and cholesterol. The genetic defect is located on chromosome 4q24, which produces microsomal triglyceride transfer proteins. Findings include minimal early pigmentary retinal changes, angioid streaks, ataxia, steatorrhea, erythrocyte acanthocytosis, growth retardation, and neuropathy. Treatment consists of vitamin supplementation with vitamin A (15 000 IU PO qd), vitamin E (100 IU/kg PO qd), vitamin K (0.15 mg/kg PO qd), omega-3 fatty acids (0.10 g/kg PO qd), and dietary fat restriction.

Alstrom's disease (autosomal recessive) is caused by a genetic defect in the *ALMS1* gene on chromosome 2p13. It causes early and profound visual loss, and is associated with cataracts, deafness, obesity, renal failure, acanthosis nigricans, baldness, and hypogenitalism.

Cockayne's syndrome consists of retinitis pigmentosa, band keratopathy, cataracts, dwarfism, deafness, intracranial calcifications, and psychosis.

Kearns–Sayre syndrome (autosomal recessive) is a form of retinitis pigmentosa associated with chronic progressive external ophthalmoplegia, ptosis, cardiac conduction defects (arrhythmias, heart block, cardiomyopathy), and other abnormalities (Figures 17–66 and 17–67). Muscle biopsy shows "ragged red" fibers.

Bardet–Biedl syndrome (polydactyly in 75% and syndactyly in 14%) and **Laurence–Moon syndrome** (spastic paraplegia, no polydactyly/syndactyly) produce minimal pigmentary retinal changes early (Figure 17–68). Both syndromes are associated with short stature, congenital obesity, hypogenitalism (50%), partial deafness (5%), renal abnormalities, and

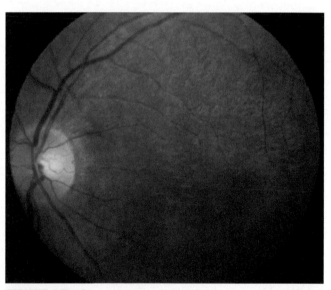

FIGURE 17–68
Diffuse pigmentary changes in a patient with Laurence–Moon syndrome.

mental retardation (85%). The genetic defect is linked to genes on multiple chromosomes.

Batten disease (**neuronal ceroid lipofuscinosis** (autosomal recessive)) causes lipofuscin to accumulate in neurons, resulting in retinal and central nervous system degeneration. The disease can have infantile (Hagberg–Santavuori syndrome), juvenile, or adult onset, with seizures, dementia, ataxia, and mental retardation. A conjunctival biopsy shows granular inclusions with autofluorescent lipopigments.

Refsum's disease (autosomal recessive) is produced by a defect in fatty acid metabolism due to phytanic acid oxidase deficiency. This causes elevated plasma phytanic acid, pipecolic acid, and very long-chain fatty acid levels. The disease is notable for minimal early pigmentary retinal changes, ichthyosis, electrocardiogram abnormalities, anosmia, deafness, progressive peripheral neuropathy, cerebellar ataxia, hypotonia, hepatomegaly, mental retardation, and elevated cerebrospinal fluid protein. Treatment consists of restricting dietary phytanic acid (animal fats and milk products) and phytol (leafy green vegetables). Serum phytanic acid levels should be followed.

Usher's syndrome (autosomal recessive), the most common systemic syndrome associated with retinitis pigmentosa (5%), is characterized by congenital, neurosensory hearing loss. It is associated with the *USH2A* gene on chromosome 1q41 that produces usherin, a basement membrane protein in the retina and inner ear. There are numerous additional loci as well. Patients should be cautioned to protect their ears from loud noise and avoid ototoxic medications. There are four types:

- **Type I**: total deafness with no vestibular function.
- **Type II** (most common; 67%): partial deafness with normal vestibular function and better vision than other types.
- **Type III** (**Hallgren's syndrome**): deafness, vestibular ataxia, and psychosis.
- **Type IV**: deafness and mental retardation.

Note: There is controversy about whether types III and IV are forms of Usher's syndrome or rather distinct genetic diseases.

Epidemiology

Retinitis pigmentosa is the most common hereditary retinal degeneration (1:5000) and can have any inheritance pattern: autosomal recessive (25%), autosomal dominant (20%, usually with variable penatrance, later onset, milder course), X-linked (9%, more severe, carriers are also affected), isolated (38%), and undetermined (8%)

Symptoms

Retinitis pigmentosa causes nyctalopia (poor night vision), delayed dark adaptation, photophobia, progressive constriction of visual fields (tunnel vision), dyschromatopsia, photopsias, and slowly progressive decreased central vision starting at approximately age 20.

Signs

Retinitis pigmentosa produces a characteristic fundus appearance with dark pigmentary clumps in the midperiphery and perivenous areas (bone spicules), attenuated retinal vessels, CME, fine pigmented vitreous cells, and waxy optic disc pallor (Figures 17–69 and 17–70). It causes decreased visual acuity and color

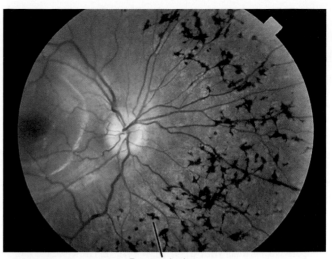

Bone spicules

FIGURE 17–69

Retinitis pigmentosa demonstrating characteristic bone spicule pigmentary changes.

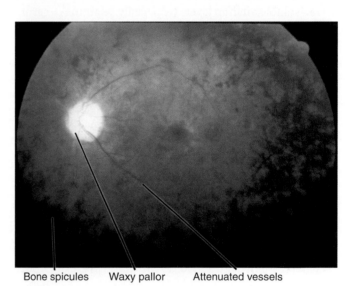

Bone spicules   Waxy pallor   Attenuated vessels

FIGURE 17–70

Retinitis pigmentosa demonstrating dense retinal pigment epithelial changes, optic disc pallor, and attenuated retinal vessels.

vision (tritanopic defect), and constricted visual fields. Retinitis pigmentosa is also associated with posterior subcapsular cataracts (39–72%), high myopia, astigmatism, keratoconus, and mild hearing loss (30%, excluding patients with Usher's syndrome). Fifty percent of female carriers with the X-linked form have a golden reflex in the posterior pole.

Differential diagnosis

The retinal pigmentary clumps that occur in retinitis pigmentosa are similar in appearance to the retinal changes in congenital rubella syndrome, syphilis, thioridazine and chloroquine drug toxicity, carcinoma-associated retinopathy, congenital stationary night blindness, vitamin A deficiency, atypical cytomegalovirus or herpesvirus chorioretinitis, trauma, diffuse unilateral subacute neuroretinitis, gyrate atrophy, and congenital hypertrophy of the RPE.

Evaluation

- The **history** should concentrate on family history of eye problems and early blindness, consanguinity, and hearing problems.
- The **eye exam** is performed with attention to visual acuity (normal or decreased), color vision (normal or decreased), visual field testing (mid peripheral ring scotoma progressing to total field loss, except for central islands that disappear late in the disease), lens (may have posterior subcapsular cataracts), vitreous (pigmented cells), and ophthalmoscopy (dark pigmentary clumps, bone spicules, vascular attenuation, disc pallor).
- Consider **lab tests**, including plasma ornithine levels, fat-soluble vitamin levels (especially vitamin A), serum lipoprotein electrophoresis (for Bassen–Kornzweig syndrome), cholesterol, triglycerides, VDRL, FTA-ABS, peripheral blood smears (acanthocytosis), and phytanic acid levels (for Refsum's disease).
- Consider **electrophysiologic testing**. The electro-retinogram is markedly reduced or absent and decreases 10% per year. It is abnormal in 90% of female carriers with the X-linked form. In addition, the electro-oculogram is abnormal, and dark adaptation causes elevated rod and cone thresholds.

Management

- There is no effective treatment for retinitis pigmentosa except in forms with treatable systemic diseases (see above).
- Correct any refractive error and prescribe dark glasses.
- Low-vision consultation for visual aids.
- For common forms of retinitis pigmentosa in patients >18 years of age, consider high-dose vitamin A therapy (15 000 IU PO qd of palmitate form slows the reduction of electroretinogram amplitudes) but avoid vitamin E. Liver function tests and serum retinol levels must be checked annually. This treatment is controversial and has not been tested in atypical forms of retinitis pigmentosa. The use of vitamin A in younger patients is even more controversial (age 6–10 years (vitamin A 5000 IU PO qd), age 10–15 years (vitamin A 10 000 IU PO qd)) and should be done in conjunction with a pediatrician.

Prognosis

The prognosis is usually poor, and patients become legally blind by the fourth decade of life.

Angioid Streaks

Definition

Angioid streaks are full-thickness breaks in a calcified, thickened Bruch's membrane that produce disruption of the overlying RPE.

Etiology

Angioid streaks can be idiopathic or associated with systemic diseases in 50% of cases. Systemic associations include pseudoxanthoma elasticum (60%; redundant skin folds in the neck, gastrointestinal bleeding, and hypertension), Paget's disease (8%; extraskeletal calcification, osteoarthritis, deafness, vertigo, increased serum alkaline phosphatase and urine calcium levels), senile elastosis, calcinosis, abetalipoproteinemia, sickle-cell disease (5%), thalassemia, hereditary spherocytosis, and Ehlers–Danlos syndrome (blue sclera, hyperextensible joints, and elastic skin). Angioid streaks are also associated with optic disc drusen, acromegaly, lead poisoning, Marfan's syndrome, and retinitis pigmentosa.

Symptoms

Angioid streaks are usually asymptomatic. Patients may have decreased vision or metamorphopsia if a CNV develops.

Signs

Angioid streaks appear as linear, irregular, deep, dark red-brown streaks radiating from the optic disc in a spoke-like pattern (Figure 17–71). The retina may also have a "peau d'orange" pigmentation, peripheral salmon spots, "histo-like" scars, and pigmentation around the

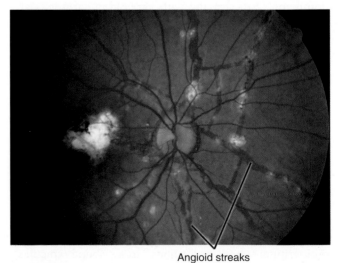

Angioid streaks

FIGURE 17–71
Angioid streaks appear as dark-red branching lines radiating from the optic nerve.

streaks. Patients with angioid streaks usually have normal vision. Decreased visual acuity and central or paracentral scotomas are seen with CNV that also produces sub-retinal hemorrhage/fluid and retinal pigment epithelial detachments.

Differential diagnosis

Angioid streaks can be confused with lacquer cracks seen in myopic degeneration, and choroidal rupture. The CNV can be mistaken for AMD.

Evaluation

- The **history** must focus on systemic diseases.
- The **eye exam** is performed with attention to visual acuity (normal or decreased), Amsler grid (usually normal, may have central distortion with CNV), and ophthalmoscopy (angioid streaks, may have CNV).
- Consider **lab tests** to rule out systemic associations, including sickle-cell prep, hemoglobin electrophoresis, serum alkaline phosphatase, serum lead levels, urine calcium, stool guaiac, and skin biopsy.
- Consider a **fluorescein angiogram** to evaluate for CNV if suspected clinically. If CNV is present, it usually occurs along the track of an angioid streak and has a granular pattern of hyperfluorescence.
- Consider **medical consultation** to rule out associated systemic diseases.

Management

- Most cases do not require any treatment and can be observed.
- Patients should be counseled to wear polycarbonate safety glasses because even mild, blunt trauma can cause hemorrhages or choroidal rupture.
- Treat CNV with focal laser photocoagulation similar to the MPS guidelines for juxta- and extrafoveal lesions, and PDT or anti-VEGF therapy for subfoveal lesions (see section on age-related macular degeneration, above).
- Treat any underlying medical condition.

Prognosis

The prognosis is good unless CNV develops, and then it is very poor because of the high recurrence rate. Minor trauma can cause rupture of Bruch's membrane, leading to hemorrhage or CNV.

Intermediate Uveitis/Pars Planitis

Definition

Intermediate uveitis is an inflammation of the pars plana and ciliary body. Pars planitis is a form of intermediate uveitis.

Epidemiology

Intermediate uveitis represents roughly 5–8% of all uveitis cases, with an incidence between 2 and 5:100 000. It primarily affects young adults and children, and is associated with multiple sclerosis (up to 15%) and sarcoidosis. The disease is rare in African Americans and Asians.

Symptoms

Most cases of intermediate uveitis present with bilateral decreased vision and floaters. Patients generally do not have a red eye, pain, or photophobia.

Signs

Intermediate uveitis primarily involves the vitreous cavity, producing fibrovascular exudates especially along the inferior pars plana ("snow-banking"), extensive vitreous cells (100% of cases), vitreous cellular aggregates ("snowballs") inferiorly, peripheral vasculitis, and CME (85% of cases), and minimal anterior-chamber cell and flare (Figure 17–72). Patients may develop neovascularization and vitreous hemorrhage in the pars plana exudate.

Differential diagnosis

The inflammatory exudates that occur in intermediate uveitis are similar to those seen in sarcoidosis, multiple sclerosis, Lyme disease, Behçet's disease, masquerade syndromes (especially lymphoma), syphilis, posterior uveitis, amyloidosis, familial exudative vitreoretinopathy, Irvine–Gass syndrome (CME following cataract surgery), toxocariasis, toxoplasmosis, candidiasis, fungal endophthalmitis, Eales' disease, Vogt–Koyanagi–Harada syndrome, and retinoblastoma.

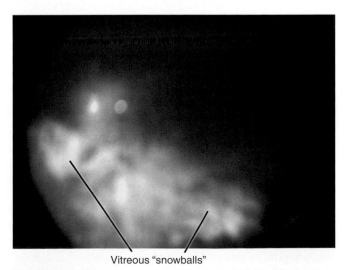

Vitreous "snowballs"

FIGURE 17–72

Pars planitis, demonstrating "snowballs" in the vitreous cavity.

Evaluation

- When gathering the **history** the patient should be questioned about systemic diseases and any previous episodes of inflammation.
- During the **eye exam**, specific attention should be directed to the anterior chamber (cell and flare), anterior vitreous (extensive cells), and ophthalmoscopy (snowballs, snowbanking, retinal vasculitis, CME).
- **Lab tests**, to narrow the differential diagnosis, include ACE, chest radiographs, chest CT scan, and serum lysozyme to rule out sarcoidosis; CBC to rule out masquerade syndromes; and VDRL, FTA-ABS, Lyme titers, toxocariasis and toxoplasmosis IgG and IgM serology to rule out infection.
- In patients with CME, the **fluorescein angiogram** demonstrates a petalloid pattern of late leakage.

Management

- Treatment is with steroids in multiple forms, including posterior subTenon's injection, systemic, and topical. The indication to administer steroids is when vision is reduced by CME or severe inflammation.
- Consider immunosuppressive agents for recalcitrant cases (i.e., cyclosporine, azathioprine, methotrexate, cytoxan).

Prognosis

The prognosis is variable since the visual outcome depends on the presence and degree of macular edema. Aggressive treatment of active inflammation is a key factor in determining a good outcome. Fifty-one percent of patients achieve 20/30 or better vision; however, 40–60% of cases will have a smoldering, chronic course with episodic exacerbations and remissions.

Posterior Uveitis

Posterior uveitis, by definition, is inflammation of the choroid. However, this term is generally used to describe any inflammation of the posterior segment, including vitritis, retinitis, and choroiditis. Posterior uveitis is caused by infections and inflammatory diseases, and can be mimicked by other disorders, known as masquerade syndromes.

INFECTIONS

Acute retinal necrosis

Acute retinal necrosis produces a fulminant retinitis and vitritis due to herpes zoster virus, herpes simplex virus, or, rarely, cytomegalovirus in healthy, as well as immunocompromised, individuals. Patients experience pain, decreased vision, and floaters often after a recent herpes simplex or zoster infection. Acute retinal necrosis

begins with small, well-demarcated areas of retinal necrosis outside the vascular arcades that enlarge very rapidly and circumferentially into large areas of white, retinal necrosis with retinal vascular occlusions and small satellite lesions (Figures 17–73 and 17–74). In the later cicatricial phase (after 1–3 months), retinal detachments with multiple holes and giant tears occur. Treatment consists of systemic or local antiviral agents, but even with treatment, acute retinal necrosis carries a poor visual prognosis (only 30% achieve >20/200 vision).

Candidiasis

Candida species (*C. albicans* and *C. tropicalis*) cause endogenous endophthalmitis in IV drug abusers and debilitated or immunocompromised individuals. These

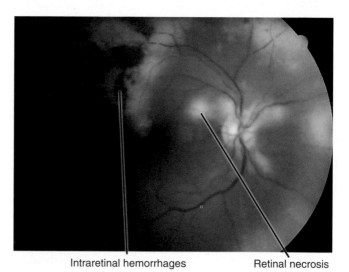

Intraretinal hemorrhages   Retinal necrosis

FIGURE 17–73
Acute retinal necrosis, demonstrating hemorrhage and yellow-white patches of necrosis.

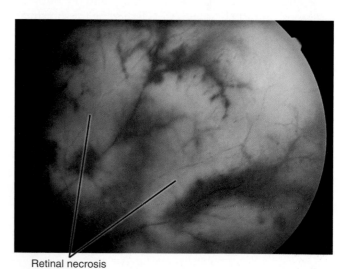

Retinal necrosis

FIGURE 17–74
Same patient as shown in Figure 17–73, 2 days later, demonstrating rapid progression with confluence of lesions.

patients note decreased vision and floaters. The infection produces white, fluffy, chorioretinal infiltrates and overlying vitreous haze, vitreous "puff-balls," anterior-chamber cell and flare, hypopyon, Roth spots, and hemorrhages (Figures 17–75 and 17–76). The eye infection is treated with vitrectomy and intraocular injection of antifungal medication and steroid. Systemic antifungal agents are used to treat disseminated disease.

Cytomegalovirus

Cytomegalovirus causes the most common retinal infection in AIDS (15–46%), especially when the CD4 count is <50 cells/mm^3. Patients are usually asymptomatic, but may have floaters, paracentral scotomas, metamorphopsia, and decreased acuity. The characteristic finding is a hemorrhagic retinitis with thick, yellow-white retinal necrosis, vascular sheathing, retinal hemorrhages, mild anterior-chamber cell and flare, and vitreous cells (Figures 17–77 and 17–78). This clinical appearance has been termed "pizza-pie" fundus. Cytomegalovirus retinitis can also have a "brush-fire" appearance with an indolent, granular, yellow advancing border and peripheral atrophic region. Retinal detachments due to small, peripheral breaks often occur in the

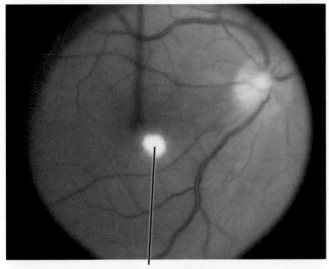

Candida albicans chorioretinal infiltrate
FIGURE 17–75
Candidiasis, demonstrating white, fluffy, chorioretinal infiltrate.

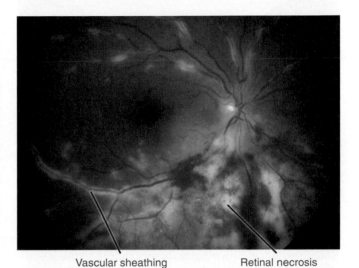

Vascular sheathing   Retinal necrosis
FIGURE 17–77
Cytomegalovirus retinitis, demonstrating patchy necrotic lesions, hemorrhage, and vascular sheathing.

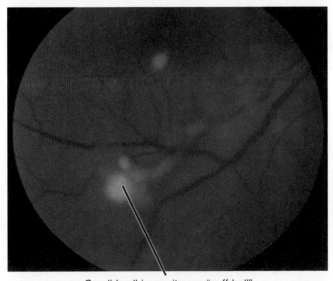

Candida albicans vitreous "puff-ball"
FIGURE 17–76
Vitreous "puff-ball" due to *Candida albicans* endogenous endophthalmitis.

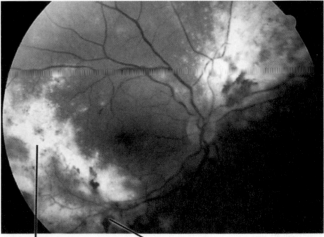

Retinal necrosis   Retinal hemorrhage
FIGURE 17–78
Cytomegalovirus retinitis with larger areas of necrosis and hemorrhage.

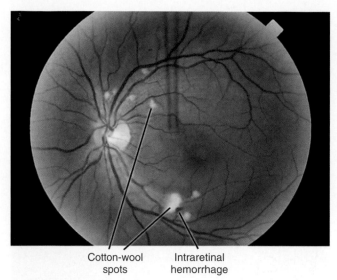

Cotton-wool   Intraretinal
spots   hemorrhage

FIGURE 17–79
Human immunodeficiency virus retinopathy, demonstrating cotton wool spots and one intraretinal hemorrhage.

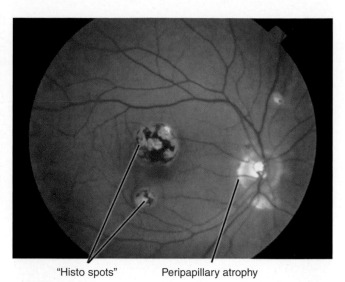

"Histo spots"   Peripapillary atrophy

FIGURE 17–80
Presumed ocular histoplasmosis syndrome, demonstrating macular and peripapillary lesions.

atrophic areas. Treatment consists of systemic or local ganciclovir, foscarnet, and/or cidofovir.

Human immunodeficiency virus

Human immunodeficiency virus infection can produce an asymptomatic, non-progressive microangiopathy characterized by multiple cotton wool spots (50–70%), Roth spots (40%), retinal hemorrhages, and microaneurysms in the posterior pole that resolves without treatment within 1–2 months (Figure 17–79). It is seen in up to 50% of patients and is not related to opportunistic infections. No treatment is necessary.

Presumed ocular histoplasmosis syndrome

Presumed ocular histoplasmosis syndrome is caused by the dimorphic fungus *Histoplasma capsulatum*, which is endemic in the Ohio and Mississippi river valleys. The condition produces small, round, yellow-brown, punched-out chorioretinal lesions ("histo spots") in the midperiphery and posterior pole, and juxtapapillary atrophic changes (Figures 17–80 and 17–81). It is usually asymptomatic and does not require treatment unless a CNV develops.

Syphilis (luetic chorioretinitis)

Secondary syphilis (6 weeks to 6 months after primary infection), due to the spirochete *Treponema pallidum*, produces an extensive iritis, retinitis, and vitritis (panuveitis). Signs of infection include anterior-chamber cell and flare, keratic precipitates, vitritis, multifocal, yellow-white chorioretinal infiltrates, salt-and-pepper pigmentary retinal changes, flame-shaped retinal hemorrhages, and vascular sheathing (Figures 17–82 and 17–83). Syphilis has been called the "great mimic,"

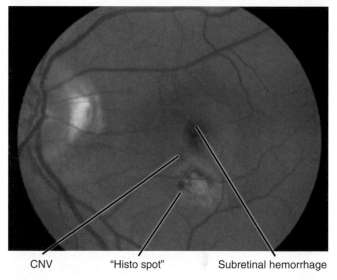

CNV   "Histo spot"   Subretinal hemorrhage

FIGURE 17–81
Presumed ocular histoplasmosis syndrome, demonstrating choroidal neovascular membrane and "histo spot".

because it can resemble many other diseases. Standard syphilis treatment with penicillin G (2.4 million U IV q4h for 10–14 days, then 2.4 million U IM every week for 3 weeks) should be instituted and serum rapid plasma reagin or VDRL can be used to monitor treatment efficacy.

Toxoplasmosis

Toxoplasmosis infection can either be acquired (eating poorly cooked meat) or congenital (transplacental transmission, which accounts for 90% of ocular disease (see Ch. 6)). In the eye, the parasite *Toxoplasma gondii* produces a necrotizing retinitis. Acquired toxoplasmosis

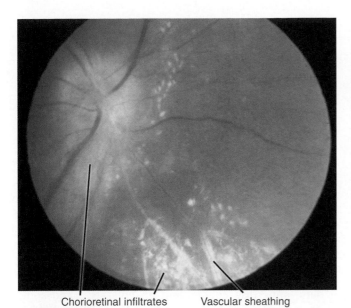

Chorioretinal infiltrates   Vascular sheathing

FIGURE 17–82
Multifocal, yellow-white chorioretinal infiltrates and vascular sheathing in a patient with luetic chorioretinitis.

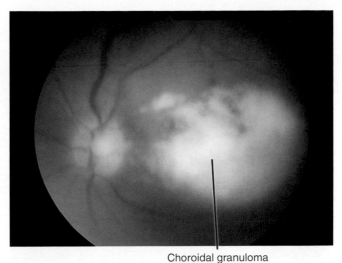

Choroidal granuloma

FIGURE 17–84
Tuberculosis with choroidal tubercle appearing as a large white subretinal mass.

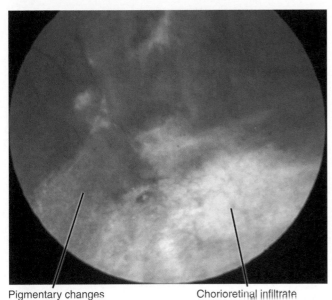

Pigmentary changes   Chorioretinal infiltrate

FIGURE 17–83
Late luetic chorioretinitis with pigmentary changes and resolving chorioretinal infiltrate.

(especially in immunocompromised patients) and reactivated congenital lesions produce decreased vision, photophobia, floaters, vascular sheathing, full-thickness retinal necrosis, a fluffy yellow-white retinal lesion (solitary in acquired and adjacent to old scars in congenital) with overlying vitreous reaction, and anterior-chamber cell and flare (see Figure 6–19 in Ch. 6). Treatment, which is typically reserved for vision-threatening lesions, consists of pyrimethamine (Daraprim), folinic acid (leucovorin), and one of the following: sulfadiazine, clindamycin, clarithromycin, azithromycin, or atovaquone. For periph-

eral or non-sight-threatening lesions, clindamycin and trimethoprim–sulfamethoxazole (Bactrim) can be used. There is a poorer prognosis with larger lesions, recurrence, longer duration, and proximity to the fovea and optic nerve.

Tuberculosis

Tuberculosis, due to the *Mycobacterium tuberculosis* bacilli, produces multifocal, light-colored choroidal granulomas (Figure 17–84). Ocular infection is commonly associated with constitutional symptoms such as malaise, night sweats, and pulmonary symptoms. Treatment is with standard antituberculosis medications, including isoniazid and rifampin for 6–9 months.

INFLAMMATORY SYNDROMES

White dot syndromes

The white-dot syndromes are a group of inflammatory disorders that result in discrete yellow-white retinal lesions, usually in young adults. They are differentiated by history, appearance, laterality, and diagnostic imaging findings.

Acute posterior multifocal placoid pigment epitheliopathy produces multiple, round, discrete, large, flat gray-yellow lesions throughout the posterior pole that become well-demarcated scars (Figure 17–85). The condition is usually bilateral and there is minimal vitreous cell. It causes a rapid loss of central or paracentral vision in 20–30-year-old, healthy adults after a viral prodrome. There is no sex predilection. Rarely, there is associated disc edema, cerebral vasculitis, head-

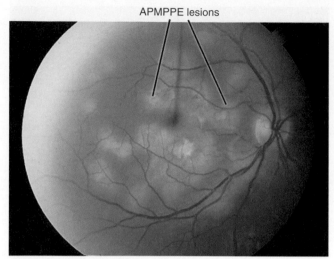

FIGURE 17–85
Acute posterior multifocal placoid pigment epitheliopathy, demonstrating multiple posterior pole lesions.

ache, dysacousia, and tinnitus. There is no effective treatment, but the syndrome resolves spontaneously and visual recovery occurs within 6 months (80% of patients achieve better than 20/50 vision).

Birdshot choroidopathy (vitiliginous chorioretinitis) produces multiple, small, discrete, ovoid, creamy yellow-white spots scattered like a birdshot blast from a shotgun in the midperiphery of the retina that spares the macula (Figure 17–86). It is associated with mild vitritis, mild anterior-chamber cell and flare (in 25% of cases), CME, and disc edema and is usually bilateral. It occurs in 50–60-year-old females (70%) and almost exclusively in Caucasians. It is associated with human leukocyte antigen (HLA)-A29 (90–98%). Patients notice mild blurred vision and floaters. Birdshot is a chronic, slowly progressive, recurring disease that has a variable visual prognosis. Treatment with steroids and other immunosuppressive agents is reserved for patients with decreased visual acuity, significant inflammation, or complications such as CME, CNV, epiretinal membranes, or macular holes.

Multiple evanescent white-dot syndrome produces multiple, small, discrete, gray-white spots at the level of the RPE in the posterior pole, sparing the fovea (Figure 17–87). The syndrome presents with sudden unilateral acute visual loss, paracentral or central scotomas, and photopsias, mainly in 20–30-year-old, healthy females (4:1) after a viral prodrome (seen in 50% of cases). Patients may also have a positive RAPD, mild vitritis, mild anterior-chamber cell and flare, optic disc edema, and an enlarged blind spot. This condition usually resolves spontaneously with recovery of vision in 3–10 weeks and disappearance of the white dots, so treatment is not required.

Behçet's disease

Behçet's disease classically presents with a triad of signs, including aphthous oral ulcers, genital ulcers, and bilateral non-granulomatous uveitis (Figure 17–88). It produces a severe and recurring uveitis with hypopyon, iris atrophy, posterior synechiae, optic disc edema, attenuation of arterioles, severe vitritis, CME, and an occlusive retinal vasculitis with retinal hemorrhages and edema (Figures 17–89 and 17–90). Patients note photophobia, pain, red eye, and decreased vision. Lab tests are positive for Behçetine skin test (prick the skin with a sterile needle, and the formation of a pustule within a

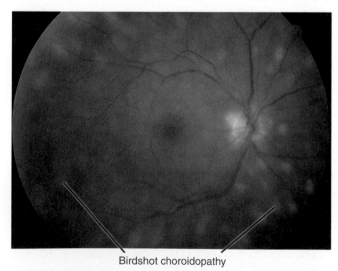

FIGURE 17–86
Birdshot choroidopathy/vitiliginous chorioretinitis, demonstrating scattered fundus lesions.

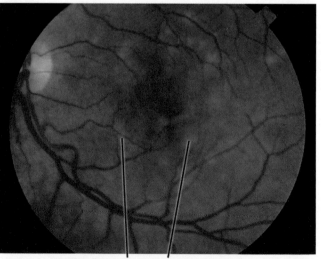

FIGURE 17–87
Multiple evanescent white-dot syndrome, demonstrating faint white spots.

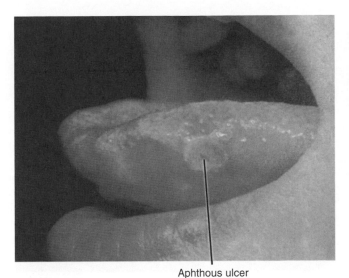

FIGURE 17–88
Behçet's disease, demonstrating aphthous oral ulcers on tongue.

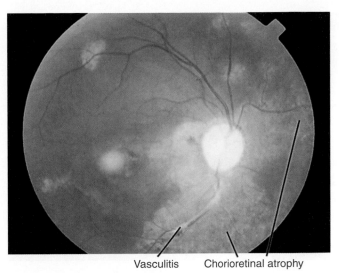

Vasculitis   Chorioretinal atrophy

FIGURE 17–90
Behçet's disease, demonstrating old vasculitis with sclerosed vessels and chorioretinal atrophy.

few minutes is a positive result), ANA, elevated ESR, C-reactive protein, acute-phase reactants, and serum proteins, but are not diagnostic. Treatment with steroids and immunosuppressive drugs is often not successful. The visual prognosis is poor, and frequent relapses are common.

Sarcoidosis

Sarcoidosis is a common cause of granulomatous panuveitis. It is more severe in young African Americans, but can affect elderly, Caucasian women. There is a bimodal age distribution with peaks between 20–30 years and 50–60 years. Most patients are asymptomatic, but the disease follows a chronic, relapsing course and is

potentially fatal. Ocular findings include retinal vasculitis, vascular sheathing, periphlebitis (candle wax drippings), vitreous snowballs (string of pearls), yellow-white retinal/choroidal granulomas, anterior-chamber cell and flare, mutton-fat keratic precipitates, Koeppe and Busacca iris nodules, and macular edema (Figures 17–91 and 17–92). Systemic findings consist of hilar adenopathy, pulmonary parenchymal involvement, pulmonary fibrosis, erythema nodosum, subcutaneous nodules, lupus pernio (purple lupus), and lymphadenopathy. The pathologic hallmark of sarcoidosis is non-caseating granulomas. Lab tests include ACE, serum lysozyme, chest radiographs, and gallium scan. Treatment consists of steroids and immuno-suppressive agents.

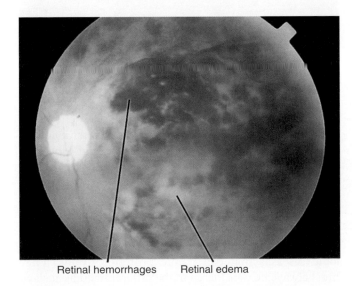

Retinal hemorrhages   Retinal edema

FIGURE 17–89
Behçet's disease, demonstrating acute vasculitis with hemorrhage.

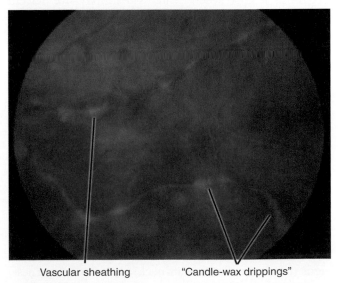

Vascular sheathing   "Candle-wax drippings"

FIGURE 17–91
Sarcoidosis with periphlebitis and vascular sheathing.

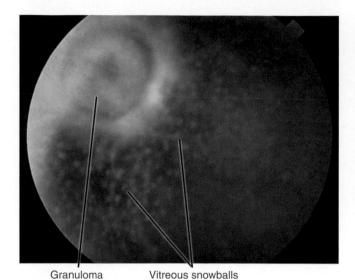

Granuloma   Vitreous snowballs

FIGURE 17–92

Sarcoidosis, demonstrating peripheral granuloma with overlying vitritis and vitreous snowballs.

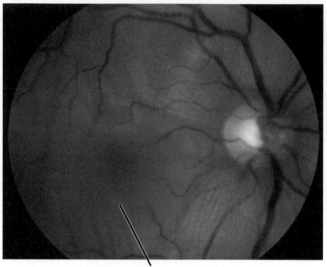

Serous retinal detachment

FIGURE 17–93

Early sympathetic ophthalmia, demonstrating serous retinal detachment.

Sympathetic ophthalmia

Sympathetic ophthalmia is a rare, bilateral, immune-mediated, mild to severe granulomatous uveitis that occurs 2 weeks to 3 months (80%) after penetrating eye trauma or surgery. Fundus exam is notable for scattered, multifocal, yellow-white subretinal infiltrates (Dalen–Fuchs' nodules, 50%) with overlying serous retinal detachments, vitritis, and papillitis (Figures 17–93 and 17–94). Patients report transient obscuration of vision, photophobia, pain, and blurred vision. Treatment consists of steroids and immunosuppressive agents. Sympathetic ophthalmia has a chronic, recurring course, but the prognosis is good when treated early. Sixty-five percent of patients regain >20/60 vision after treatment.

Vogt–Koyanagi–Harada syndrome/ Harada's disease

Vogt–Koyanagi–Harada syndrome is a bilateral inflammatory disorder that occurs mainly in pigmented individuals (Native Americans, African Americans, Asians, and Hispanics) 20–40 years old. The ocular findings (**Harada's disease**) include yellow-white exudates at the level of the RPE, bullous serous retinal detachments (75%), and focal retinal pigment epithelial detachments (Figure 17–95). It is also associated with anterior-chamber cell and flare, mutton-fat keratic precipitates, posterior synechiae, vitritis, choroidal folds, choroidal thickening, Dalen–Fuchs'–like nodules, and optic disc hyperemia. Systemic manifestations such as meningeal signs (headache, nausea, stiff neck), dysacousis (deafness, tinnitus), and skin changes (poliosis, alopecia, vitiligo) may occur (**Vogt–Koyanagi–Harada syndrome**). Treat-

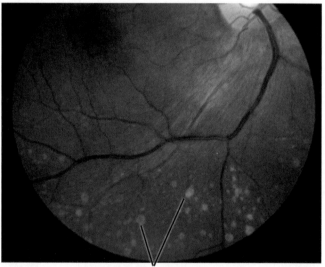

Dalen-Fuchs' nodules

FIGURE 17–94

Dalen–Fuchs' nodules in a patient with sympathetic ophthalmia.

ment consists of steroids and immunosuppressive agents. Although recurrences are common, the visual prognosis is good.

Masquerade Syndromes

Masquerade syndromes are systemic and ophthalmologic diseases that can mimic posterior uveitis. They must always be considered in the differential diagnosis of uveitis since they can be life-threatening. The masquerade syndromes can be divided by etiology.

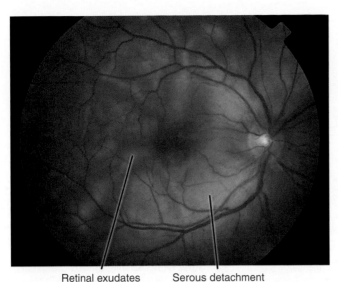

Retinal exudates   Serous detachment

FIGURE 17–95
Vogt–Koyanagi–Harada syndrome with multiple serous retinal detachments.

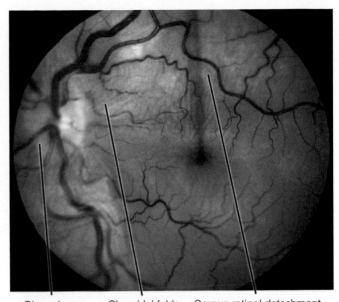

Disc edema   Choroidal folds   Serous retinal detachment

FIGURE 17–96
Posterior scleritis with orange-red choroidal elevation superiorly, serous retinal detachments, vitritis, and mild optic disc edema.

MALIGNANCIES

Intraocular lymphoma

This rare, lethal malignancy is typically a non-Hodgkin's large B-cell lymphoma of the eye and central nervous system. It usually affects older adults (median age of 50–60 years) and presents with blurred vision and floaters due to vitritis. On examination, the vitreous contains large clumps of cells and there are multifocal, large, yellow, subretinal infiltrative lesions. If this diagnosis is suspected, then a diagnostic pars plana vitrectomy and vitreous biopsy to obtain tissue samples should be performed by a retina specialist (see primary intraocular lymphoma section, below).

Other malignancies

Leukemia, malignant melanoma, retinoblastoma, and metastatic tumors can also masquerade as uveitis.

ENDOPHTHALMITIS

Both chronic postoperative endophthalmitis and endogenous endophthalmitis can present as a masquerade syndrome (see Ch. 12).

NON-MALIGNANT/NON-INFECTIOUS DISORDERS

These masquerade syndromes are characterized by the presence of intraocular cells secondary to non-inflammatory conditions. Although rare, these disorders include rhegmatogenous retinal detachment, retinitis pigmentosa, intraocular foreign body, ocular ischemic syndrome, and juvenile xanthogranuloma.

Posterior Scleritis

Posterior scleritis is an inflammation of the sclera that usually occurs in 20–30-year-old females and is associated with collagen vascular diseases, rheumatoid arthritis, relapsing polychondritis, inflammatory bowel disease, Wegener's granulomatosis, and syphilis. Patients note pain, photophobia, and decreased vision. The scleral thickening produces an orange-red elevation of the choroid and RPE with overlying serous retinal detachments, choroidal folds, vitritis, and optic disc edema (Figure 17–96). Posterior scleritis can also cause induced hyperopia, proptosis, limitation of ocular motility, and angle-closure glaucoma due to anterior rotation of the ciliary body with forward displacement of the lens. B-scan ultrasonography shows a characteristic appearance of diffuse scleral thickening (echolucent space between the choroid and Tenon's capsule) and the "T-sign" in the peripapillary region from scleral thickening around the echolucent optic nerve (Figure 17–97). Treatment consists of steroids and NSAIDs. Immunosuppressive agents may be required in refractory cases.

Tumors

CHOROIDAL HEMANGIOMA

A choroidal hemangioma is a vascular tumor that is usually asymptomatic. It occurs in two forms:

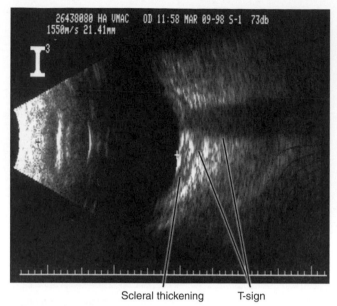

Scleral thickening   T-sign

FIGURE 17–97

B-scan ultrasound of same patient as shown in Figure 17–96, demonstrating scleral thickening and the characteristic peripapillary T-sign.

1. The tumor is usually unilateral, well circumscribed, solitary, round, slightly elevated (<3 mm), and orange-red in appearance (Figure 17–98). It is typically located in the posterior pole with an overlying serous retinal detachment. There are no extraocular associations.

2. The tumor produces a diffuse, reddish, choroidal thickening described as "tomato-catsup" fundus that occurs in patients with Sturge–Weber syndrome (Figure 17–99).

Both types can cause exudative retinal detachments (50%). Patients may have reduced vision, meta-

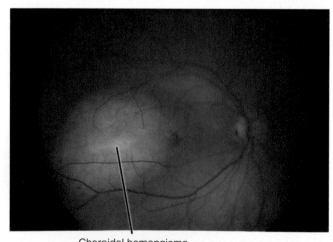

Choroidal hemangioma

FIGURE 17–98

Choroidal hemangioma (discrete type) appearing as an elevated orange lesion in the macula.

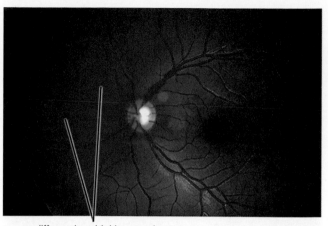

diffuse choroidal hemangioma

FIGURE 17–99

Encephalotrigeminal angiomatosis demonstrating tomato-catsup fundus appearance of a diffuse choroidal hemangioma.

morphopsia, micropsia from foveal distortion due to an underlying tumor or accumulation of subretinal fluid. On B-scan ultrasonography, the mass has moderate elevation and high internal reflectivity, often with an overlying serous retinal detachment. The fluorescein angiogram shows early filling of intrinsic tumor vessels or feeder vessels, progressive hyperfluorescence during the transit views, and late leakage in a multiloculated pattern. Patients should be observed if asymptomatic, especially if the tumor is located extrafoveally and there is no subretinal fluid. In addition, long-standing subfoveal lesions with a poor chance of visual recovery are also observed. The decision to treat with laser photocoagulation, PDT with verteporfin, transpupillary thermotherapy, or I-125 plaque brachytherapy is individualized based on the extent of symptoms, loss of vision, and potential for visual recovery. The aim of treatment is to induce tumor atrophy with resolution of subretinal fluid and tumor-induced foveal distortion without destroying function of the overlying retina. The goal is not to obliterate the tumor.

CHOROIDAL NEVUS

A choroidal nevus is a dark gray-brown pigmented, flat or slightly elevated lesion (<2 mm). It often exhibits overlying drusen and a hypopigmented ring around the base (Figures 17–100 and 17–101). A nevus is usually non-progressive, but can grow during puberty. B-scan ultrasonography demonstrates a flat or minimally elevated mass with medium to high internal reflectivity. Growth in an adult should be monitored carefully, and the patient should be reevaluated frequently with serial photographs, ultrasonography, and clinical examination for any growth that would be suspicious for malignant melanoma at 1, 3, 6, 9, and 12 months, and then on an annual or semi-annual basis if there is no growth.

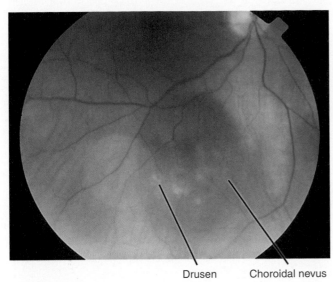

Drusen   Choroidal nevus

FIGURE 17–100
Large choroidal nevus (nevoma) with overlying drusen.

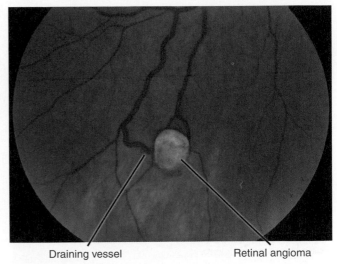

Draining vessel   Retinal angioma

FIGURE 17–102
Retinal angioma with feeder and draining vessels in patient with von Hippel–Lindau syndrome.

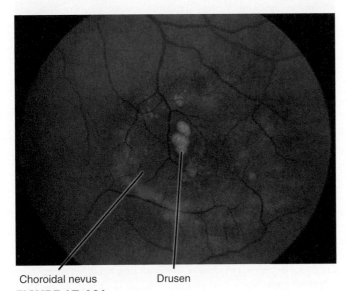

Choroidal nevus   Drusen

FIGURE 17–101
Flat choroidal nevus with overlying drusen indicating chronicity

Multiple nevi may be seen in patients with neurofibromatosis. Characteristics of suspicious nevi include growth, tumor thickness (>2 mm), visual symptoms, overlying orange pigment, subretinal fluid, and proximity to the optic nerve head. Ten percent of suspicious lesions become malignant melanoma.

CAPILLARY HEMANGIOMA

A capillary hemangioma is a benign vascular neoplasm arising from the inner retina and extending toward the retinal surface. There are two forms of capillary hemangioma:

1. The tumor is sporadic, non-hereditary, and unilateral with no systemic associations. There are usually no feeder vessels.
2. The tumor is hereditary, bilateral (50%), multifocal, and associated with multiple systemic abnormalities (von Hippel–Lindau syndrome). Classically, it has dilated feeder and draining vessels. Patients should have a medical consultation to evaluate for systemic capillary hemangiomas.

Both types appear as a red, pink, or gray lesion that enlarges as capillary channels within the tumor proliferate. These new vessels leak fluid, causing exudates around the tumor and often an overlying serous retinal detachment (Figures 17–102 and 17–103). The fluorescein angiogram shows early filling of the tumor with late leakage. No treatment is recommended for sporadic tumors unless vision is affected, then cryotherapy, photocoagulation, and/or plaque brachytherapy can be considered.

CAVERNOUS HEMANGIOMA

A cavernous hemangioma is a rare vascular tumor containing saccular, intraretinal aneurysms filled with dark venous blood ("cluster-of-grapes" appearance) (Figure 17–104). Fine epiretinal membranes may grow over the tumor. It is usually unilateral and develops in the second to third decade of life with a slight female predilection (60%). There is usually no fluid exudation. The fluorescein angiogram demonstrates characteristic hyperfluorescent saccules with fluid levels. The tumor is usually asymptomatic and non-progressive, so treatment is not required.

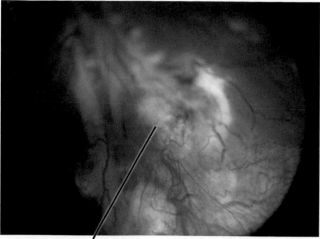

Retinal angioma

FIGURE 17–103
Capillary hemangioma in a patient with von Hippel disease, demonstrating the characteristic pink lesion with a dilated, tortuous feeder vessel; there is also some surrounding exudate.

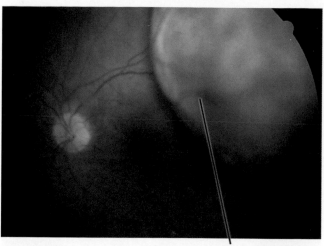

Choroidal malignant melanoma

FIGURE 17–105
Choroidal malignant melanoma, demonstrating elevated dome-shaped tumor.

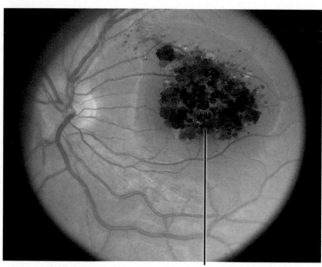

Cavernous hemangioma

FIGURE 17–104
Cavernous hemangioma with "cluster-of-grapes" appearance.

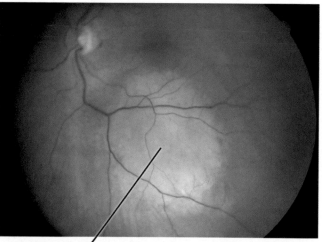

Choroidal malignant melanoma

FIGURE 17–106
Choroidal amelanotic melanoma, demonstrating hypopigmented subretinal mass.

CHOROIDAL MALIGNANT MELANOMA

A choroidal malignant melanoma is the most common primary intraocular malignancy in adults. It has a focal, darkly pigmented or amelanotic, dome- or collar-button-shaped (after breaking through Bruch's membrane) appearance that is frequently associated with an overlying serous retinal detachment and lipofuscin (orange spots) (Figures 17–105 and 17–106). Most melanomas have episcleral sentinel vessels visible on external examination. The **Collaborative Ocular Melanoma Study (COMS)** distinguished the lesions by size: small, medium, and large (Box 17–1). B-scan ultrasonography should be performed in all patients and shows a dome-shaped (60% in COMS) or collar-button-shaped (27% in COMS) mass that is usually >2.5 mm (95%) in thickness with low to medium internal reflectivity, regular internal structure, solid consistency, echo attenuation, acoustic hollowness within the tumor, choroidal excavation, and orbital shadowing (Figure 17–107). A fluorescein angiogram can also be performed and reveals a characteristic double circulation due to the intrinsic tumor circulation in large tumors and late staining of the lesion with multiple pinpoint hyperfluorescent hot spots. All patients should have medical and oncology consultations to rule out metastasis, which is most commonly to the liver, lung, bone, skin, and central nervous system.

Collaborative Ocular Melanoma Study (COMS)

- **Small lesions** (1–3 mm apical height, 5–16 mm basal diameter): patients with tumors not large enough to be randomized to treatment in the study were followed. There was a 6% all-cause mortality at 5 years and 14.9% all-cause mortality at 8 years. There was a 1% melanoma mortality at 5 years and 3.8% at 8 years.
- **Medium lesions** (2.5–10 mm apical height and ≤16 mm longest basal diameter): patients with medium tumors were randomized to enucleation versus iodine-125 brachytherapy. There was a 34% all-cause mortality for enucleation and 34% all-cause mortality for iodine-125 brachytherapy at 10 years. Metastatic mortality occurred in 17% after enucleation and 17% after iodine-125 brachytherapy at 10 years.
- **Large lesions** (apical height ≥2 mm and >16 mm longest basal diameter *or* >10 mm apical height, regardless of basal diameter *or* >8 mm apical height if <2 mm from the optic disc): patients with large tumors all received enucleation and were randomized to either pre-enucleation external-beam radiation therapy (PERT) or not. There was a 61% all-cause mortality for enucleation and 61% all-cause mortality for PERT/enucleation at 10 years. Metastasis occurred in 62%. There was an additional 21% suspected based on imaging and ancillary testing. Metastatic mortality was seen in 39% after enucleation and 42% after PERT/enucleation at 10 years.

Factors predictive of metastasis include the presence of epithelioid cells, high number of mitoses, extrascleral extension, increased tumor thickness, ciliary body involvement, tumor growth, and proximity to the optic disc.

CHOROIDAL METASTASES

Choroidal metastases are the most common intraocular malignancy in adults. They appear as creamy yellow-white lesions with mottled pigment clumping (leopard spots) with low to medium elevation (Figures 17–108 and 17–109). There is often an overlying serous retinal detachment. Choroidal metastases have a predilection for the posterior pole and can be multifocal and bilateral (20%). B-scan ultrasonography should be performed in all patients and reveals flat or mildly elevated mass(es) with irregular surface, medium to high internal reflectivity, overlying serous retinal detachment, no orbital shadowing or acoustically silent zone. A fluorescein angiogram can be considered and shows early hypofluorescence with pinpoint hyperfluorescence that increases in later views. Two-thirds of metastatic lesions originate from a known primary. The most common primary tumors for females are breast (metastasize late), lung, gastrointestinal tract and pancreas, skin melanoma, and other rare sources. The most common primary tumors for males are lung (metastasize early), unknown primary, gastrointestinal tract and pancreas, prostate, renal cell, and skin melanoma. Ocular involvement is from hematogenous spread. Thus, all patients must have an oncology consultation for a metastatic work-up and lab tests, including liver function tests, serum chemistry analysis, isotope bone scan, and chest radiographs. Treatment depends on the clinical situation, and options

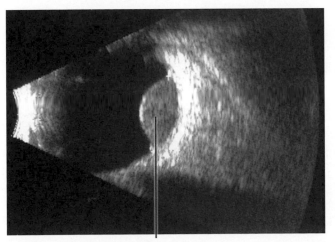

Choroidal malignant melanoma

FIGURE 17–107
B-scan ultrasound of same patient as shown in Figure 17–106, demonstrating dome-shaped choroidal mass.

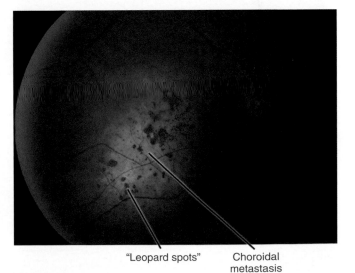

"Leopard spots"   Choroidal metastasis

FIGURE 17–108
Choroidal metastasis with leopard-spot appearance (lung carcinoma).

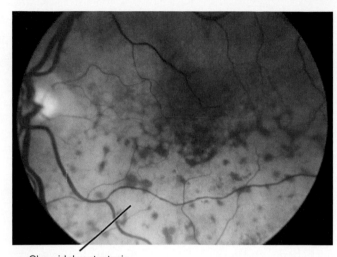

Choroidal metastasis

FIGURE 17–109
Metastatic breast carcinoma with yellow, creamy posterior pole lesion.

include enucleation, laser photocoagulation, radiation therapy, brachytherapy, and chemotherapy. The prognosis is very poor due to rapid growth, with a median survival of 8.5 months from the time of diagnosis.

PRIMARY INTRAOCULAR LYMPHOMA

Primary intraocular lymphoma produces anterior uveitis, vitritis, retinal vasculitis, CME, creamy yellow pigment epithelial detachments, hypopigmented retinal pigment epithelial lesions with overlying serous retinal detachments, and disc edema. Most cases are bilateral and usually occur in the sixth to seventh decade of life. Patients present with decreased vision and floaters. Primary intraocular lymphoma is associated with central nervous system involvement and dementia. Medical and oncology consultations should be obtained in all patients with lumbar puncture for cytology, head magnetic resonance imaging scan, and if the diagnosis is in doubt a diagnostic pars plana vitrectomy to obtain a vitreous biopsy for histopathologic and cytologic analysis. Treatment consists of chemotherapy and radiation. This malignancy carries a poor prognosis, with death within 2 years of diagnosis.

Differential Diagnosis of Common Ocular Symptoms

Blurred vision: there are many causes of blurred or decreased vision, so to narrow the differential diagnosis, it is important to characterize further the visual loss in terms of rapidity of onset, duration, central versus peripheral vision, distance versus near vision, monocular versus binocular, and other associated symptoms (i.e., none, pain, red eye, tearing, flashes of light, headache, other neurologic symptoms).

- **Sudden loss of vision**: ophthalmic artery occlusion, retinal vascular occlusion (central will cause profound loss, branch will cause visual field defect), wet macular degeneration (usually central loss, peripheral vision preserved), macular hole (usually central loss, peripheral vision preserved), retinal detachment, vitreous hemorrhage, hyphema, acute angle closure (painful), central corneal epithelial defect (blurry vision and very painful; i.e., abrasion, recurrent erosion, herpes simplex keratitis).
- **Gradual loss of vision**: optic neuropathy, optic neuritis (pain with eye movements), glaucoma, dry macular degeneration, macular edema, diabetic retinopathy, central serous retinopathy, chronic retinal detachment, uveitis (mild pain/photophobia), cataract (may also cause glare from bright lights), corneal edema, corneal dystrophy, change in refractive error.
- **Transient loss of vision (<24 hours)**: amaurosis fugax (transient ischemic attack), vertebrobasilar insufficiency, migraine, papilledema, presyncopal episode.
- **Visual field defect**: stroke, optic neuropathy, branch retinal vascular occlusion, chronic glaucoma, retinal detachment.

Eye pain: patients with ocular discomfort must be asked about the character of their pain.

- **Superficial/foreign-body sensation/itch/burn**: usually due to anterior ocular structures, including corneal or conjunctival foreign body, pingueculitis, inflamed pterygium, corneal abrasion, recurrent erosion, keratitis, dry-eye syndrome, conjunctivitis, blepharitis.
- **Deep/ache**: uveitis, angle closure, scleritis, myositis, optic neuritis, cranial nerve palsy, orbital lesion (idiopathic orbital inflammation, cellulitis, mass).

Tearing: dry eye, trichiasis, ectropion, conjunctivitis, nasolacrimal duct obstruction, dacryocystitis, keratitis, corneal or conjunctival foreign body, blepharitis.

Discharge: conjunctivitis, nasolacrimal duct obstruction, dacryocystitis, canaliculitis, corneal ulcer, blepharitis.

Flashes of light: retinal tear/detachment, posterior vitreous detachment, migraine, optic neuritis.

Red eye: the common causes and associated findings of a red eye are listed in Table A.1.

TABLE A–1

Common Causes and Associated Findings of a Red Eye							
Diagnosis	Vision	Redness	Pain	Discharge	Cornea	Intraocular pressure	Pupil
Conjunctivitis	Normal	Diffuse, superficial	Itch or foreign body	Watery, sticky, or purulent	May have punctate staining	Normal	Normal
Subconjunctival hemorrhage	Normal	Bright red, confluent	None	None	Normal	Normal	Normal
Corneal abrasion	May be blurred	Diffuse or ciliary flush	Sharp, foreign body	Tearing	Staining defect	Normal	Normal
Episcleritis	Normal	Often sectoral	Irritation	None	Normal	Normal	Normal
Scleritis	Normal	Deep, violaceous	Tender, deep ache	None	Normal	Normal	Normal
Angle-closure glaucoma	Decreased	Ciliary flush	Severe	None	Cloudy, edema	Very high	Mid dilated
Uveitis	May be blurred	Ciliary flush	Ache, photophobia	None	May have keratic precipitates	Normal, low, or high	Small

Further Reading

General Texts

Albert D M, Jakobiec F A. Principles and practice of ophthalmology, 2nd edn. W B Saunders, Philadelphia.

Friedman N J, Trattler W B, Kaiser P K. 2005 Review of ophthalmology. Elsevier, Philadelphia.

Goldberg S, Trattler W. 2005 Ophthalmology made ridiculously simple, 3rd edn. MedMaster, Miami.

Kaiser P K, Friedman N J. 2004 The Massachusetts Eye & Ear Infirmary's illustrated manual of ophthalmology, 2nd edn. W B Saunders, Philadelphia.

Kanski J J. 2003 Clinical ophthalmology, 5th edn. Butterworth-Heinemann, Philadelphia.

Mannis M J, MacSai M S, Huntley A C. 1996 Eye and skin disease. Lippincott-Raven, Philadelphia.

Newell F W. 1996 Ophthalmology principles and concepts, 8th edn. Mosby, St Louis.

Roy F H. 2002 Ocular differential diagnosis, 7th edn. Lippincott-Williams and Wilkins, Philadelphia.

Spaeth G L. 2003 Ophthalmic surgery: principles and practice, 3rd edn. W B Saunders, Philadelphia.

Spalton D J, Hitchings R A, Hunter P A. 1994 Atlas of clinical ophthalmology, 2nd edn. Mosby, St Louis.

Tabbara K F. 1995 Infections of the eye, 2nd edn. Little, Brown Medical Division, Boston.

Tasman W, Jaeger E A. 2001 Duane's clinical ophthalmology. W B Saunders, Philadelphia.

Vaughan D, Asbury T. 2003 General ophthalmology, 16th edn. Appleton-Lange, Norwalk.

Weingeist T A, Gold D H. 2001 Color atlas of the eye in systemic disease, 3rd edn. Lippincott-Williams and Wilkins, Philadelphia.

Yanoff M, Duker J S. 2004 Ophthalmology, 2nd edn. Mosby, St Louis.

Chapter 1: Ocular Anatomy, Physiology, and Embryology

American Academy of Ophthalmology. 2006 Fundamentals and principles of ophthalmology, vol. 2. AAO, San Francisco.

Kaufman P L, Alm A. 2003 Adler's physiology of the eye, 10th edn. Mosby, St Louis.

Mann I. 1964 Development of the human eye. Grune & Stratton, New York.

Chapter 2: Basic Optics

American Academy of Ophthalmology. 2006 Clinical optics, vol. 3. AAO, San Francisco.

Benjamin W J. 1998 Borish's clinical refraction. W B Saunders, Philadelphia.

MacInnes B J. 1994 Ophthalmology Board Review: optics and refraction. Mosby, St Louis.

Milder B, Rubin M L, Weinstein G W. 1991 The fine art of prescribing glasses without making a spectacle of yourself. Triad Scientific Publications, Gainesville.

Rubin M L. 1993 Optics for clinicians. Triad Scientific Publications, Gainesville.

Chapter 3: Ocular Pharmacology

Doughty M J. 2001 Ocular pharmacology and therapeutics: a primary care guide. Butterworth-Heinemann, Philadelphia.

Fraunfelder F T, Fraunfelder F W. 2001 Drug-induced ocular side effects, 5th edn. Butterworth-Heinemann, Philadelphia.

Fraunfelder F T, Roy F H. 2000 Current ocular therapy, 5th edn. W B Saunders, Philadelphia.

Greenbaum S. 1997 Ocular anesthesia. W B Saunders, Philadelphia.

Schuman J S, Grant W M. 1993 Toxicology of the eye, 4th edn. Charles C. Thomas, Springfield.

Thomson P D R. 2003 Physicians' desk reference for ophthalmic medicines. Medical Economics, Montvale.

Zimmerman T J. 1997 Textbook of ocular pharmacology. Lippincott-Raven, Philadelphia.

Chapter 4: The Eye Exam

Kaiser P K, Friedman N J. 2004 The Massachusetts Eye & Ear Infirmary's illustrated manual of ophthalmology, 2nd edn. W B Saunders, Philadelphia.

Richard J M. 1980 A manual for the beginning ophthalmology resident, 3rd edn. American Academy of Ophthalmology, San Francisco.

Chapter 5: Neuro-Ophthalmology

American Academy of Ophthalmology. 2006 Neuro-ophthalmology, vol. 5. AAO, San Francisco.

Burde R M, Savino P J, Trobe J D. 2002 Clinical decisions in neuro-ophthalmology, 3rd edn. Mosby, Philadelphia.

Kline L B, Bajandas F. 2001 Neuro-ophthalmology review manual, 5th edn. Slack, Thorofare.

Liu G T, Volpe N J, Galetta S. 2001 Neuro-ophthalmology: diagnosis and management. W B Saunders, Philadelphia.

Loewenfeld I E, Lowenstein O. 1999 The pupil: anatomy, physiology, and clinical applications, 2nd edn. Butterworth-Heinemann, Philadelphia.

Milder B, Rubin M L, Weinstein G W. 1991 The fine art of prescribing glasses without making a spectacle of yourself. Triad Scientific Publications, Gainesville.

Miller N R. 1999 Walsh & Hoyt's clinical neuro-ophthalmology, 5th edn. Lippincott-Williams and Wilkins, Baltimore.

Chapter 6: Pediatric Ophthalmology and Strabismus

American Academy of Ophthalmology. 2006 Pediatric ophthalmology and strabismus, vol. 6. AAO, San Francisco.

Harley R D, Nelson L B. 1998 Harley's pediatric ophthalmology, 4th edn. W B Saunders, Philadelphia.

Nelson L B, Catalano R A. 1997 Atlas of ocular motility. W B Saunders, Philadelphia.

Netland P A, Mandal A K. 2003 Pediatric glaucoma. Butterworth-Heinemann, Philadelphia.

Von Noorden G K. 1983 Atlas of strabismus, 4th edn. Mosby, St Louis.

Chapter 7: Orbit

American Academy of Ophthalmology. 2006 Orbit, eyelids and lacrimal system, vol. 7. AAO, San Francisco.

Dutton J S. 1994 Atlas of clinical and surgical orbital anatomy. W B Saunders, Philadelphia.

Levine M R. 2003 Manual of oculoplastic surgery, 3rd edn. Butterworth-Heinemann, Philadelphia.

Nesi F A, Levine M R, Lisman R D. 1998 Smith's ophthalmic plastic and reconstructive surgery, 2nd edn. Mosby, St Louis.

Rootman J. 2002 Diseases of the orbit, 2nd edn. Lippincott-Williams and Wilkins, Philadelphia.

Chapter 8: Lids and Adnexa

American Academy of Ophthalmology. 2006 Orbit, eyelids and lacrimal system, vol. 7. AAO, San Francisco.

Collin J R O. Manual of systematic eyelid surgery, 3rd edn. Butterworth-Heinemann, Philadelphia.

Putterman A M. 1999 Cosmetic oculoplastic surgery: eyelid, forehead, and facial techniques, 3rd edn. W B Saunders, Philadelphia.

Chapter 9: Conjunctiva

Abelson M B. 2001 Allergic diseases of the eye. W B Saunders, Philadelphia.

American Academy of Ophthalmology. 2006 External disease and cornea, vol. 8. AAO, San Francisco.

Mackie I A. 2003 External eye disease. Butterworth-Heinemann, Boston.

Chapter 10: Sclera

American Academy of Ophthalmology. 2006 External disease and cornea, vol. 8. AAO, San Francisco.

Watson P, Hazleman B, Pavesio C. 2003 Sclera and systemic disorders. Butterworth-Heinemann, Philadelphia.

Chapter 11: Cornea

American Academy of Ophthalmology. 2006 External disease and cornea, vol. 8. AAO, San Francisco.

Arffa R C. 1998 Grayson's diseases of the cornea, 4th edn. Mosby, St Louis.

Brightbill F S. 1999 Corneal surgery: theory, technique and tissue, 3rd edn. Mosby, St Louis.

Kaufman H E, Barron B A, McDonald M B. 1997 The cornea, 2nd edn. Butterworth-Heinemann, Philadelphia.

Krachmer J H, Mannis M J, Holland E J. 1995 Cornea. Mosby, St Louis.

Krachmer J H, Palay D A. 1995 Cornea color atlas. Mosby, St Louis.

Leibowitz H M, Waring G O. 1998 Corneal disorders: clinical diagnosis and management, 2nd edn. W B Saunders, Philadelphia.

Smolin G, Thoft R A. 1994 The cornea: scientific foundations and clinical practice, 3rd edn. Little Brown, Boston.

Chapter 12: Anterior Chamber

American Academy of Ophthalmology. 2006 Intraocular inflammation and uveitis, vol. 9. AAO, San Francisco.

Foster C S, Vitale A. 2002 Diagnosis and treatment of uveitis. W B Saunders, Philadelphia.

Jones N P. 1998 Uveitis: an illustrated manual. Butterworth-Heinemann, Philadelphia.

Michelson J B. 1992 Color atlas of uveitis, 2nd edn. Mosby, St Louis.

Nussenblatt R B, Whitcup S M, Palestine A G. 2003 Uveitis: fundamentals and clinical practice, 2nd edn. Mosby, Philadelphia.

Pepose J S, Holland G N, Wilhelmus K R. 1996 Ocular infection and immunity. Mosby, St Louis.

Chapter 13: Glaucoma

American Academy of Ophthalmology. 2006 Glaucoma, vol. 10. AAO, San Francisco.

Campbell D G, Netland P A. 1998 Stereo atlas of glaucoma. Mosby, St Louis.

Higginbotham E J, Lee D A. 2003 Clinical guide to glaucoma management. Butterworth-Heinemann, Amsterdam.

Ritch R, Shields M B, Krupin T. 1996 The glaucomas, 2nd edn. Mosby, St Louis.

Shields M B. 1998 Textbook of glaucoma, 4th edn. Lippincott-Williams and Wilkins, Philadelphia.

Chapter 15: Lens

American Academy of Ophthalmology. 2006 Lens and cataract, vol. 11. AAO, San Francisco.

Boruchoff S A. 2001 Anterior segment disorder: a diagnostic color atlas. Butterworth-Heinemann, Boston.

Jaffe N S, Jaffe M S, Jaffe G F. 1997 Cataract surgery and its complications, 6th edn. Mosby, St Louis.

Chapter 16: Vitreous

American Academy of Ophthalmology. 2006 Retina and vitreous, vol. 12. AAO, San Francisco.

Chapter 17: Retina

American Academy of Ophthalmology. 2006 Ophthalmic pathology and intraocular tumors, vol. 4. AAO, San Francisco.

American Academy of Ophthalmology. 2006 Retina and vitreous, vol. 12. AAO, San Francisco.

Bell W J, Stenstrom W J. 1998 Atlas of the peripheral retina. W B Saunders, Philadelphia.

Gass J. 1997 Stereoscopic atlas of macular diseases: diagnosis and treatment, 4th edn. Mosby, St Louis.

Guyer D R, Yannuzzi L A, Chang A, Shields J A, Green W R. 1999 Retina–vitreous–macula. W B Saunders, Philadelphia.

Ryan S J. 2001 Retina, 3rd edn. Mosby, St Louis.

Shields J A, Shields C L. 1992 Intraocular tumors: a text and atlas. W B Saunders, Philadelphia.

Tabbara K F, Nussenblatt R B. 1994 Posterior uveitis: diagnosis and management. Butterworth-Heinemann, Philadelphia.

Yannuzzi L A, Guyer D R, Green W R. 1995 The retina. Mosby, St Louis.

Index